# ADVANCING THE NATION'S
# HEALTH
# NEEDS

Committee for Monitoring the Nation's Changing Needs for Biomedical, Behavioral, and Clinical Personnel

Board on Higher Education and Workforce
Policy and Global Affairs

NATIONAL RESEARCH COUNCIL
*OF THE NATIONAL ACADEMIES*

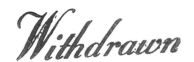

THE NATIONAL ACADEMIES PRESS
Washington, D.C.
**www.nap.edu**

**THE NATIONAL ACADEMIES PRESS**   500 Fifth Street, N.W.   Washington, DC 20001

NOTICE: The project that is the subject of this report was approved by the Governing Board of the National Research Council, whose members are drawn from the councils of the National Academy of Sciences, the National Academy of Engineering, and the Institute of Medicine. The members of the committee responsible for the report were chosen for their special competences and with regard for appropriate balance.

**This study was supported by Contract/Grant No. N01-OD-4-2139, TO#104, between the National Academy of Sciences and the National Institutes of Health, Department of Health and Human Services. Additional support was provided by the Agency for Healthcare Research and Quality** Any opinions, findings, conclusions, or recommendations expressed in this publication are those of the Committee for Monitoring the Nation's Changing Needs for Biomedical, Behavioral, and Clinical Personnel and do not necessarily reflect the views of the organizations or agencies that provided support for the project.

International Standard Book Number 0-309-09427-5
Library of Congress Catalog Card Number 2005928995

Additional copies of this report are available from the National Academies Press, 500 Fifth Street, N.W., Lockbox 285, Washington, DC 20055; (800) 624-6242 or (202) 334-3313 (in the Washington metropolitan area); Internet, http://www.nap.edu

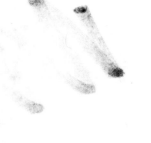

# THE NATIONAL ACADEMIES
*Advisers to the Nation on Science, Engineering, and Medicine*

The **National Academy of Sciences** is a private, nonprofit, self-perpetuating society of distinguished scholars engaged in scientific and engineering research, dedicated to the furtherance of science and technology and to their use for the general welfare. Upon the authority of the charter granted to it by the Congress in 1863, the Academy has a mandate that requires it to advise the federal government on scientific and technical matters. Dr. Ralph J. Cicerone is president of the National Academy of Sciences.

The **National Academy of Engineering** was established in 1964, under the charter of the National Academy of Sciences, as a parallel organization of outstanding engineers. It is autonomous in its administration and in the selection of its members, sharing with the National Academy of Sciences the responsibility for advising the federal government. The National Academy of Engineering also sponsors engineering programs aimed at meeting national needs, encourages education and research, and recognizes the superior achievements of engineers. Dr. Wm. A. Wulf is president of the National Academy of Engineering.

The **Institute of Medicine** was established in 1970 by the National Academy of Sciences to secure the services of eminent members of appropriate professions in the examination of policy matters pertaining to the health of the public. The Institute acts under the responsibility given to the National Academy of Sciences by its congressional charter to be an adviser to the federal government and, upon its own initiative, to identify issues of medical care, research, and education. Dr. Harvey V. Fineberg is president of the Institute of Medicine.

The **National Research Council** was organized by the National Academy of Sciences in 1916 to associate the broad community of science and technology with the Academy's purposes of furthering knowledge and advising the federal government. Functioning in accordance with general policies determined by the Academy, the Council has become the principal operating agency of both the National Academy of Sciences and the National Academy of Engineering in providing services to the government, the public, and the scientific and engineering communities. The Council is administered jointly by both Academies and the Institute of Medicine. Dr. Ralph J. Cicerone and Dr. Wm. A. Wulf are chair and vice chair, respectively, of the National Research Council.

**www.national-academies.org**

# Preface

This report is the twelfth assessment of the National Institutes of Health National Research Service Awards program. The research training needs of the country in basic biomedical, clinical, and behavioral and social sciences are considered. Also included are the training needs of oral health, nursing, and health services research. The report has been broadly constructed to take into account the rapidly evolving national and international health care needs. The past and present are analyzed, and predictions with regard to future needs are presented.

This report represents a team effort of a diverse group of people. The primary committee consisted of experts from the basic biomedical sciences, clinical sciences, behavioral and social sciences, and demographics. In addition, subcommittees were constituted to assess research training in oral health and nursing, and an expert in health services research was consulted. Information was obtained from many different groups and individuals, including experts within the National Institutes of Health. The final report is a composite of the many viewpoints that were expressed. Although we attempted to base the final recommendations solely on factual information, we found that the data available were incomplete. Moreover, even with the best data, the research training venue is dependent on unpredictable events such as international politics and the federal budget. Consequently, the bases for the recommendations in the report are a combination of factual data and expert opinion. It is our general consensus that although the research training establishment is doing well, implementation of the recommendations would significantly improve research training. In addition, we believe that a process allowing continuous monitoring of the research training system would permit more rapid and well-tuned responses to a changing external environment.

This report was made possible by funding from the National Institutes of Health and the Agency for Healthcare Research and Quality. In addition, staff members from each of these agencies were very helpful in providing information about their training programs. From the National Institutes of Health, Walter Schaffer and Walter Goldschmidts, the program officers for this project, Sharon Gordon, and Bill McGarvey provided details on their training support and other data relevant to the committee's deliberations. Data and information about training in health services research were provided by Karen Rudzinski at the Agency for Healthcare Research and Quality and Pamela Flattau from Flattau Associates. A commissioned paper by Donald Steinwachs was also very helpful in addressing issues in health services research. The committee is also indebted to a number of people who made presentations at committee meetings: Ruth Kirschstein, Raynard Kington, Wendy Baldwin, Judith Greenberg, Patricia Grady, and Lawrence Tabak from the National Institutes of Health; Francis Chesley from the Agency for Healthcare Research and Quality; Marguerite Barratt, and Joann Roskoski from the National Science Foundation; Alan Kraut from the American Psychological Society; and Norman Anderson from the American Psychological Association.

The committee also appreciates the work of the expert staff of the National Research Council. In particular, Jim Voytuk, the study director, did a magnificent job of gathering data, organizing the committee activities, and doing much of the writing. He was ably assisted by Herman Alvarado with the data collection, Elizabeth Scott with the arrangement of meetings and editing of the committee report, and Patricia Santos whose work in preparing and editing the manuscript, researching material for the committee, and general oversight of project activities was invaluable. We also greatly appreciate the work of Rodolfo Bulatao in analyzing the demographics of the workforce and drafting Appendix D of this report. As part of the normal procedure, this report was reviewed by a group of experts and was greatly improved as a result. In the final analysis, however, responsibility for the report resides with the primary committee. We trust that the recommendations presented will receive serious consideration from the National Institutes of Health and associated agencies.

A list of the committee, panel, and staff members who contributed directly to this report is given at the beginning of the report. As the committee chair, I commend and thank them all for their contributions. This report has been reviewed in draft form by individuals chosen for their diverse perspectives and technical expertise, in accordance with procedures approved by the National Research Council's Report Review Committee. The purpose of this independent review is to provide candid and critical comments that will assist the institution in making its published report as sound as possible and to ensure that the report meets institutional standards for objectivity, evidence, and responsiveness to the study charge. The review comments and draft manuscript remain confidential to protect the integrity of the deliberative process.

We wish to thank the following individuals for their review of this report: Irwin Arias, Tufts University; David Breneman, University of Virginia; Gerard Burrow, Yale University; Thomas Carew, University of California, Irvine; Susan Fiske, Princeton University; Maureen Henderson, University of Washington; Hedvig Hricak, Memorial Sloan-Kettering Cancer Center; Peter Barton Hutt, Covington and Burling; Paul Kincade, University of Oklahoma; Ruth McCorkle, Yale University; Michael Teitelbaum, Alfred P. Sloan Foundation; Richard Valachovic, American Dental Education Association; Bailus Walker, Howard University; and Nancy Fugate Woods, University of Washington.

Although the reviewers listed above provided many constructive comments and suggestions, they were not asked to endorse the conclusions or recommendations, nor did they see the final draft of the report before its release. The review of this report was overseen by Charles Phelps, University of Rochester. Appointed by the National Research Council, he was responsible for making certain that an independent examination of this report was carried out in accordance with institutional procedures and that all review comments were carefully considered. Responsibility for the final content of this report rests entirely with the authoring committee and the institution.

Gordon G. Hammes
*Chair*

# Contents

# Figures, Tables, and Boxes

## FIGURES

## TABLES

## BOXES

# Summary

## INTRODUCTION

This report is the twelfth in a series on monitoring the changing needs for biomedical and behavioral research personnel in the United States. The task of assessing and predicting the status of research personnel over the entire spectrum of health sciences is daunting. The need for improved health care in the nation remains a priority. This need can only be met by research in health areas over a broad and continually expanding venue. Research and research training are national as well as international in scope and personnel.

The Statement of Task for the committee is as follows: "A committee will advise the National Institutes of Health (NIH) on issues regarding research personnel needs in the basic biomedical sciences, behavioral and social sciences, clinical sciences, oral health, nursing, and health services. The committee will gather and analyze information on the employment of research scientists in these fields and on the need for educating additional researchers. The committee will deal broadly with the training needs and direction of the Ruth L. Kirschstein National Research Service Award (NRSA) program, as dictated by congressional legislation and with the process to assess the needs. The report will examine long-range trends and identify training needs through 2010."

The research enterprise is divided into three major areas: basic biomedical, behavioral and social sciences, and clinical research. The scope of these areas is discussed in the body of the report and will not be dwelt on here. In addition, oral health, nursing, and health services are considered separately because of their special needs. However, it should be recognized that these divisions are arbitrary and broad. The boundaries are not sharp and are continually evolving. Furthermore, the crossing of these boundaries is crucial for the development of new ideas and fields. For this reason, a separate chapter is devoted to interdisciplinary and emerging fields. Finally, major advances in research require a con-

tinual input of new personnel with fresh ideas, so career development is an essential part of the overall picture.

## FINDINGS AND RECOMMENDATIONS

For the three major areas considered, workforce models were developed that include extrapolations of new Ph.D.s and M.D.s entering the market and job availability through 2011. The results of this modeling cannot be taken literally. First, the data available to analyze the current situation are approximate at best. Second, extrapolation into the future requires information that exists only up to 2003: the world and national economy; the budget available for research; the state of the world in general with regard to war, disease, and immigration policies; and unanticipated advances in science. A particularly speculative issue is the role of foreign scientists in the health research enterprise, due to recent changes in immigration policy in this country and changes in research support in foreign countries. However, the research workforce tends to adapt to changing conditions, a tendency that in the long run works to bring the workforce's needs and demands into equilibrium. Taking into account workforce models and all other known factors, this committee finds the following: (1) the system is currently in reasonable balance, and (2) despite the emergence of new and unanticipated factors over the next six years, the system will adapt toward a balanced state unless major policy changes are made in the patterns of federal research support. This means that unemployment among trained researchers should remain low and that most of the trained personnel will remain in science.

A quantitative assessment does not ensure a successful research enterprise. Quality is an essential ingredient for progress. In this regard, the NRSA program plays a unique role. Although these awards support only a small fraction of the students and postdoctorals being trained, they set the standards for the entire research training establishment. In addition, they attract high-quality students into research and into fields of particular need. The record of success of

NRSA holders in obtaining research funding is impressive. The results of the training efforts in the nation are self-evident: this country continues to be a world leader in health-related research.

While recognizing the success of these awards in promoting research, it is important to maintain a diverse support pattern for training. Research grants not only provide a viable alternative, they also fill a special niche in their own right. They provide personnel to carry out the research specified by funding agencies. These personnel may not be eligible for the NRSA, and research grants provide an alternate entry into the research enterprise. The most obvious examples are foreign scientists. Many foreign scientists remain in this country and make important contributions to training and research. This is beneficial to both the research community and the nation. In this regard, the committee is greatly concerned that current immigration policies will make the interchange of scientists and students with the rest of the world increasingly difficult.

Based on the balance with regard to output of trained personnel, job opportunities, and overall quality, **the committee's primary recommendation for the three major areas is that the total number of NRSA positions awarded should remain at least at the fiscal year 2002 level. Furthermore, the committee recommends that future increases be commensurate with the rise in the total extramural research funding at NIH in the biomedical, clinical, and behavioral and social sciences.** The year 2002 is specified because it is the most recent year for which data were available to the committee. Despite this single recommendation for the three areas, the committee recognizes that each area has considerations that merit special mention. For example, in the basic biomedical and behavioral and social sciences, it is important to maintain focus on basic research. Although the ultimate goal of NIH is improved health care, the committee believes that critical breakthroughs are usually founded on basic research rather than highly applied research. Clearly applied research has an important place in the research training portfolio, but broad training in basic concepts is essential.

The application of lessons learned from basic science to health-related problems requires training in translational areas, and this should be a focus of the clinical sciences. Ideally, physicians are best equipped to do this research but may be unlikely to pursue research because of the heavy debt load M.D.s incur in medical school. To alleviate some of the above concerns, **the committee recommends that the size and scope of the Medical Scientist Training Program (MSTP) be expanded at least 20 percent and that the scope be expanded to include the clinical, health services, and behavioral and social sciences.** This program has proved remarkably successful in attracting outstanding physicians into research. Although the program is expensive, a modest expansion would serve the nation well. Furthermore, expansion of the scope would permit the be-

havioral and social sciences, for example, to participate more fully in the program. The expansion of scope should not be at the expense of the current MSTP support for basic biomedical research. **In addition, the committee recommends that training grants be established for physicians to learn the skills necessary for clinical investigation.** These programs can be part-time programs for physicians that would lead to a master's degree. The shortage of physicians to carry out clinical research is already critical and will worsen if positive steps are not taken.

The behavioral and social sciences receive considerably less research funding from NIH than the basic biomedical sciences and correspondingly less research training support. Many of the nation's health problems are not just physiological in nature and need to be addressed by research in the behavioral and social sciences as well. Consequently, **the committee recommends that each NIH institute and center incorporate the behavioral and social sciences into its training portfolio, including institutes and centers that have not emphasized these disciplines in the past.**

Although the need for research in oral health and nursing is apparent, both areas have difficulty providing an environment that fosters research as a career and in finding high-quality trainees interested in pursuing a research career. The long-term solution to this problem will require significant changes in traditional schools of dentistry and nursing. To attract trainees into oral health research, **the committee recommends that all required years of the D.D.S./Ph.D. program be funded by the National Institute for Dental and Craniofacial Research (NIDCR) (analogous to the highly successful MSTP) and that the loan forgiveness program require documentation of time spent in research and scholarly success. This committee also recommends that the NIDCR design and implement programs intended to increase the number and quality of dental school applicants who are committed to careers in oral health research. In the case of nursing, the committee recommends that a new institutional research training grant (T32) program be established that focuses on rapid progression into research careers. Criteria might include predoctoral trainees who are within eight years of high school graduation, not requiring a master's degree before commencing with a Ph.D., and postdoctoral trainees who are within two years of their Ph.D.** These modest recommendations for oral health and nursing are intended only as starting points for these professions to move more strongly into research and research training.

A growing need exists to shorten the interval between research advances in biomedical science and the ability to apply these advances effectively to improve the health of the public. Thus, more effective health care delivery practices are required. Because of this need, **health services research training should be expanded and strengthened within each NIH institute and center.** In addition, **the training programs of the Agency for Healthcare Re-**

search and Quality should be expanded, commensurate with the growth in total spending on health services research.

Thus far this report has been somewhat restrictive in its definition of research fields. However, the committee recognizes that many important advances occur at the boundaries of traditional fields, and indeed the boundaries themselves are continually shifting. It is essential that NIH adopt a proactive stance in encouraging training in interdisciplinary and emerging fields. Given the importance of the institute structure of NIH, research training should be better integrated across all of the NIH institutes and centers. Broadly based research training should be an essential effort for all institutes and centers, rather than concentrated narrowly in a few. NIH itself must serve as a paragon for interdisciplinary research and training. Most importantly, training must be broad and deep so that trainees are equipped to move both within and between traditional fields. Several specific recommendations are made here to address some of the important issues in this regard.

**The NIH should target individual NRSAs in emerging fields, interdisciplinary areas, and specific fields of interest. Such applications should be given priority in the awards process, and special review panels should be used as needed. Furthermore, quantitative subject matter should be integrated into and required for training programs in all areas. Quantitative subjects include statistics, mathematics, physics, physical chemistry, computer science, and informatics.** In this age of genomics and computers, the large amount of new information generated requires all scientists to be well versed in quantitative reasoning. Finally, the difficulty in identifying emerging fields and the importance of encouraging these fields as they emerge are noted. **The committee recommends that a standing committee (proposed later in this summary) provide recommendations to NIH as to the identity of emerging research.**

The career development of research personnel requires serious attention. The time to degree is increasing, as is the age at which individuals enter the job market as independent investigators. This trend does not appear to be abating but may change if the research personnel system remains in balance in terms of output and job placement. The decline in the postdoctoral pool suggests this may be occurring. NIH should be proactive in promoting career development. In this regard the intent of the K awards program, which has the goal of supporting the development of scientists into independent investigators, including a period of supervised research, is applauded. However, the current system is sufficiently complex to discourage applicants. **The committee recommends that career development grants (currently K awards) be maintained but be restructured such that fewer mechanisms are established and consistently implemented across NIH. Furthermore, the committee recommends that the restructured K awards include the**

following: **(1) a transition award to span senior postdoctoral status and an independent research position; (2) beginning faculty awards to free certain classes of investigators from nonresearch duties; (3) senior scientist awards for the purpose of faculty moving into new research areas; (4) awards to allow faculty and other researchers to maintain research careers during periods when personal demands (e.g., child rearing) prevent full employment status; and (5) clinical science awards to provide research training for clinical faculty/personnel.** There is particular concern that talented researchers are being lost from the pool because career development opportunities are not available for women during their child-rearing years. Although the number of women in medical research has increased, this has not been uniform across fields, and continual vigilance and encouragement are required.

The status of individuals in nonfaculty positions needs to be improved, in general. Since the report on the status of postdoctorals, *Enhancing the Postdoctoral Experience for Scientists and Engineers: A Guide for Postdoctoral Scholars, Advisers, Institutions, Funding Organizations, and Disciplinary Societies*, was released in 2000 by the National Academies Committee on Science, Engineering, and Public Policy and because other groups are exploring this issue, it is not handled in detail here. However, employee benefits are a particularly important issue, especially health insurance. Therefore, **the committee recommends that NIH develop a mechanism for support such that NRSA postdoctoral fellows receive the normal employee benefits of the institutions at which they are located.**

The number of underrepresented racial and ethnic minorities entering research across the entirety of medicine is disappointing. Since this subject is currently being reviewed in depth by another National Academies committee, detailed recommendations with regard to this issue are not provided in this report. However, it is the unanimous opinion of the committee that intervention must occur well before graduate/professional school. To assist in this process, **the committee recommends that supplements to existing training grants be made available for the purpose of developing outreach programs for undergraduates and high school students from underrepresented minorities and for the secondary school teachers serving them.** The general solution to this problem clearly will require action across all of society as well as the research establishment.

The committee is greatly concerned with the decline in preparation and interest in science students have in the early stages of their education. If this trend continues, the supply of Ph.D. scientists may be insufficient to carry out vital health-related research. Therefore, **it is recommended that NIH work with other federal agencies to find ways to encourage students at precollege levels to pursue training in technical, computational, mathematical, and scientific areas that are necessary precursors for careers in science.**

Finally, the need for research in health areas is of sufficient importance, from health and economic perspectives, to the nation is discussed. The external environment changes rapidly, including job availability, crises in health care, and emerging fields. **The committee recommends that a standing independent committee be created to monitor biomedical, clinical, and behavioral and social science research personnel needs, to evaluate the training of such personnel, to assess the number and nature of research personnel that will be required in the future, to assist in the collection and analysis of appropriate data, and to make recommendations concerning these matters to NIH.** Such a committee would be established by and be advisory to NIH. In particular, there is a lack of data with regard to tracking career outcomes for individuals supported by NIH. **The committee recommends that NIH implement a data collection system for tracking the career outcomes of its recipients of research training support. A minimum set of outcomes would include employment sector, involvement in research, and subsequent NIH awards.**

By necessity, this summary is brief; the points raised here are discussed in detail in the full report. Although continual monitoring and development are required, the medical research training establishment is in good health and the NRSA program has been critical for past accomplishments and will continue to be critical for achieving future goals.

# 1

# Introduction

The work of the National Institutes of Health (NIH)—a U.S. research establishment whose agenda ranges from the very basic to the highly applied—has long been recognized as critical to advancing the quality of health care in the nation and the world. The virtual elimination of polio resulted from basic and applied research in virology; the development of blood pressure–lowering drugs came from an understanding of the fundamental regulation of the underlying biological process; the development of cholesterol-lowering drugs is due to studies of the transport and enzymes controlling cholesterol flux in humans; the development of new imaging techniques has led to improved diagnostic procedures; and improved treatments of mental disease are due to a better understanding of brain function. As a result of NIH research, major diseases such as AIDS, stroke, congestive heart failure, and diabetes are treated more successfully each year. The net result has been a dramatic increase in Americans' longevity. At the turn of the 20th century, life expectancy for women and men was 53 and 50, respectively; in the year 2000 it was 80 and 74.[1]

Virtually all of these improvements in health care were derived from basic research that led to an understanding of human physiology. In many cases the basic research occurred decades before its application, often with little or no obvious expectation that an application to health care might develop. Who could have imagined, for example, that being able to orient hydrogen nuclei in a magnetic field would lead to today's magnetic resonance imaging techniques? Or that understanding the basis of enzyme action and regulation in bacteria would lead to specific drugs? One might go so far as to say that a greater understanding of basic physiology is the key to successful medical applications and that this knowledge can only come from research.

The work goes on, in new and constantly evolving ways, to keep improving the methods and outcomes of health care. The sequence of the human genome and the linkage of spe-

cific genome sequences with diseases such as Alzheimer's, cystic fibrosis, and many others are intriguing developments. Similarly, the linkage of genome sequences with mental disorders promises greater understanding—and, ultimately, improved treatment—of such diseases as major depressive disorders, which affect 5 percent of the population (9.9 million Americans) annually.[2] Meanwhile, the addition of computer science and bioinformatics to the arsenal of biomedical, social and behavioral, and clinical research holds enormous promise and is stirring considerable excitement among scientists. Further research will undoubtedly lead to better medical therapies.

To continue to derive these benefits, a highly trained workforce is required. This workforce must have a steady infusion of highly trained people with new approaches if it is to be successful. Support of this workforce's training, therefore, is an investment in the health of the country.

The National Research Council has been evaluating workforce needs in the biomedical, social and behavioral, and clinical sciences on a continuing basis since 1975, as mandated by Congress. This report and its predecessors monitor the current workforce of these areas and attempt to predict their necessary size and composition for the future. It also makes recommendations on how the National Research Service Award program in particular can optimally contribute to overall training efforts for the biomedical, social and behavioral, and clinical sciences.

## HISTORICAL CONTEXT

### Research Training and the National Institutes of Health

The origins of research training at NIH date to 1930, when the Ransdell Act changed the name of the Hygienic Laboratory to the National Institute of Health (a single institute at that time) and authorized the establishment of fellowships

---

[1]National Center for Health Statistics. 2003.

[2]National Institute for Mental Health. 2001.

for research into basic biological and medical problems. While the harsh economic realities of the Great Depression imposed constraints, this legislation marked a new commitment to public funding of medical research and training. The National Cancer Act of 1937, which established the National Cancer Institute (NCI) within the Public Health Service (PHS), funded the first training programs targeting a specific area. This legislation supported training facilities and the award of fellowships to outstanding individuals for studies related to the causes and treatment of cancer. In 1938, 17 individuals received fellowships in cancer-related research fields such as biochemistry, physiology, and genetics.

NCI became part of NIH with the passage of the Public Health Services Act of 1944—the legislative basis for NIH's wartime and postwar expansion of research and training programs and more generally for a major federal commitment to support biomedical research. This expansion was supported by legislative actions that converted existing divisions within NIH to institutes and centers and the establishment of new institutes or centers, each with field-specific training and research missions. In particular, the first of these laws—the National Heart Act of 1947—established the National Heart Institute and changed the name of the National Institute of Health to the National Institutes of Health.

Throughout the 1940s, 1950s, and 1960s there was substantial growth in the NIH budget, with annual increases averaging 40 percent from 1957 to 1963 (with dollar increases ranging from $98 million to $930 million). This funding raised the number of grants to academic institutions and enabled greater federal assistance in both the construction of research facilities and the establishment of fellowship and training programs for research personnel; this generous funding even allowed for limited investment to support research in foreign countries. The growth in research and training support slowed in the late 1960s, to about 6 percent annually, with a consequent decline in the number of research grants, both foreign and domestic, and a curtailment of facilities construction.

Support in the 1970s reflected public and congressional interest in specific diseases. Research areas such as cancer and pulmonary and vascular disorders were identified by legislation for increased funding, and the eleventh institute on the NIH campus, the National Institute on Aging (NIA), was established in 1974. The NIA also brought a new perspective to NIH in that it was authorized to support not only biological research but also social and behavioral research. While funding for research in targeted areas was welcomed at NIH, this also meant that research in less visible areas tended to decline. Institutes such as the National Institute for General Medical Sciences (NIGMS) and the National Institute of Allergy and Infectious Diseases saw annual average reductions of about 10 percent.

By the early 1970s, training support was authorized through the different institutes and centers by 11 separate pieces of legislation. However, in its FY 1974 budget rec-

ommendations, the administration proposed the phasing out of research training and fellowship programs over a five-year period by making no new awards and honoring only existing commitments. The reasons it cited for this proposal were as follows: the need for such programs and the manpower trained by them had never been adequately justified; people trained in these programs earned incomes later in life that made it reasonable to ask them to bear the cost of their training; large numbers of those trained did not enter biomedical research or continue their training; alternative federal programs of support for this training were available; and the programs were not equitable because support was not available equally to all students.[3]

The administration's proposal met with virtually universal opposition by members of the nation's biomedical research community. As a result, the administration revised its position and proposed a new, but smaller, fellowship program at the postdoctoral level. This proposal also met with objections, and in 1974 Congress enacted the National Research Act (P.L. 93-348), which amended the Public Health Services Act by repealing existing research training and fellowship authorities and consolidating them into the National Research Service Award (NRSA) program. The legislation authorized support for individual and institutional training grants at the predoctoral and postdoctoral levels, with the stipulation that an individual could be supported for no more than 3 years. Moreover, to safeguard against some of the cited abuses of the former programs, it restricted training support on the basis of subject-area shortages and imposed service obligations and payback requirements.

In the years since the National Research Act was signed, the law governing the NRSA program has been modified several times in order to include new areas of research training and establish funding levels for selected disciplines. The first change came in 1976, when Congress extended the program to encompass research training in nursing.[4] Then, in 1978, Congress expanded the NRSA program to cover training in health services research.[5] In 1985 the program was enlarged once again to include training in primary care research.[6]

Specific funding targets for training in health services and primary care research were established with the Health Research Extension Act of 1985, when Congress required that 0.5 percent of NRSA funds be allocated to each of the two fields.[7] The same law directed that funds for training in health services research be administered by the Agency for Health Care Policy and Research (AHCPR) and its successor, the Agency for Healthcare Research and Quality (AHRQ). Research training in primary care originally came

---

[3]U.S. Congress, Senate. 1973.
[4]U.S. Congress. 1976.
[5]U.S. Congress. 1978.
[6]U.S. Congress. 1985.
[7]Ibid.

under the purview of NIH but was delegated to the Health Resources and Services Administration by Congress in 1988 after concerns were raised that NIH was interpreting the meaning of "primary care" too broadly.[8,9] Funding levels for training in health services and primary care research were increased to 1 percent of the NRSA budget with the passage of the NIH Revitalization Act of 1993, and these two fields remain the only ones for which specific funding levels have been established by law.[10]

## Minority Programs at NIH

The recruitment of underrepresented minorities into research careers has been a long-standing activity at NIH. In 1972, about the time the NRSA program was established, the Minority Schools Biomedical Support program—under the administration of the NIH Division of Research Resources—began awarding grants to faculty and students at minority institutions. That same year research awards were made to minority faculty under the Minority Access to Research Careers (MARC) Visiting Scientist and Faculty Fellowship program; and in 1974, MARC was officially established within NIGMS as a formal program to stimulate undergraduates' interest in biomedical research and to assist minority institutions in developing strong undergraduate curricula in the biomedical sciences. In 1977 the MARC Honors Undergraduate Research Training (HURT) program was established, and in 1981 the MARC Predoctoral Fellowship program was created to provide further incentive for graduates of the HURT program to obtain research training in the nation's best graduate programs.

These programs continue today with some modifications, such as the replacement of the MARC HURT program with the MARC Undergraduate Student Training in Academic Research program, designed to help meet the need for continual improvement in institutional offerings. Other additions have included the Post-Baccalaureate Research Education Program Award, MARC Faculty Predoctoral Fellowships, MARC Faculty Senior Fellowships, MARC Visiting Scientist Fellowships, and MARC Ancillary Training Activities.

Concurrent with the growth of the MARC programs, the Minority Schools Biomedical Support program also has been evolving. When eligibility for the program was expanded in 1973, it was renamed the Minority Biological Support program; its name was changed again in 1982 to the Minority Biological Research Support (MBRS) program in order to reflect its research scope. This MBRS program was transferred to NIGMS from the Division of Research Resources in 1988, and the NIGMS established the Minority Opportunities in Research (MORE) program branch to serve as the focal point for efforts across NIH to increase the number and capabilities of minority individuals engaged in biomedical research and teaching. In 1996 the MORE Faculty Development and Initiative for Minority Student Development awards were established, and in 1998 the Institutional Research and Academic Career Development Award was announced to encourage postdoctoral candidates' progress toward research and teaching careers in academia. Both the MARC and the MBRS programs have benefited from their coordination in NIGMS and the regular conferences that are held to promote program activities.

In 1989, NIH introduced the Research Supplements for Underrepresented Minorities program. This program allows principal investigators interested in mentoring minorities to add students or researchers to an existing grant by applying for a supplement. Individuals from the high school to junior faculty level are eligible, but nearly 90 percent of the awards are for training at the predoctoral, postdoctoral, and faculty levels. Like others offered by NIH, this program provides an opportunity for promising minority researchers to gain experience that will help them build a research career—but it is not a vehicle for attracting minorities into science, as seen by the low participation rate at the precollege level. The fact that minority candidates initiate the process by expressing their interest to a principal investigator may be the reason for the focus at the higher career levels; about 35 percent of the program's funding is for faculty support.

Another action that helped increase minority participation was an NIH directive in the mid-1990s to encourage training directors to support more minorities on their grants. As a result, the percentage of minorities on training grants more than quadrupled from the 1990s (2 percent) to 2003 (9 percent).

## Career Development Programs

While the education and training of graduate students or postdoctoral researchers prepare individuals for research careers, in the 1980s NIH recognized the need for programs to help individuals establish strong and productive research careers. To that end, it began programs to facilitate the transition from trainee to research status and give established scientists the opportunity to pursue new research directions.

One such mechanism, referred to as the K award, has the goal of providing Ph.D. scientists with the advanced research training and additional experiences needed to become independent investigators and holders of clinical degrees with the research training needed to conduct patient-oriented research. Over 20 different K award types have existed over the years, though the number at any one time has varied—with some being replaced by other awards or combined to make administration more efficient and others being created to address special needs. Currently, there are 15 K awards, which target different parts of the research population with different forms of support and training features. Not all NIH institutes or centers offer K awards. However, for those that

---

[8]U.S. General Accounting Office. 1987.
[9]U.S. Congress. 1988.
[10]U.S. Congress. 1993.

do, they are only for research training in areas that are consistent with the mission of that particular institute or center.

### Dual-Degree Training

The NIGMS established the Medical Scientist Training Program (MSTP) in 1964 to encourage research training that would lead to the combined M.D./Ph.D. degree. The program was designed to train investigators who could better bridge the gap between basic science and clinical research by providing both graduate training in the biomedical sciences and clinical training offered through medical schools. Students receive a combined M.D./Ph.D. in an average time of about 8 years. The impact of this specialized training program on increasing the productivity of physician-scientists is noteworthy: M.D./Ph.D.s make up about 2.5 percent of medical school graduates each year, yet they hold approximately 33 percent of the NIH grants going to physician-scientists.

What began in 1964 with three programs—at the Albert Einstein College of Medicine, Northwestern University, and New York University—has now grown to 32 MSTP programs, and almost all of the programs have had continuous funding from their beginning. There were 66 trainees in the program in 1964, and by 2000 the number had grown to over 900 and about 300 program graduates. The establishment of these programs has also prompted institutions to develop additional dual-degree programs that are not MSTP funded.

Since the inception of the MSTP, several assessments documenting the success of the programs have been conducted. The most recent study in 1998 included graduates of all of the funded MSTP programs, graduates of non-MSTP programs, and graduates of MSTP programs with either an M.D. or a Ph.D. Over a range of measures, the study showed that MSTP graduates appear to have been successful in establishing research careers, and their recent publication records suggest that members of all cohorts continue to be productive researchers. While the program has clearly been a success, the level of funding for it has not kept pace with the overall NIH budget.

## NATIONAL RESEARCH SERVICE AWARD PROGRAM

In its nearly 30-year history, the NRSA program has provided research training in the biomedical, clinical, and behavioral and social sciences to more than 140,000 students and young investigators. It has done so through a combination of individual fellowship awards and institutional training grants to some 465 universities, research institutes, and teaching hospitals. Moreover, as the NIH and the PHS have grown over the last quarter-century, the NRSA program has evolved to encompass new fields in the basic biomedical sciences such as genome research and neuroscience. NRSA has also expanded in breadth to include research training in

fields such as communication disorders, health services research, primary care, and nursing.

Since 1980, when the NRSA program was well under way, the number of individual training positions has increased by over 4,500, or about 40 percent—from 5,884 predoctoral and 6,173 postdoctoral positions (for a total of 12,057) to 9,308 predoctoral and 7,457 postdoctoral positions (for a total of 16,765) in 2003, as shown in Figure 1-1. Over the same period, the training budget at NIH increased from about $196 million to $681 million, though in 1980 dollars the 2003 expenditure for training was just a little over $230 million.[11] Although the NIH training budget grew slightly over that period, it did not kept pace with the overall NIH budget. Between 1980 and 1998, for example, while the NIH budget went from $3 billion to $5.6 billion (in 1980 dollars), the training budget declined from $196 million to $177 million. By another measure, the NIH training budget declined from a high in 1981 of 7.9 percent of the extramural research grant funding (that is, for work done in institutions outside the NIH campus) to 4.3 percent in 1998. The training budget leveled off at 3.8 percent in 2003.

There was significant change, however, from 1998 to 2003, during which time the training budget increased by about $253 million, or 59 percent, in current dollars. This gain resulted in part from growth in the number of predoctoral and postdoctoral awards (about 1,000 and 500, respectively) as well as from a significant increase in the NRSA stipends. These recent increases in the training budget are more in line with the total NIH budget, which doubled—from $13.6 billion to $27.2 billion—during those 5 years.

Data on the number of awards for 2004 are not complete, but the FY 2004 budget for NIH sets the full-time NRSA training positions at 17,197. This marks an increase of 80 budgeted positions over 2003 and a training budget of $716 million, up 3.9 percent over 2003.[12] The president's budget request for FY 2005 again has a proposed increase for NRSA training. The request for training positions at the individual and institutional levels is up by 225 from 2004, with a budget of $764 million, and the budget proposes to hold the stipends at 2004 levels for both predoctoral and postdoctoral positions. However, no information is currently available on the actual number of positions that will be supported for 2005. In these difficult budgetary times, with many agencies receiving cuts, NIH and health-related research is still in a preferential position, but it is unclear what affect the small increases in the NIH budget will have on research training or even research in general in the future.

Institutional training grants, which funded the education

---

[11]National Institutes of Health Office of Extramural Research.

[12]The number of positions and the amount allocated for those positions, as budgeted by Congress, includes a 1 percent set-aside each for the Agency for Healthcare Research and Quality (AHRQ) and the Health Resources and Service Administration (HRSA).

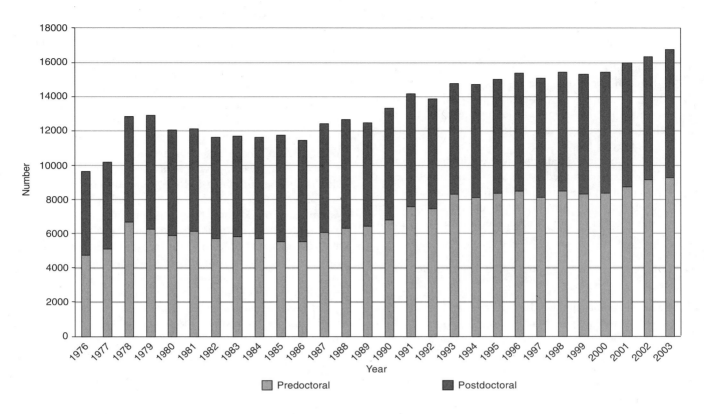

FIGURE 1-1 NRSA training and fellowship grants, 1975–2003.
SOURCE: NIH IMPACII Database.

of about 84 percent of NRSA participants in 2003, are widely regarded as one of the best vehicles for learning the theories and techniques of biomedical and behavioral research.[13,14] The NIH, as well as the AHRQ and the Health Resources and Services Administration, make such awards only after competitive review; institutions are assessed and compared on their previous records in research training, the objectives and designs of their programs, the caliber of their preceptors, their ability to recruit high-quality trainees, their institutional environment, and their commitment to research training. Over the past few years the success rate of proposals for T32 training grants has averaged 62 percent, with the rate dropping to 53 percent in 2003 as the result of a significant increase in the number of proposals. The number of proposals went from an average of 570 between 1996 and 2001 to 666 in 2002 and 753 in 2003.

The remaining 16 percent of the awards in 2003 were individual fellowships, which are also awarded on a competitive basis and provide what is often a first step toward professional independence. Fellows at the predoctoral and postdoctoral levels develop their own proposals and, once an

award has been made, are generally accorded a great deal of autonomy in pursuing their educational and research goals. Through much of the 1990s, the majority of these awards—about 73 percent—were at the postdoctoral level, but in 2003 the percentage dropped to 64 percent. For example, applications for F32[15] postdoctoral fellowships declined from 2,556 in 1996 to 1,552 in 2002; in turn, the number of awards also declined—from 968 to 614. The reasons for these declines are unclear but could possibly have resulted from the low NRSA stipends before the NIH increases that set $45,000 as a five-year goal. A recent turnaround in the number of applications brought the 2003 total to 1,949 and the 2004 level to more than 2,000, thus possibly supporting the stipend-level conjecture. As a result of these increased application levels, the number of F32 awards increased from 614 in 2002 to 713 in 2003. Meanwhile, applications for F31 predoctoral awards increased steadily between 1990 and 2003 (from 275 to over 972, respectively), and the number of grants awarded grew from 141 to 414.

The NRSA program accounts for only 22 percent of NIH's total funding for graduate education in the biomedical, behavioral, and clinical sciences. Nevertheless, the pro-

[13]National Research Council. 1995.
[14]National Research Council. 1998c.

[15]See Appendix B for a complete explanation of the NRSA awards.

gram occupies a leadership role in research training in these fields. NRSA awards are important as they:

- Serve to attract quality people into biomedical research. Perhaps the best example of this phenomenon is the MSTP, which has a well-established track record for launching physicians into outstanding research careers.
- Help direct training into specific research areas, such as cell biology or biophysics.
- Establish training standards—the requirements imposed on individuals supported by NRSA training grants are also imposed on trainees supported by other means.
- Offer the possibility of providing support for training in emerging areas for which other mechanisms may not be available.
- Provide graduate students, during the early years of their training, the opportunity to explore different areas of research.

While NRSA grants are awarded with the expressed purpose of providing research training, not all supported graduate students or postdoctorates actually pursue research careers as independent investigators or researchers. This is documented by the 1998 analysis of the career progression of NRSA predoctoral trainees[16] and may be even more the case in the current employment market, where few tenure-track faculty positions are available to new doctorates and postdoctorates.

Over the years the NRSA program has been responsible for several improvements and new developments in research training. For example, NIGMS has focused on multidisciplinary research training right from its first NRSA training grant awards in 1975. As a result, almost all universities now structure the education of basic biomedical scientists in a way that cuts across disciplinary and departmental lines. Similarly, after the NRSA program required (in 1990) that institutional training grants provide education in the responsible conduct of research, most universities began to offer such instruction to all students and fellows engaged in health research training, regardless of the source of their financial support. Finally, although M.D./Ph.D. training had been introduced by NIH prior to the passage of the National Research Act in 1974, dual-degree training programs have grown considerably since; they are now supported not only by NRSA funds but by private and institutional sources as well. In addition, dual-degree training has been extended to the oral health sciences. In 1996 the National Institute of Dental Research established a D.D.S./Ph.D. program.

To lessen the sizable personal investment required of those who pursue careers in biomedical, behavioral, or clinical research, the NRSA program provides its fellows and trainees with stipends and tuition subsidies. For predoctoral NRSA recipients, at least, the results have been measurable. Graduate students with NRSA support are more likely to

begin their careers without education debt than their fellow Ph.D.s in the life and social sciences. The effects of education debt are particularly striking for those who participate in NIH-sponsored M.D./Ph.D. programs: in 1996 their median debt was $1,000, in contrast to their medical school classmates who graduated with a single degree and whose median debt approached $60,000.

Beyond the financial differences, there are a number of other distinctions. A 1984 evaluation of formal NIH-sponsored research training, which included programs predating the establishment of the NRSA, found that participants in the programs were more likely than their counterparts to complete their doctoral programs and go on to NIH-supported postdoctoral training. Further, those supported by NIH during their predoctoral studies applied for and received NIH research grants with greater success, authored more articles, and were cited more often by their peers. At the postdoctoral level, regardless of whether trainees were appointed to institutional training grants or had received individual fellowship awards, they were more likely to pursue research careers than their colleagues without formal NIH research training. These differences were true for M.D.s with postdoctoral research training as well as Ph.D.s.

A follow-up to the 1984 evaluation of the NRSA predoctoral program was conducted in 1998 to examine the characteristics of doctorates from three groups between 1981 and 1992: NRSA-supported doctorates, Ph.D.s at institutions with NRSA training grants who did not receive this type of support, and doctorates at institutions without NRSA grants.[17] Many of the same conclusions were reached as in the 1984 study. In particular, it revealed the following:

- As an indicator of the high quality of the NRSA program, 80 percent of the NRSA trainees or fellows received their Ph.D.s from 50 institutions in the top quarter of the biomedical sciences programs, and nearly 60 percent received their degrees from the top 25 institutions.
- The completion rate for students supported by the NRSA program was an estimated 76 percent, a figure comparable to those of other merit-based national fellowship programs and students in high-quality doctoral programs.
- NRSA trainees and fellows spent less time enrolled in graduate school than their non-NRSA-supported counterparts—three months less than doctorates without NRSA support at their institutions and seven months less than those at institutions without NRSA grants.
- Nearly 58 percent of the NRSA trainees and fellows received their doctorates by the age of 30, compared to 38.9 and 32.3 percent, respectively, for the non-NRSA-supported doctorates from NRSA institutions and non-NRSA institutions.
- Following graduate school, NRSA recipients were, by some measures, more likely to make progress toward re-

---

[16]National Institutes of Health. 1998.

[17]Ibid.

search careers. In fields in which postdoctoral study is very common, 93 percent of the NRSA trainees and fellows reported definite postdoctoral commitments, compared to 84 and 80 percent, respectively, at NRSA institutions and non-NRSA institutions.

• NRSA trainees and fellows appeared to be more likely to move into faculty or research positions. About 37 percent of the NRSA recipients held faculty positions seven to 8 years past the doctorate, compared to 24 and 16 percent, respectively, for their non-NRSA-supported counterparts at NRSA institutions and non-NRSA institutions. Similarly, 87 percent of the NRSA trainees and fellows, compared to 77 and 72 percent, respectively, for the NRSA and non-NRSA institutions, were in research-related positions in academia, industry, or other research settings.

• NRSA trainees and fellows were more likely to have grants. For example, among the doctorates who received their degrees between 1981 and 1988 and applied to NIH by 1994 for research grant support, the success rate for NRSA recipients was 67 percent, compared to 55 and 47 percent, respectively, for the NRSA and non-NRSA institution graduates.

• NRSA trainees and fellows had more publications—another indicator of productivity.

• NRSA predoctoral trainees and fellows in the 1981–1982 cohort had a median number of publications (8.5) that was more than twice that of doctorates from institutions without NRSA grants (4) and 70 percent more than that of non-NRSA-supported Ph.D.s at NRSA institutions (5).

Such studies do not explain whether the success of former NRSA trainees and fellows reflects the training they re-ceived, the selection process, or other factors. Nonetheless, these findings do suggest some of the strengths and achievements of the NRSA program.

## STUDY ORIGINS AND RELATED ACTIVITIES

In the legislation that established the NRSA program, Congress decreed that awards be made only in areas for which "there is a need for personnel," and it directed that the National Academy of Sciences provide periodic guidance on the fields in which researchers were likely to be needed and the numbers that should be trained (see Box 1-1). In response, the National Research Council (NRC)—the operating arm of the National Academy of Sciences, Institute of Medicine, and National Academy of Engineering—has issued regular reports since 1975 on the supply of biomedical and behavioral researchers in the United States and the likely demand for new investigators. The present study is the twelfth one completed by the NRC.

## PAST REPORTS

In each of the 11 assessments of national need for research personnel in the biomedical and social and behavioral sciences submitted thus far by the NRC, the congressional committees adhered to the purpose of those assessments and forwarded the information to NIH and Congress for their use in making budgetary decisions. However, the manner in which the assessments should be conducted and the scope of the investigations were left to the discretion of the NRC. As a result, in many of the reports the characteristics, mecha-

---

**BOX 1-1**
**National Research Act of 1974 (P.L. 93-348)**

Sec. 472. (a) (3) Effective July 1, 1975, National Research Service Award may be made for research or research training in only those subject areas for which, as determined under section 473, there is a need for personnel.

Sec. 473. (a) The Secretary shall, in accordance with subsection (b), arrange for the conduct of a continuing study to—
(a) establish (A) the Nation's overall need for biomedical and behavioral research personnel, (B) the subject areas in which such personnel are needed and the number of such personnel needed in each such area, and (C) the kinds and extent of training which should be provided such personnel;
(b) assess (A) current training programs available for the training of biomedical and behavioral research personnel which are conducted under this Act at or through institutes under the National Institutes of Health and the Alcohol, Drug Abuse, and Mental Health Administration, and (B) other current training programs available for the training of such personnel;
(c) identify the kinds of research positions available to and held by individuals completing such programs;
(d) determine, to the extent feasible, whether the programs referred to in clause (B) or paragraph (2) would be adequate to meet the needs established under paragraph (1) if the programs referred to in clause (A) of paragraph (2) were terminated; and
(e) determine what modifications in the programs referred to in paragraph (2) are required to meet the needs established under paragraph (1).

(c) A Report on the results of the study required under subsection (a) shall be submitted by the Secretary to the Committee on Energy and Commerce of the House of Representatives and the Committee on Labor and Human Resources of the Senate at least once every four years.

nisms, and quality of NRSA training programs were also addressed.

Prior to the first assessment, the NRC conducted a feasibility study in late 1974 to determine if it was possible to collect the data, perform the analyses, and determine the need for biomedical and behavioral research personnel as outlined in the legislation. In early 1975 the committee for this study returned a report[18] which recommended that a follow-on study be conducted. While it recognized the difficulties of the task, the committee viewed it as necessary and feasible. Shortly after conclusion of the feasibility study, a committee was formed to conduct the first study. This study was preliminary and was to be completed in 90 days. The committee viewed its task as one of bringing readily available data and professional judgment to bear on the study requirements and looked to the 1976 study and beyond to provide the basis on which the effectiveness of continuing studies can be judged. The 1975 assessment limited its scope to the demand for faculty, basing findings on federal support for university-based research and enrollments in higher education.[19] With this information, it recommended that the training levels in FY 1976 be the same as in FY 1975, while emphasizing the importance of vesting quality in a smaller number of training programs and the need for a balance between supply and demand. It also set a precedent for later reports by broadly interpreting the research areas to include the basic biomedical sciences, the behavioral and social sciences, the clinical sciences and health services research and by providing training levels in each field. This committee, as well as later committees, noted the difficulties of making personnel projections on the basis of the available data; it singled out in particular the lack of data on medical doctors doing either basic biomedical or clinical research. It also drew attention to the growing postdoctoral pool in the early 1970s; while this population seemed to fall within reasonable bounds, the committee expressed concerns about its future size.

Initially the studies were conducted on an annual basis by a standing committee. In its first full-length report in 1976 the committee concluded that Ph.D. production in most areas was more than adequate to meet existing demand, though it recommended some changes from the 1975 level—in particular, that the number of predoctoral training positions in the biomedical sciences be reduced by 10 percent in 1976 and remain at that level through 1978. In the behavioral and social sciences, the committee recommended a dramatic shift from predoctoral to postdoctoral institutional training positions. While in 1975 the apportionment was about 90 percent predoctoral and 10 percent postdoctoral, the committee suggested that the proportion in the behavioral and social sciences instead be 30 percent predoctoral and 70 percent postdoctoral. Its reasoning was based on the perceived need

for research in special areas of health and the belief that individuals with a Ph.D. or an M.D. are better able to address those needs. The change was not to affect the funding level and was to take place over time, with an annual reduction of 250 to 350 predoctoral positions and an increase of 150 to 200 postdoctoral positions. Over the next few years NIH partially implemented this recommendation by cutting support at the predoctoral level from 1,754 in 1975 to 653 in 1980, but it increased support at the postdoctoral level from 212 in 1975 to only 349 in 1980. In addition, because the committee believed that the clinical area was one where there was a need for more support to increase the flow of M.D.s into clinical research careers, it recommended a 10 percent annual growth rate through 1978 at both the predoctoral and postdoctoral levels.

In the 1977, 1978, and 1979 studies the committee continued to express concerns about the increased number of doctorates, and the growing postdoctoral pool, in the biomedical sciences. In 1977 it recommended another 10 percent decrease in predoctoral support. In 1978 and 1979 it did not recommend additional decreases due to a concern that the loss of or a reduction in the size of training programs would seriously affect their quality. Each of these studies also reaffirmed the shift from predoctoral to postdoctoral support in the social and behavioral sciences. While recommendations on the number of positions were made for each of the four broad fields—the basic biomedical sciences, the social and behavioral sciences, the clinical sciences, and health services research—the committee in 1978 did draw attention to subfields in the biomedical sciences, such as toxicology and biostatistics, and presented reasons why they should have increased support. The 1979 assessment was the last of the annual reports. In 1978, amendments to the original NRSA Act of 1974 changed the report cycle to every 2 years.

The findings from the next study in 1981 were similar to those of the earlier studies. It expressed concern for career prospects in the biomedical sciences, a "soft" job market in the nonclinical social and behavioral sciences, and a continued need for physician-scientists in health-related research. Thus the committee's recommendations followed those of earlier studies: no change regarding the biomedical sciences, a shift from predoctoral to postdoctoral support in the social and behavioral sciences, and increases in predoctoral clinical support. The committee also focused on two other needs: to increase minority participation and to stabilize federal support of research training. The committee's report contained a rather complete list of federal programs aimed at increasing minority participation and recommended that assessments be made of these programs in order to determine their effectiveness. The committee's concern on the stability issue was that sharp fluctuations in training support could have serious consequences; it therefore suggested that a core level of support, independent of short-term demand, be maintained.

[18]National Research Council. 1975b.
[19]National Research Council. 1975a.

The reports in 1983 and 1985 found signs of increased demand for biomedical research personnel, such as the leveling off of the postdoctoral pool and a decline in the number of graduate students in this area. These committees also believed that recent biological discoveries would create a demand for researchers in industry, government, teaching hospitals, and other settings, and they incorporated employment trends in those sectors into their analyses of national need. By 1985 the biotechnology industry indeed began to recruit significant numbers of Ph.D.s, and that committee called for additional research training in the basic biomedical sciences. In the social and behavioral sciences, the 1983 and 1985 reports restated the need for increased training at the postdoctoral level in clinically related subfields and the return of predoctoral support to the 1981 level. With regard to clinical awards, there was an increase in 1981 over the numbers in the late 1970s, and committees in 1983 and 1985 supported this increase and recommended that it be maintained through 1987. But because they saw a need for increased training of physicians at the postdoctoral level, they stipulated that 85 percent of the positions at this level should go to physicians.

The next (1989) committee report, citing a decline in predoctoral biomedical positions from about 4,000 in 1985 to less than 3,700 in 1987, recommended a significant increase to 5,200 positions by 1995. For the social and behavioral sciences, the committee projected a fairly stable job market and recommended no change in current support levels. With regard to clinical fields, it did expect an increased demand for physician-scientists, but given the lack of reliable data it recommended no change in current support levels.

By 1994 demand for personnel in the biotechnology industry appeared to be slowing, and that year's committee recommended that NRSA training support in the basic biomedical sciences be maintained at the present levels—5,175 predoctoral and 3,835 postdoctoral trainees—through 1999. The committee also called for a gradual increase in research training in the social and behavioral sciences—at the predoctoral level from 673 positions in 1993 to 900 by 1996 and at the postdoctoral level from 323 to 500. This recommendation was not based on an increased demand for faculty but rather on the continuing gains being made by behavioral scientists in areas of national interest and thus on an *anticipated* demand for mental health–related research. In the clinical sciences the committee recommended an increase in MSTP grantees from 822 in 1993 to 1,020 in 1996 and a decrease in other clinical programs to offset the MSTP increase. The committee's 1994 report also expanded the scope of its investigation by highlighting several issues of particular concern to the administration of the NRSA program. These included the growth of the Ph.D. population in the biomedical sciences, the decline in the number of physician-researchers, the recognition that the social and behavioral sciences should play a more important role in health care, the decline in the proportion of graduate students funded by

training grants, and the lack of promising research career options for young scientists. These and related issues have subsequently been addressed in later NRSA reports and other policy studies (as discussed below).

In response to the major recommendations put forth by the 1994 study committee, NIH focused on increasing the stipends for trainees and fellows and on evaluating the NRSA program. The committee's suggestions for maintaining training levels in the basic biomedical sciences and for attracting underrepresented minorities also were pursued. However, recommendations for increasing the number of NRSA training grants and fellowships in the behavioral and clinical sciences, oral health, nursing, and health services research were not acted on; this prompted Congress to request a report on NIH's implementation of the 1994 study.[20] In explaining its actions to Congress, NIH indicated that it had focused on the highest-priority recommendations: it was likely to continue to direct additional research training monies to NRSA stipends until their levels were comparable to those of other sources. The level of support for the social and behavioral sciences, however, was a point of controversy, and this issue appeared again in a minority report in the next study.

The most recent committee to assess the need for research personnel began its work in 1997, concentrating its attention on the three broad fields of biomedical, behavioral, and clinical research, with dental, nursing, and health services research included in the latter category. Two major changes from earlier reports were this committee's movement away from detailed recommendations on the number of individuals who should be trained under the NRSA program and its use of a demographic life-table model, proposed in the 1994 report, to estimate the size of the workforce each year up to 2005. The life-table model was adopted in 1997 because previous models of supply and demand could not be relied on for valid forecasts. This report's analysis considered such factors as the average age of current investigators in the biomedical and behavioral sciences, the number of Ph.D.s expected to join the workforce in the years ahead, and the likely effect of retirements and deaths. The committee supplemented this analysis by reviewing indicators of short-term demand—trends in faculty and industry hiring, for example, and perceptions of the job market by recent Ph.D.s.

Implemented for the biomedical and social and behavioral sciences, the model showed that the supply of doctorates, even if at a low level, would be much greater than the demand for researchers during the projection period. This result prompted the committee to suggest that degree production be maintained at current levels in all three broad fields. However, it did recommend increases in clinical research related to patient care and in interdisciplinary research. Many of the committee's recommendations concerned administration of the NRSA program, and NIH

---

[20]National Institutes of Health. 1997.

responded by establishing new guidelines for stipends at the predoctoral and postdoctoral levels, encouraging early completion of education and training and establishing limitations on the period of NRSA support at the predoctoral and postdoctoral levels.

## A PERSPECTIVE ON RESEARCH TRAINING ACTIVITIES

Since the establishment of the NRSA program, several reports—other than those mandated by the NRSA Act of 1974—have addressed the state of health-related training, either in general or from the perspective of individual fields. Particular attention has been paid to clinical research and the need to train more physician-scientists. For example, a 1976 study[21] by the NRC found that postdoctoral training was essential to the research productivity of M.D.s. Similar results were obtained in a 1986 study by NIH.[22] The research activities of medical school faculty were addressed in a 1987 report,[23] which found that only 29.5 percent of the M.D.s in departments of medicine devoted 40 percent or more of their time to research and almost 30 percent of the M.D.s spent no time in research at all. These and related clinical research issues were also described in detail by Ahrens in 1992.[24]

In 1994 the Institute of Medicine (IOM) issued a report, *Careers in Clinical Research: Obstacles and Opportunities*,[25] that made the following recommendations for research training:

• Further evaluate clinical research training programs.
• Redirect funds to the most effective forms of clinical research training.
• Emphasize training programs that provide opportunities to earn advanced degrees in the evaluative sciences.
• Increase the number of M.D./Ph.D. and D.D.S./Ph.D. programs that train investigators with expertise in patient-oriented research.
• Expand initiatives that reduce education debt, either through tuition subsidies (as in the case of dual-degree programs) or loan forgiveness.

This report was followed in the spring of 1995 by the convening of an NIH director's panel to review the status of clinical research in the United States and to consider, among other topics, the recruitment and training of future clinical researchers. When the panel presented its report in late 1997, a number of the suggestions for clinical research training

paralleled those put forth by the IOM in 1994.[26] It included the following recommendations:

• Initiate clinical research training programs, such as M.D./Ph.D. programs specifically for clinical research, aimed at medical students.
• Ensure that postdoctoral training grants include formal training in clinical research.
• Provide new support mechanisms for young and mid-term clinical investigators.
• Take steps to reduce the education debt of clinical investigators.

Even before the panel issued its recommendations, NIH made a number of changes to support the training of clinical investigators. These included a program to bring medical and dental students to its Maryland campus for a one- to two-year clinical research training experience and new guidelines from the NIGMS to assure that its M.D./Ph.D. training grants would encourage research training in fields such as computer science, social and behavioral sciences, economics, epidemiology, public health, bioengineering, biostatistics, and bioethics. In response to the panel's recommendation regarding support mechanisms for young and midcareer investigators, NIH established three new career development awards aimed at advancing careers in clinical research.

Despite these efforts, the issues surrounding clinical research training remained unresolved, so in 1999 the Association of American Medical Colleges, in conjunction with several other organizations, convened a clinical research summit. The resulting report outlined nine core problems and made recommendations for each. For example, it cited the lack of a comprehensive clinical research agenda and suggested that the solution might lie in the formation of a National Clinical Research Roundtable. Such a roundtable was in fact formed by the IOM in 2000, and it has met on a regular basis since then to conduct workshops and discuss issues. Recent workshop reports have addressed topics ranging from the needs of the education infrastructure to engaging the public in the clinical research enterprise.

In 1995 another IOM committee published the results of a study in a related area—the training and supply of health services researchers—and the report[27] endorsed the recommendation of the 1994 NRSA "needs" study to substantially increase the number of training positions in health services research. The IOM report also encouraged the AHCPR, now the AHRQ, to focus its training funds on areas in which research was needed—such as outcomes measurement, biostatistics, epidemiology, health economics, and health policy—and to set up institutional training grants for innovative

[21]National Research Council. 1976.

[22]National Institutes of Health. 1986. *Effects of the National Research Service Award Program on Biomedical Research and Teaching Careers.* Bethesda, MD: NIH.

[23]Gentile, N. D., et al. 1987.

[24]Ahrens, E. H. Jr. 1992.

[25]Institute of Medicine. 1994.

[26]National Institutes of Health. 1997.

[27]Institute of Medicine. 1995.

research training programs. In response, AHCPR made "innovation awards" to 10 institutions in 1998 in order to support the design and implementation of new models of health services research training.[28]

One of the primary concerns in many of the NRSA "needs" studies for the biomedical sciences was the possible oversupply of researchers, as indicated at various times by the increasing number of doctorates being awarded and the growing size of the postdoctoral pool. While many books and articles, such as *In Pursuit of the PhD*, discussed the quality of doctoral education,[29] it was not until 1995 that the NRC published the findings of a major study directed at graduate training's effects on career progression. The report, *Reshaping the Graduate Education of Scientists and Engineers*, reviewed graduate education across the biological, physical, and social and behavioral sciences and engineering and called on universities to offer programs that allow for a broader range of career options; it also called on federal agencies to encourage this trend by supporting graduate education through training grants.[30] The report urged universities, government, industry, and professional organizations to work together to develop a national human resources policy for scientists and engineers.

In response to a congressional inquiry about how NIH was planning to adapt its policies to conform with the 1995 NRC report's recommendations, the agency noted that it would take steps to require institutions with training grants to expose their students to a range of career options. The NIGMS in particular announced new guidelines in 1997 for biomedical sciences graduate programs, so interested trainees might be able to take internships in industry as well as gain experience in teaching. In addition, graduate programs were urged to supply trainees with information on the career histories of previous graduates and to offer workshops on employment opportunities and career counseling.

A 1995 examination of supply and demand regarding Ph.D. scientists, published by Massy and Goldman (RAND Corp.), suggested that U.S. universities were producing more Ph.D.s than necessary in engineering, mathematics, and fields such as the biological and geological sciences.[31] Their paper maintained that this overproduction would create a group of chronically underemployed doctorates. An expansion in research funding, furthermore, would likely worsen future job prospects even further as more Ph.D.s were produced. Contending that enrollment of doctoral students in fields such as the biosciences was driven more by the need for research and teaching assistants than by the labor market, Massy and Goldman called for academic restructuring to bring the production of Ph.D.s into balance with demand. The authors noted that improvements in the development

and dissemination of data on the scientific and engineering labor market could help restrain production rates, but they ultimately concluded that Ph.D. overproduction would end only if departments were required to reduce their dependence on the research and teaching services provided by doctoral students. In a follow-up report, *The PhD Factory*,[32] in 2001 the authors predicted that without such requirements the "employment gap" (the difference between the supply and the demand) in the biosciences would exceed 25 percent into the future.

In 1996 a consensus conference sponsored by the Federation of American Societies for Experimental Biology addressed some of the issues raised by Massy and Goldman. It concluded by opposing national regulation on the size of graduate programs. However, participants called for data on employment trends to be made available to students and for universities to self-regulate the size of their graduate programs. In addition, institutions were urged to refrain from enrolling graduate students simply to meet teaching or research needs.

In 1994 an NRC report, *The Funding of Young Investigators in the Biological and Biomedical Sciences*, noted an increase in the age at which young researchers were obtaining their first R01 grant; as a result, an NRC committee was formed to examine the career paths of young investigators. The 1998 report, *Trends in the Early Careers of Life Scientists*, noted that the number of Ph.D.s awarded annually may be too high and called for restraining the rate of growth in the number of graduate students in the life sciences.[33] The report also suggested several policy options for the federal government to consider, such as restricting the number of graduate students supported by research grants and emphasizing research training via training grants and fellowships. However, in the end the committee noted that the rate of Ph.D. production was the cumulative result of individual decisions—by faculty, departments, universities, and students—and it maintained that these groups should bear the primary responsibility for implementing the committee's recommendations.

As the annual number of new doctorates in the biomedical sciences continued to grow during the 1980s and the 1990s, so did the postdoctoral pool. Aside from concerns about size, the working conditions of postdoctorates and the career guidance they were receiving also became serious issues. The NRC was prompted to release, in 2000, a widely distributed guide that set down a body of principles for advisors, institutions, funding organizations, and disciplinary societies to follow in addressing these issues.[34] At that time a number of institutions recognized the problems their postdoctorates were encountering and at a minimum began to count and keep track of postdoctoral appointments. Dedi-

[28]Agency for Healthcare Research and Quality. 1998.
[29]Bowen, W. G., and N. L. Rubenstine. 1992.
[30]National Research Council. 1995.
[31]Massy, W. F., and C. A. Goldman. 1995.

[32]Massy, W. F., and C. A. Goldman. 2001.
[33]National Research Council. 1994.
[34]National Research Council. 1998c.

cated offices were established, and local postdoctoral organizations were formed. Eventually, a national association was founded to provide a central voice in helping policymakers address postdoctoral employment and training issues.

It was not the size alone of the postdoctoral pool that has been of concern but the fact that postdoctorates are not independent researchers and cannot in most cases develop their own research agendas. This is a particular issue at NIH, which conducted a workshop in the fall of 2003 to investigate possible mechanisms for moving researchers it would normally support as postdoctorates into positions of independent research status. NIH also sponsored a meeting at the NRC in June 2004 to address the same subject. The report of that meeting will be published in early 2005.

The significant growth in the number of postdoctorates in the biomedical sciences may have been fueled in part by the growth in the NIH budget. The doubling of the NIH R&D budget—from $13.6 billion in 1998 to $27.2 billion in 2003—resulted in an increased number of new, competing, and noncompeting research grants (33,570 in 1998 to 45,922 in 2003) and an increase in the amount for these grants (from $9.58 billion to $18.04 billion). Although grant amounts have almost doubled, the number of awards has only increased by 36 percent, indicating that more personnel at the graduate and postdoctoral levels will be able to be supported on them. Now that the NIH budget has returned to relatively modest single-digit increases, graduate enrollment and the size of the postdoctoral pool may be reduced—though these effects are yet to be determined. It is also interesting to note that the number of Type I or new awards increased by 45 percent and that the amount of these awards more than doubled during the growth in the NIH budget, but a return to normal growth may have serious consequences for young investigators obtaining independent research status.

A new initiative at NIH that may have an impact on research training is the NIH Roadmap, developed during 2002 and 2003 at the urging of NIH Director Elias A. Zerhouni. This program, resulting from a process of internal discussions and consultation with leaders of the biomedical community, has three major themes:

- *New Pathways to Discovery*—a set of proposals that will create and develop new tools and technologies for bench scientists.
- *Research Teams of the Future*—a set of initiatives to promote public-private partnerships and to train investigators to work in interdisciplinary and multidisciplinary teams.
- *Reengineering the Clinical Research Enterprise*—a complete reorganization, expansion, and streamlining of clinical research in the United States.

NIH has been criticized in the past for its conservative approach—for funding research that may incrementally add to results already in hand. The NIH Roadmap is designed to break with this image and allow for greater innovation. Each of these themes encourages programs that cut across the NIH institutes and centers, with the aim of fostering new interdisciplinary areas of research.

Of the Requests for Applications (RFAs) issued so far, several are for research training. One of these, the Curriculum Development Award in Interdisciplinary Research, supports the creation of courses or curricula at the undergraduate, graduate, or postdoctoral levels that integrate the principles and conceptual approaches of diverse disciplines in emerging areas of biomedical research. Another RFA, Short Programs for Interdisciplinary Research Training, will support grants to develop 8- to 10-week training programs that combine lectures with lab experience. These courses are targeted at not only trainees but also established scientists seeking to develop interdisciplinary research projects. The program is open to a broad spectrum of the scientific community, including foreign as well as domestic institutions.

Using the NRSA mechanism, the National Institute of Mental Health is sponsoring an initiative that seeks to support as many as 40 postdoctoral scientists under an institutional training grant to integrate behavior, environment, and biology into a single discipline. Possibly, the most novel approach is a program called Training for a New Interdisciplinary Research Workforce, which uses a new funding mechanism (the T90) and seeks to capitalize on existing multidisciplinary and interdisciplinary research programs. This new training program, which combines aspects of research grants and NRSA training into a single mechanism, is open to all organizations, foreign and domestic. Trainees can be at any level, from undergraduate to postdoctoral, and do not need to be U.S. citizens or permanent residents.

## THE PRESENT STUDY

The purpose of the current study is to advise NIH and Congress on the appropriate level of training for the NRSA program. The committee for this study, in much the same spirit as the preceding study committee, has interpreted its charge more broadly and examined the contributions of the NRSA and career development programs in the general context of health-related research training.

The committee began its work in September 2002 and over the next 28 months held five meetings, drawing on members' own expertise—as well as information provided by government agencies and disciplinary professional organizations that support health-related research—to determine this study's findings and recommendations. The committee's objectives were to:

- Estimate future needs for biomedical, behavioral, and clinical research personnel.
- Make recommendations about the size and composition of the NRSA program and other NIH research training

and career development programs, using its estimates of future needs as well as information about the rate of Ph.D. production.

• Assess the quality of existing NIH research training and career development programs.

• Recommend modifications in the existing programs so that they may better prepare the research workforce to meet anticipated needs.

The committee's initial attention was focused on the biomedical, behavioral, and clinical fields, but it expanded its analysis to include oral health, nursing, and health services research. These three new fields were not addressed in the last report, nor were they initially identified for consideration in the current study. However, the corresponding NIH institutes and centers and the AHRQ asked the committee to examine training in these fields, given an apparent shortage of research personnel in oral health and nursing and a need for more training in health services research.

For this report a life-table model was developed to simulate the changing characteristics of the research workforce in the biomedical, behavioral, and clinical sciences and to assess the future need for personnel in each of these fields. Data from various sources were used to estimate the input of research personnel into the model and to estimate the outputs with mortality and retirement data. In assessing the results of this analysis, several qualifications are in order. First, the model is necessarily fairly simple. Second, available data for the model are incomplete, since it is difficult to determine what proportion of the workforce is actually engaged in research, the number of foreign training scientists that are researchers, and whether available data represent current trends. Third, the models base projections only on the current situation—or, to be more precise, the situation for which the data were valid (typically 2–3 years earlier). Fourth, extrapolation to the future depends in large part on unknown variables, such as the strength of the economy and the amounts of federal spending for research. This analysis was not conducted for oral health, nursing, or health services research for the same reasons as above, and in addition, the results would be even more questionable, since the size of the workforce is small.

It should be noted that the life-table model and much of the analysis in this report address the supply side for research personnel. Metrics for the demand side of the analysis are either unknown or are difficult to quantify. The demand for research personnel could depend on the state of the U.S. economy, the speed at which discovery takes place, levels of research support from government and foundations, the outsourcing of research to foreign countries or the growth of research in foreign countries, and the importance of a field of research in the general scientific and engineering enterprise. The unprecedented growth in the biomedical research workforce in the 1980s and 1990s was fueled by the important discoveries during and before this period and the financial resources that were available to support the research. Predicting this growth in the 1970s on the basis of the current workforce and degree production would have been difficult.

When developing recommendations for the future, it should be remembered that workforce models are only part of the necessary considerations. As shown in the data presented earlier in this chapter, NRSAs support only a relatively small fraction of the total number of people being trained in the biomedical, social and behavioral, and clinical sciences. This is a significant addition to the pool of trained personnel, but the primary role of the NRSA program is not to just add numbers to the pool. It serves several other more important roles. The NRSA program serves as a beacon to attract quality people into biomedical, behavioral, and clinical research. Perhaps the best example of this is the MSTP, which has a well-established track record for launching physicians into outstanding research careers. The program also serves to facilitate training in specific research areas, such as molecular and cell biology and biophysics. These awards also establish training standards that affect not only NRSA awardees but all trainees. Generally, the requirements imposed on individuals supported by training grants, for example, are also imposed on trainees supported by other means. Finally, they offer the possibility of providing support for training in emerging areas for which other mechanisms may not be available. This has been particularly important in promoting multi- and interdisciplinary training.

Because the NRSA program's leadership role in research training is so vital to the health of the biomedical, behavioral, and clinical research establishments, a regular assessment is important. Moreover, in formulating this report the committee tried to weigh all of the above factors not only to assess the situation but also to arrive at a set of recommendations for *optimizing* the NRSA program in the future. In that way the committee anticipates that the NRSA program will continue to be the bellwether for improved health care through research.

Following this introductory and background discussion, Chapters 2, 3, and 4 focus on research workforce considerations in the biomedical sciences, behavioral and social sciences, and clinical sciences, respectively. The next three chapters examine in succession the training issues in oral health, nursing, and health services research. In Chapter 8 the committee addresses aspects of training for emerging fields and interdisciplinary research. Chapter 9 discusses various stages in the career progression of biomedical, behavioral, and clinical researchers, as well as the impact—or lack of it—of foreign-trained scientists and underrepresented minorities. Chapter 10 offers some final overarching comments and recommendations.

# 2

# Basic Biomedical Sciences Research

Basic biomedical research, which addresses mechanisms that underlie the formation and function of living organisms, ranging from the study of single molecules to complex integrated functions of humans, contributes profoundly to our knowledge of how disease, trauma, or genetic defects alter normal physiological and behavioral processes. Recent advances in molecular biology techniques and characterization of the human genome, as well as the genomes of an increasing number of model organisms, have provided basic biomedical researchers with the tools to elucidate molecular-, cellular-, and systems-level processes at an unprecedented depth and rate.

Thus basic biomedical research affects clinical research and vice versa. Biomedical researchers supply many of the new ideas that can be translated into potential therapies and subsequently tested in clinical studies, while clinical researchers may suggest novel mechanisms of disease that can then be tested in basic studies using animal models.

The tools also now exist to rapidly apply insights gained from model organisms to human health and disease. For example, gene mutations known to contribute to human disease can be investigated in model organisms, whose underlying characteristics lend them to rapid assessment. Resulting treatment strategies can then be tested in mammalian species prior to the design of human clinical trials.

These and other mutually supportive systems suggest that such interactions between basic biomedical and clinical researchers not only will continue but will grow as the two domains keep expanding. But the two corresponding workforces will likely remain, for the most part, distinct.

Similarly, there is a symbiosis between basic biomedical and behavioral and social sciences research (covered in Chapter 3) and an obvious overlap at the interface of neuroscience, physiological psychology, and behavior. The boundary between these areas is likely to remain indistinct as genetic and environmental influences that affect brain formation and function are better understood. Consequently, such investigations will impact the study of higher cognitive functions, motivation, and other areas traditionally studied by behavioral and social scientists.

Basic biomedical research will therefore undoubtedly continue to play a central role in the discovery of novel mechanisms underlying human disease and in the elucidation of those suggested by clinical studies. As an example, although a number of genes that contribute to disorders such as Huntington's, Parkinson's, and Alzheimer's disease have been identified, the development of successful therapies will require an understanding of the role that the proteins encoded by these genes play in normal cellular processes. Similarly, realizing the potential of stem cell–based therapies for a number of disorders will require characterization of the signals that cause stem cells to differentiate into specific cell types. Thus a workforce trained in basic biomedical research will be needed to apply current knowledge and that gained in the future toward the improvement of human health. Since such research will be carried out not only in academic institutions but increasingly in industry as well, the workforce must be sufficient to supply basic biomedical researchers for large pharmaceutical companies as well as smaller biotech and bioengineering firms, thereby contributing to the economy as well as human health.

The role of the independent investigator in academe, industry, and government is crucial to this research enterprise. They provide the ideas that expand knowledge and the research that leads to discovery. The doubling of the NIH budget has increased the number of research grants and the number of investigators but not at a rate commensurate to the budget increases. Grants have become bigger and senior investigators have received more of them. While this trend has not decreased the nation's research capacity, there may be things that will affect the future pool of independent researchers, such as a sufficient number of academic faculty that can apply for research grants, an industrial workforce that is more application oriented, and most important, a decline in doctorates from U.S. institutions.

## BIOMEDICAL RESEARCH WORKFORCE

The research workforce for the biomedical sciences is broad and diverse. It is primarily composed of individuals who hold Ph.D.s, though it also includes individuals with broader educational backgrounds, such as those who have earned their M.D.s from the Medical Scientist Training Program (MSTP) or other dual-degree programs. In addition, some individuals with M.D.s but without Ph.D.s have acquired the necessary training to do basic biomedical research. But although the analysis in this report should ideally be based on the entire workforce just defined, there are no comprehensive databases that identify the research activities of M.D.s. Therefore much of the analysis will be restricted to holders of a Ph.D. in one of the fields listed in Appendix C, with the assumption that an individual's area of research is related to his or her degree field. A separate section in this chapter is devoted to M.D.s doing biomedical research, and an analysis of the clinical research M.D. workforce is given in Chapter 4.

It should also be noted that the discussion in this chapter does not include individuals with doctorates in other professions, such as dentistry and nursing even if they hold a Ph.D. in addition to their professional degrees. However, there are important workforce issues in these two fields, and they are addressed separately in Chapters 5 and 6 of this report.

## EDUCATIONAL PROGRESSION

The major sources of Ph.D. researchers in the biomedical sciences are the U.S. research universities, but a substantial number also come from foreign institutions. These scientists, whether native or foreign born, enter the U.S. biomedical research workforce either directly into permanent assignments or via postdoctoral positions.

For most doctorates in the biomedical sciences, interest in the field begins at an early age, in high school or even grade school. In fact, almost all high school graduates (93 percent) in the class of 1998 took a biology course—a rate much greater than other science fields, for which the percentages are below 60 percent.[1] Even in the early 1980s, over 75 percent of high school graduates had taken biology, compared to about 30 percent for chemistry, which had the next-highest enrollment. This interest in biology continues into college, with 7.3 percent of the 2000 freshman science and engineering (S&E) population having declared a major in biology. This was an increase from about 6 percent of freshman majors in the early 1980s but less than the high of about 9.5 percent in the mid-1990s. Overall, the number of freshman biology majors increased from about 50,000 in the early 1980s to over 73,000 in 2000.[2] In terms of actual

bachelor's degrees awarded in the biological sciences, there was a decrease from about 47,000 in 1980 to 37,000 in 1989 and then a relatively sharp rise to over 67,000 in 1998. This was followed by a slight decline to about 65,000 in 2000.

There is attrition, however, in the transition from undergraduate to graduate school. In the 1980s and 1990s only about 11,000 first-year students were enrolled at any one time in graduate school biology programs. Percentage-wise, this loss of students is greater than in other S&E fields but is understandable: many undergraduates obtain a bachelor's degree in biology as a precursor to medical school and have no intention of graduate study in biology per se. The total graduate enrollment in biomedical sciences at Ph.D.-granting institutions grew in the early 1990s and was steady at a little under 50,000 during the latter part of the decade. However, there was some growth in 2001, of about 4 percent over the 2000 level, and the growth from 2000 to 2002 was about 10 percent (see Figure 2-1), driven in large part by an 18.9 percent increase of temporary residents. The overall growth may not continue, however, as the first-year enrollment for this group slowed from 8.9 percent in 2001 to 3.0 percent in 2002.

The tendency for graduate students to receive a doctorate in a field similar to that of their baccalaureate degree is not as strong in the biomedical sciences as it is in other fields, where it is about 85 percent. From 1993 to 2002, some 68.4 percent of the doctorates in biomedical programs received their bachelor's degree in the same field and another 8.4 percent received bachelor's degrees in chemistry.[3] This relative tendency to shift fields should not be viewed negatively, however, as doctoral students with exposure to other disciplines at the undergraduate level could provide the opportunity for greater interdisciplinary training and research.

## EARLY CAREER PROGRESSION IN THE BIOMEDICAL SCIENCES

Advances in biomedical research and health care delivery, together with a strong economy in the 1990s and increased R&D support, drove the growth of academic programs. Total academic R&D expenditures in the biological sciences, in 2001 dollars, began to rise dramatically in the early 1980s. They started from a base of about $3 billion and reached a plateau of almost $5 billion in the mid-1990s. As seen in Figure 2-2, this increase of about $2 billion was virtually repeated in the much shorter period from the late 1990s to 2002, as the NIH budget doubled. Although the increases in R&D support during the earlier period were reflected in the increased graduate enrollments of the 1980s and mid-1990s (seen in Figure 2-1), the enrollments since then have not kept pace with fast-growing R&D expenditures. This

---

[1]U.S. Department of Education. 2000.

[2]Tabulations from the Higher Education Research Institute and the U.S. Department of Education.

[3]Unpublished tabulation from the Survey of Earned Doctorates, 2001. Available from the National Academies.

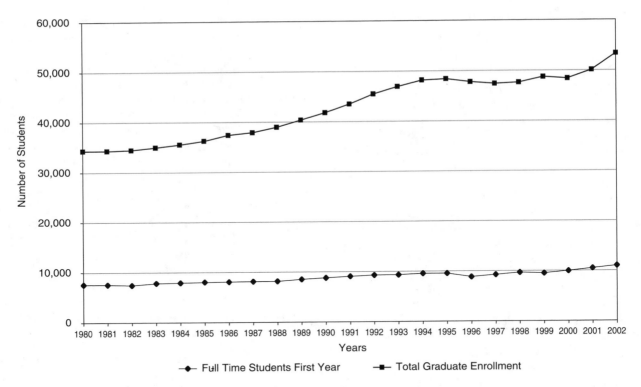

FIGURE 2-1  First-year and total graduate enrollment in the biomedical sciences at Ph.D.-granting institutions, 1980–2002.
SOURCE: National Science Foundation Survey of Graduate Students and Postdoctorates in Science and Engineering.

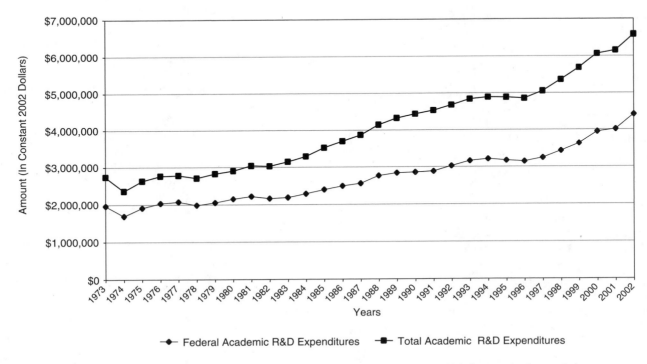

FIGURE 2-2  Academic research and development expenditures in the biological sciences. (All dollars are in thousands.)
SOURCE: National Science Foundation R&D Expenditures at Universities and Colleges, 1973–2002. Adjusted to 2002 dollars by the Biomedical R&D Price Index.

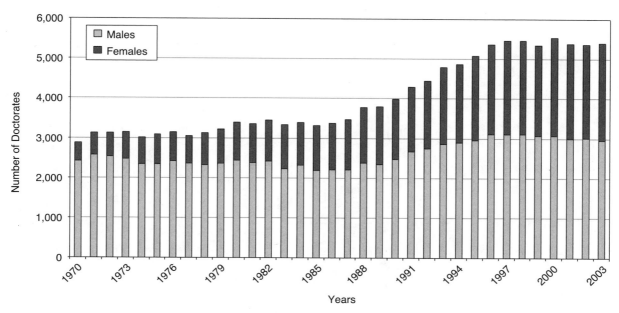

FIGURE 2-3 Number of doctorates in the biomedical sciences, 1970–2003.
SOURCE: National Science Foundation Survey of Earned Doctorates, 2001.

disconnect between research funding and enrollment in the late 1990s is difficult to explain but could in part be due to the unsettled career prospects in the biomedical sciences. In a report[4] from the American Society for Cell Biology, the authors examined the data on enrollment and surveyed both undergraduate and graduate students and postdoctorates on their career goals and found that students were aware of and concerned about the problem young people were having in establishing an independent research career. This ASCB report, as well as in the National Research Council report, *Trends in the Early Careers of Life Scientists,*[5] express concern for the future of biomedical research, if the best young people pursue different career paths. This slowdown in graduate enrollment in the late 1990s might have also contributed to the expansion of the postdoctoral and non-tenure-track faculty pool of researchers, since there was an increasing need for research personnel.

The increase in funding and enrollments in the early 1990s did lead to an increase in doctoral degrees awarded in the late 1990s, as seen in Figure 2-3. Since the 1970s, Ph.D.s awarded by U.S. institutions in the biomedical sciences increased from roughly 3,000 then to 5,366 in 2002. Most of the increase occurred in the mid-1990s and has since remained fairly constant. The year with the largest number of doctorates was 2000, when 5,532 degrees were awarded. The number of degrees in 2000 may be an anomaly, since the

number in 2001 (5,397 Ph.D.), 2002 (5,375 Ph.D.), and 2003 (5,412 Ph.D.) are more in line with the number in the late 1990s (see Appendix Table E-1).

Increases in doctorates were seen among women, temporary residents, and underrepresented minorities. Notably, since 1986 much of the increase in the number of doctorates has come from increased participation by women. In 1970 only 16 percent of doctorates were awarded to women; by 2003 the percentage had grown to 45.2. Temporary residents earned about 10 percent of the doctorates in 1970, and although this had increased to almost one-quarter in the early 2000s, it was still lower than the percentage awarded in many other fields in the physical sciences and engineering. Participation by underrepresented minorities in 2003 stood at 9.4 percent—as in many other S&E fields, substantially below their representation in the general population.

The percentage of doctorates with definite postdoctoral study plans increased from about 50 percent in the early 1970s to a high of 79 percent in 1995. It then declined to 71 percent in 2002 but increased to 75 percent in 2003. The changes in doctorates electing postdoctoral study are reflected in those choosing employment after they received their degrees (from 20 percent in 1995 to 28 percent in 2002 and 25 percent in 2003). It is difficult to find reasons for these changes in career plans. Prior to 2003 it may be the result of more diverse and attractive employment opportunities generated by recent advances in the applied biological sciences, especially in industry, or a conscious choice not to pursue an academic research career, where postdoctoral training is required since an academic position may not be

---

[4]Freeman, R. B., et. al. 2001.
[5]National Research Council. 1998c.

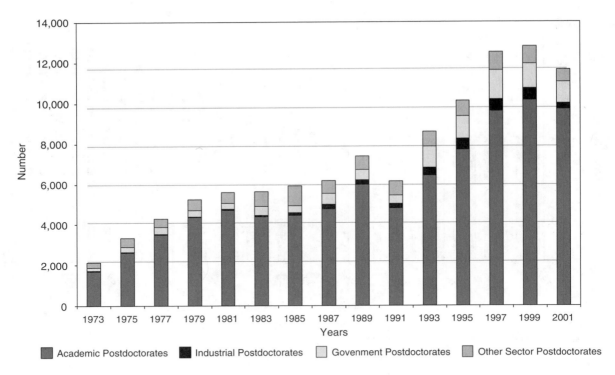

FIGURE 2-4  Postdoctoral appointments in the biomedical sciences by sector, 1973–2001.
SOURCE: National Science Foundation Survey of Doctorate Recipients.

available down the road. The increase in postdoctoral appointments in 2003 and the decline in employment might be due to poor economic conditions in the early part of this decade. Whether these changes will impact the quality of the biomedical workforce and its research should be monitored.

Time to degree, age at receipt of degree, and the long training period prior to reaching R01 research status have been cited as critical issues in the career progression of biomedical researchers.[6] Graduate students are taking longer and longer periods of time to earn their Ph.Ds. The median registered time in a graduate degree program gradually increased from 5.4 years in 1970 to 6.7 years in 2003, and the median age of a newly minted degree holder in the biomedical sciences grew during the same period—from 28.9 in 1970 to 30.6 in 2003 (see Appendix E). It should be noted that this time to degree is shorter than those of such fields as physics, computer science, and the earth sciences. Only chemistry, mathematics, and engineering have a lower median age at time of degree. While shortening the time in graduate school would reduce the age at which doctorates could become independent investigators, it may not significantly affect their career paths since postdoctoral training is required of almost

all researchers in the biomedical sciences, and the time spent in these positions seems to be lengthening.

With the growth of research funding and productivity in the biomedical sciences, the postdoctoral appointment has become a normal part of research training. From the 1980s to the late 1990s, the number of postdoctoral appointments doubled for doctorates from U.S. educational institutions (see Figure 2-4). The rapid increase in the postdoctoral pool from 1993 to 1999 in particular appears to be the result of longer training periods for individuals and not the result of an increase in the number of individuals being trained since Table E-1 shows a decline in the number of new doctorates planning postdoctoral study and the number of doctorates has remained fairly constant over recent years.

The lengthening of postdoctoral training is documented by data collected in 1995 on the employment history of doctorates.[7] Of the Ph.D.s who pursued postdoctoral study after graduating in the early 1970s, about 35 percent spent less than two years and about 65 percent spent more than 2 years in a postdoctoral appointment. By contrast, of Ph.D.s who received their degrees in the late 1980s and completed postdoctorates in the 1990s, 80 percent spent more than two

[6]Goldman, E. and E. Marshall. 2002.

[7]National Science Foundation. 1997.

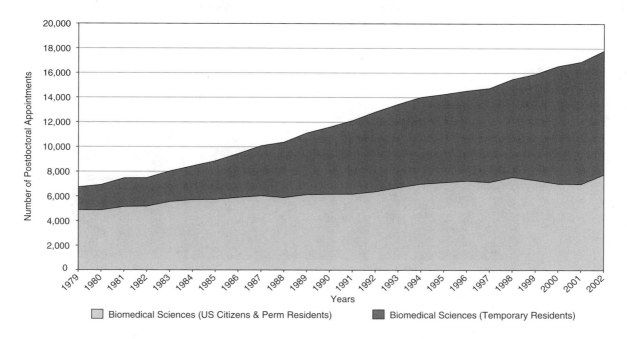

FIGURE 2-5 Postdoctoral appointments in academic institutions in the biomedical sciences.
SOURCE: National Science Foundation Survey of Graduate Students and Postdoctorates in Science and Engineering.

years and 20 percent spent less than 2 years in such appointments. More indicative of the change in postdoctoral training was the increase in the proportion that spent more than 4 years in a position, from about 20 percent to nearly 40 percent.

In 2001 the number of postdoctoral appointments actually declined across all employment sectors. This decline might be the result of lower interest by new doctorates in postdoctoral study and an academic career but is probably a response to the highlighting of issues related to postdoctoral appointments, such as the long periods of training with lack of employment benefits, the general perception that the positions are more like low-paying jobs than training experiences, and the poor prospects of a follow-up position as an independent investigator. Not only is interest in postdoctoral positions declining, there appears to be more rapid movement out of them by present incumbents. (These phenomena are more fully explored in Chapter 9, Career Progression.)

The above discussion applies only to U.S. doctorates. There are also a large number of individuals with Ph.D.s from foreign institutions being trained in postdoctoral positions in U.S. educational institutions and other employment sectors. Data from another source are available for postdoctorates from this population at academic institutions,[8] but there is no source for data in the industrial, governmental,

and nonprofit sectors other than an estimate that about half of the 4,000 intramural postdoctoral appointments at NIH are held by temporary residents. Almost all of these temporary residents have foreign doctorates. The number of temporary residents in academic institutions steadily increased through the 1980s and 1990s until 2002 when the number reached 10,000 (see Figure 2-5). The data also show that the rate at which temporary residents took postdoctoral positions slowed in 2002. The decline in academic appointments in 2001 for U.S. citizens and permanent residents population that was described above is also seen in this data, but that might be temporary since there was an increase in 2002. The reasons for this change may be twofold: a tighter employment market for citizens and permanent residents and immigration restrictions. However, it is still important to recognize that foreign-educated researchers hold about two-thirds of the postdoctoral positions in academic institutions. If national security policies were to limit the flow of foreign scientists into the United States, this could adversely affect the research enterprise in the biomedical sciences.

## A PORTRAIT OF THE WORKFORCE

The traditional career progression for biomedical scientists after graduate school includes a postdoctoral position followed by an academic appointment, either a tenure-track or nonpermanent appointment that is often on "soft" research money. As shown in Figure 2-6, the total population of aca-

---

[8]National Science Foundation. 2002b.

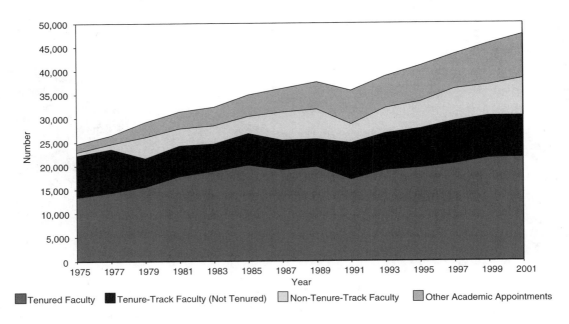

FIGURE 2-6  Academic positions for doctorates in the biomedical sciences, 1975–2001. SOURCE: National Science Foundation Survey of Doctorate Recipients.

demic biomedical sciences researchers, excluding post-doctoral positions, grew at an average annual rate of 3.1 per-cent from 1975 to 1989.[9]

Since 1995, growth slowed to about 2.5 percent, with al-most all of the growth in the non-tenure-track area. From 1999 to 2001 there was actually a decline in the number of non-tenure-track positions (by a few hundred). The fastest-growing employment category since the early 1980s has been "Other Academic Appointments," which is currently increasing at about 4.9 percent annually (see Appendix E-2). These jobs are essentially holding positions, filled by young researchers, coming from postdoctoral experiences, who would like to join an academic faculty on a tenure track and are willing to wait. In effect, they are gambling because in-stitutions are restricting the number of faculty appointments in order to reduce the possible long-term commitments that come with such positions. From 1993 to 2001, the number of tenure-track appointments increased by only 13.8 percent, while those for non-tenure-track faculty and other academic appointments increased by 45.1 percent and 38.9 percent, respectively.

The longer time to independent research status is also seen by looking at the age distributions of tenure-track faculty over the past two decades (see Figure 2-7). By comparing age cohorts in 1985 and 2001, it is observed that doctorates entered tenure-track positions at a later age in 2001.

For example, while about 1,000 doctorates in the 33 to 34 age cohort were in faculty positions in 1985, only about half that number were similarly employed in 2001, even though the number of doctorates for that cohort was greater in the late 1990s than in the early 1980s. The age cohort data also show that the academic workforce is aging, with about 20 percent of the 2001 academic workforce over the age of 58. The constraints of a rather young biomedical academic workforce and the conservative attitudes of institutions to not expand their faculties in the tight economic times of the early 1990s may have slowed the progression of young re-searchers into research positions. However, this may change in the next 8 to 10 years as more faculty members retire.

Meanwhile, over 40 percent of the biomedical sciences workforce is employed in nonacademic institutions (see Fig-ure 2-8). Researchers' employment in industry, the largest of these other sectors, has been growing at a 15 percent rate over the past 20 years. There was a lull in employment in the early 1990s, but growth since the mid-1990s has been strong. The increases in industrial employment may be due to the unavailability of faculty positions, but is more likely fueled by the R&D growth in pharmaceutical and other medical industries from $9.3 billion in 1992 to $24.6 in 2001 (con-stant 2001 dollars).[10] In 1992 almost all of this funding was from nonfederal sources, but in 2001 only 42 percent was from those sources. The result of this increase in federal

---

[9]The down turn in 1991 may be due to a change in the Survey of Doctor-ate Recipient data collection methods.

[10]National Science Foundation. 2004.

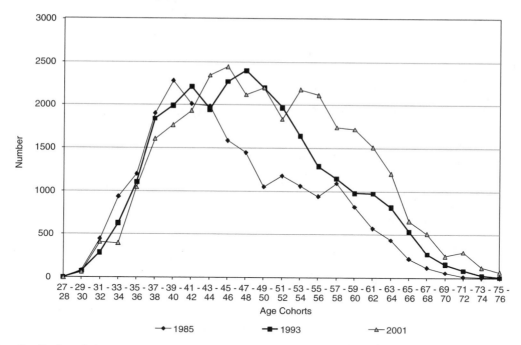

FIGURE 2-7  Age distribution of biomedical tenured and tenure-track faculty, 1985, 1993, and 2001.
SOURCE: National Science Foundation Survey of Doctorate Recipients.

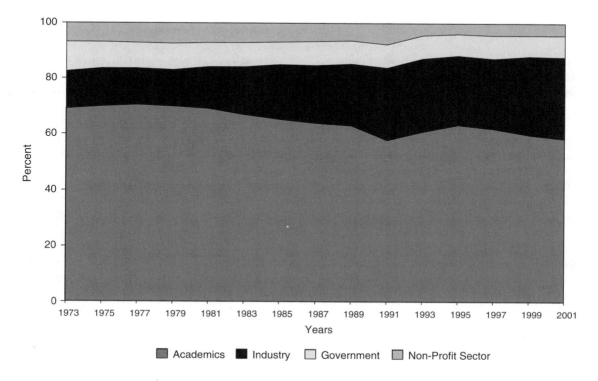

FIGURE 2-8  Employment of biomedical scientists by sector, 1973–2001.
SOURCE: National Science Foundation Survey of Doctorate Recipients.

funding has resulted in an increase in R&D employment, but not as large as would be expected. It is difficult to estimate the increase in biomedical doctorates in this industrial sector since they are drawn from many fields and are at different degree levels, but the total full-time equivalent R&D scientists and engineers increased 6.2 percent from 38,700 in 1992 to 41,100 in 2001.[11] However, there may be a trend toward increased employment in this sector, since a growing fraction of new doctorates are planning industrial employment (see Table E-1). The downturn in 2003 may be an anomaly due to the economy and not the strength of the medical industry, but data from a longer time period will be needed before definite trends in industrial employment can be determined. The government and nonprofit sectors have been fairly stable in their use of biomedical scientists, with about 8 and 4 percent growth rates, respectively, in recent years.

The number of underrepresented minorities in the basic biomedical sciences workforce increased from 1,066 in 1975 to 5,345 in 2001 and now accounts for 5.3 percent of the research employment in the field. Even though the annual average rate of growth for minorities in the workforce has been 15 percent over the past 10 years—more than twice the growth rate of the total workforce (6.5 percent)—the overall representation of minorities in biomedical research is still a small percentage of the overall workforce (see Appendix E-2). Their representation is also important from the scientific perspective, since researchers from minority groups may be better able and willing to address minority health care issues.

## PHYSICIAN-RESEARCHERS

Throughout this report Ph.D.s are considered to be researchers or potential researchers, but no such assumption is made of M.D.s because they could be practitioners. The above discussion, in particular, applies only to Ph.D.s in the fields listed in Appendix C, but it does not take into consideration physicians who are doing basic biomedical research. It is difficult to get a complete picture of this workforce because there is no database that tracks M.D.s involved in such activity, but a partial picture can be obtained from NIH files on R01 awards.

In 2001, R01 grants were awarded to 4,383 M.D.s (and to 17,505 Ph.D.s).[12] The number of R01-supported M.D. researchers has been increasing over the years (see Table 2-1) but has remained at about 20 percent. This means that the size of the biomedical workforce could be as much as one-fifth larger than indicated above. In fact, since NIH began to classify clinical research awards in 1996, it has become evident that both M.D.s and M.D./Ph.D.s supported by the agency are more likely to conduct nonclinical—that is, bio-

TABLE 2-1  Number of M.D.s and Ph.D.s with Grant Support from NIH

|  | 1993 | 1995 | 1997 | 1999 | 2001 |
|---|---|---|---|---|---|
| M.D.s with R01 Support | 3,115 | 3,123 | 3,527 | 3,762 | 4,383 |
| Ph.D.s with R01 Support | 11,230 | 10,983 | 11,621 | 13,469 | 17,505 |

SOURCE: NIH IMPACII Database.

medical—than clinical research. Because many physician-investigators approach nonclinical research with the goal of understanding the mechanisms underlying a particular disease or disorder, their findings are likely to ultimately contribute to improvements in human health.

Some data are available from the American Medical Association on the national supply of physicians potentially in research. In 2002 there were 15,316 medical school faculty members in basic science departments and 82,623 in clinical departments. Of those in basic science, 2,255 had M.D. degrees, 11,471 had Ph.D.s, and 1,128 had combined M.D./Ph.D. degrees. To identify the M.D.s in basic science departments who were actually doing research, the Association of American Medical Colleges Faculty Roster was linked to NIH records; it found that 1,261 M.D.s had been supported as principal investigators (PIs) on an R01 NIH grant at some point. This number is clearly an undercount of the M.D. research population, however, given that there are forms of NIH research support other than PI status and non-NIH organizations also support biomedical research.

## THE NATIONAL RESEARCH SERVICE AWARD PROGRAM AND BIOMEDICAL TRAINING SUPPORT

### The National Research Service Award Program

In 1975, when the National Research Service Award (NRSA) program began, 23,968 graduate students in the basic biomedical sciences received some form of financial assistance for their studies, and about 8,000 supported their own education through loans, savings, or family funds.[13] The number of fellowships and traineeships, whether institutional or from external sources, was about 8,500 in 1975 and remained at about that level into the early 1990s, increasing only recently to 12,186 in 2002 (see Figure 2-9).

In the 1970s the majority of graduate student support came from these fellowships, traineeships, and institutional teaching assistantships. The picture began to change in the early 1980s as the prevalence of research grants grew. By 2002 it represented almost 50 percent of the support for graduate study in the biomedical sciences, and NIH's fund-

---

[11]Ibid.

[12]NIH Web site: *http://grants.nih.gov/grants/award/research/rgbydgre 01.htm.* Accessed on October 22, 2004.

---

[13]Unpublished tabulation from the NIH IMPAC System.

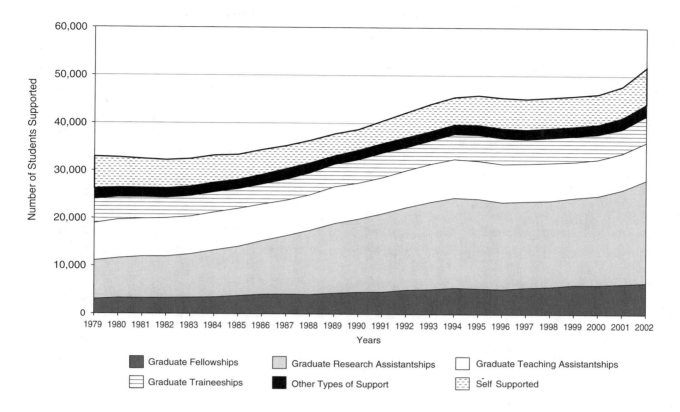

FIGURE 2-9 Mechanisms of support for full-time graduate students in the biomedical sciences, 1979–2002.
SOURCE: National Science Foundation Survey of Graduate Students and Postdoctorates in Science and Engineering.

ing of this mechanism grew as well. In the early 1980s, NIH research grants formed about 40 percent of the total, and by the early 1990s this fraction grew to 64 percent and has remained at about this level through 2002 (see Figure 2-10). Even during the years when the NIH budget doubled, there was not a shift in this balance. In fact, from 1997 to 2002 both research grant and trainee/fellowship support from NIH increased by 14 percent. NIH in its response to the 2000 assessment of the NRSA program[14] has stated that research grants and trainee/fellowship awards are not used for the control of graduate support and that it would be inappropriate to try to do so.

The NRSA program now comprises the major part of NIH's fellowship and traineeship support. It began small in 1975—with 1,046 traineeships and 26 fellowships—but quickly expanded. By 1980 the number was nearly 5,000 for the traineeships; it remained at that level until 2001, though it dropped to a little over 4,000 in 2002 (see Table 2-2). (The drop in 2002 traineeships was probably an institutional reporting issue. Given that the total number of awards by NIH

under the T32[15] mechanisms was about the same as in 2001, it is unlikely that the awards in the biomedical sciences would fall below the 2000 or 2001 levels.)

Information on funding patterns for postdoctorates in the basic biomedical sciences is not as complete as that for graduate students since academic institutions are the only sources of data. As has been the case for graduate student support, the portion of federal funds devoted to postdoctoral training grants and fellowships has diminished since the 1970s. In 1995, 1,966 (or 45.3 percent) of the 4,343 federally funded university-based postdoctorates received their training on a fellowship or traineeship. By 2002 the number had increased to 2,670 but was still only 20.3 percent of the total federal funding. The remaining 79.7 percent (or 10,514) in 2002 were supported by federal research grants. Meanwhile, the number of postdoctoral positions, funded by nonfederal institutional sources, was fairly constant at about 25 percent and grew from 1,325 in 1975 to 4,628 in 2002.

The picture for NRSA support at the postdoctoral level for the period following introduction of the NRSA program resembled that of the graduate level. However, in 2002 there was a sharp decrease in the number of postdoctoral trainee-

[14]NIH Web site: NIH Statement in Response to *Addressing the Nation's Changing Needs for Biomedical and Behavioral Scientists, http://grants. nih.gov/training/nas_report/NIHResponse.htm.*

[15]See Appendix B for a complete explanation of the awards.

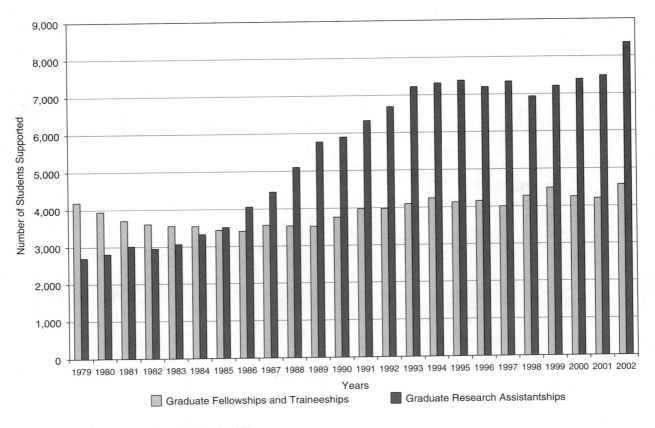

FIGURE 2-10 Graduate support for NIH, 1979–2002.
SOURCE: National Science Foundation Survey of Graduate Students and Postdoctorates in Science and Engineering.

TABLE 2-2 NRSA Predoctoral Trainee and Fellowship Support in the Basic Biomedical Sciences

|                              | 1975  | 1980  | 1985  | 1990  | 1995  | 2000  | 2001  | 2002[a] |
|------------------------------|-------|-------|-------|-------|-------|-------|-------|---------|
| Traineeships (T32)[b]        | 1,046 | 4,834 | 4,996 | 4,648 | 4,495 | 5,083 | 5,099 | 4,171   |
| Fellowships (F30, F31)[b]    | 26    | 9     | 74    | 103   | 365   | 297   | 402   | 462     |

[a]For 2002 and possibly 2001, the data are incomplete for traineeships since educational institutions report on the number of students trained in certain fields and the information was last processed in February 2003.

[b]See Appendix B for a complete explanation of the awards.

SOURCE: NIH IMPACII Database.

ships; but, as in the case for predoctoral trainees, this may be an institutional reporting issue (see Table 2-3). Since the decline from 2001 to 2002 is nearly 50 percent and the decline for predoctoral trainees was only 20 percent, there may be a real decline at the postdoctoral level. The reason for this is unclear, though factors may include the limited number of individuals who can be supported under the increased stipend levels and the general decline in the number of postdoctoral research trainees eligible for NRSA support.

The shift in the pattern of federal research training sup-

port, at both the graduate and postdoctoral levels, can be traced to a number of related trends. Over the past 25 years, the number of research grants awarded by the NIH and other agencies of the U.S. Department of Health and Human Services has more than doubled.[16] PIs have come to depend on graduate students and postdoctorates to carry out much of their day-to-day research work, and, as a result, the number

[16]NIH Web site. Available on *http://grants.nih.gov/grants/award/research/rgbydgre01.htm*. Accessed October 22, 2004.

TABLE 2-3 NRSA Postdoctoral Trainee and Fellowship Support in the Basic Biomedical Sciences

| | 1975 | 1980 | 1985 | 1990 | 1995 | 2000 | 2001 | 2002[a] |
|---|---|---|---|---|---|---|---|---|
| Traineeships (T32)[b] | 518 | 2,299 | 2,068 | 1,897 | 1,794 | 1,756 | 1,668 | 888 |
| Fellowships (F32)[b] | 936 | 1,944 | 1,501 | 1,413 | 1,574 | 1,391 | 1,383 | 1,232 |

[a]For 2002 and possibly 2001, the data are incomplete for traineeships since educational institutions report on the number of students trained in certain fields and the information was last processed in February 2003.

[b]See Appendix B for a complete explanation of the awards.

SOURCE: NIH IMPACII Database.

of universities awarding Ph.D.s in the basic biomedical sciences, as well as the quantity of Ph.D.s awarded by existing programs, has grown.

Furthermore, federal funding policies have inadvertently provided universities with an incentive to appoint students and postdoctorates to research assistantships instead of training grants or fellowships. An example given in the eleventh NRSA study[17] shows that in 1999 the NIH provided almost $9,000 more to research assistants and their institutions (largely in the form of indirect cost payments to universities) than to NRSA trainees or fellows. Because the indirect cost rate for institutional training grants is generally about 7 percent compared to the 60 to 70 percent rate on research grants, it is financially advantageous for an institution to have as many research grants as possible for the support of graduate students. However, current policies at NIH have raised the NRSA predoctoral stipend levels to $19,968 and starting postdoctoral levels to $34,200. These increases might force stipends on research grants to similar levels and reduce the number of students who can be supported on research grants.

As described earlier, the number of students and postdoctorates provided with research training through NRSA training grants and fellowships has been deliberately limited over much of the past 25 years, as a control on the number of researchers entering the workforce. No similar federal effort has been undertaken thus far to ensure an adequate supply of technically prepared support staff in research, nor is there a system for regulating the number of research assistantships. As Massy and Goldman concluded in their 1995 analysis of science and engineering Ph.D. production, the size of doctoral programs is driven largely by departmental needs for research and teaching assistants rather than by the labor market for Ph.D.s.[18]

In any case, NRSA training grants to institutions are highly prized and competitively sought. They confer prestige and add stability to graduate programs as they are usually for five years and allow for planning into the future. On the other hand, since the legislation that established the

NRSA program allows only U.S. citizens and permanent residents to be trained through these grants and fellowships, the growing number of graduate students with temporary-resident status must be supported by other mechanisms.

Another factor in the shifting pattern of federal research training support is the type of education the students receive. Since the beginning of the NRSA program, NIH has required predoctoral training grants in the basic biomedical sciences to be "multidisciplinary" in order to expose students to a range of biomedical fields and even to other branches of science. Given that research collaborations between a wide variety of scientists have been producing significant advances, this requirement is even more important. Although the level of multidisciplinary training varies from program to program, students in training grant programs with this as part of their curriculum may better be ensured of such interdisciplinary training than those on a research assistantship. The committee considers multidisciplinary training in the biomedical sciences to be very valuable and of increasing importance. (A full discussion of these issues is presented in Chapter 8, Emerging Fields and Interdisciplinary Studies.)

Although research grants provide an important base for training, data suggest that NRSA training grant participants complete training faster and go on to more productive research careers than do non-NRSA-supported students at their institution or doctorates from universities without NRSA training programs. This is supported by an assessment, completed in 1984, in which NRSA participants were found to complete their doctoral degrees faster and were more likely to go on to NIH-supported postdoctoral training than graduate students with other forms of support.[19] They also received a higher percentage of NIH research grants, authored more articles, and were cited more frequently by their peers.

Comparable outcomes were seen in a more recent study conducted by NIH.[20] Ph.D.s in the basic biomedical sciences who received NRSA support for at least one academic year spent less time in graduate school. About 57 percent of NRSA trainees and fellows received their doctorates by age

---

[17]National Research Council. 2000b.
[18]Massy, W. F., and C. A. Goldman. 1995.

[19]Coggeshall, P., and P. W. Brown. 1984.
[20]Pion, G. M. 2000.

30, while only 39 percent of their classmates and 32 percent of graduates from departments without NRSA support similarly reached that milestone.

The study also showed that NRSA trainees and fellows were more likely to move into faculty or other research positions. Nearly 40 percent of the NRSA program participants held faculty appointments at institutions ranking in the top 100 in NIH funding, as opposed to 24 and 16 percent, respectively, for non-NRSA graduates from the same institution and graduates from non-NRSA institutions. Similarly, NRSA trainees and fellows were more likely to be successful in competing for grants and had better publication records than either of the other groups.

The NRSA program is essential to training in the biomedical sciences not only for these and other direct reasons; there are also its indirect benefits, such as establishing high standards for the entire graduate program and creating a generally improved environment for all students. Also, when students are supported by a combination of NRSA and research grant support, the NRSA funding is significantly leveraged.

## The Medical Scientist Training Program

The MSTP was established at NIH in 1964 by the National Institute of General Medical Sciences (NIGMS) to support education leading to the M.D./Ph.D degree. By combining graduate training in the biomedical sciences with clinical training offered through medical schools, the program was designed to produce investigators who could better bridge the gap between basic science and clinical research. Since its inception, the Ph.D. portion of the training has been expanded to include the physical sciences, computer science, behavioral and social sciences, economics, epidemiology, public health, bioengineering, biostatistics, and bioethics, though almost all trainees receive a Ph.D. in a biomedical field.

When the MSTP began, it had only three programs, but it has since grown—in 2003 it had 41 programs involving 45 degree-granting institutions, with a total of 925 full-time training slots. This number is slightly down from the 933 slots in 2002. In addition, about 75 medical schools that do not have MSTP grants nevertheless offer opportunities for M.D./Ph.D. studies. The number of new students supported each year by MSTP funds varies from 2 or 3 at many institutions to 10 to 12 at a few exceptional ones, such as Duke University and the University of California, San Francisco. Some 170 new students nationwide are added to the program each year, with selection being highly competitive. The program provides 6 years of support for both phases of training, and institutions usually continue the awards for any additional years needed to complete the degrees. Support includes a tuition allowance, a stipend that is usually supplemented by the institution, and modest funds for travel, equipment, and supplies.

While the funds from NIH are sufficient to support only a few students in any one year of their training, institutions have been able to parlay the NIH funds by judiciously using institutional or research grant funds to support more students. A typical scenario is to support a student on MSTP funds during the first two years of medical training and again in the sixth or seventh years, when he or she returns to complete the medical degree. But during their Ph.D. studies, MSTP students are in a position to receive research grant support just like any other Ph.D. student. For example, one institution uses MSTP funds to support only 10 students during their first year and 2 during their second year in medical school, but there are 60 students in the MSTP program, with the remaining 48 receiving institutional or research grant support. This combination of funding results in the awarding of about 350 MSTP M.D./Ph.D. graduates each year. In the eyes of NIH, any student who receives MSTP funds and is supported for his or her entire course of study is considered a product of the program.

These graduates usually move on to postdoctoral, intern, and residency appointments and after completing their training tend to find academic research positions relatively easily. Another measure of the program's success is seen at the other end of the cycle—the competition among students for entry into the program. Some institutions, such as Johns Hopkins University, receive over 500 applications for the 10 or 12 available positions. Many of these students are highly qualified, and they apply for many programs simultaneously. Institutions easily fill their MSTP class, but some institutions with smaller and less well recognized programs have only a 30 percent acceptance rate. Occasionally these institutions lose students to other programs and begin the year with unfilled MSTP slots. Although not all applicants find MSTP positions, many end up pursuing a joint dual-degree program at an MSTP institution with partial or sometimes full support from non-MSTP funds. They follow the same track as the MSTP students and are indistinguishable from them.

Funding of the program is an issue at almost all MSTP institutions. While institutions are creative in the use of MSTP funds, they are unable to support many highly qualified students who have an interest in research but opt instead to attend just medical school and pursue a professional career. At a time when there is a need for more researchers with a medical background, it would be advantageous to have more M.D.s who are generally debt free and able to pursue research that requires the unique combination of biomedical and clinical training.

In addition to the advantages to biomedical and clinical research, MSTP graduates appear to have more productive research careers. In 1998 the NIGMS published a study of past recipients of MSTP support.[21] This study used résumé data of MSTP graduates with both an M.D. and a Ph.D. to

---

[21]National Institute of General Medical Sciences. 1998.

TABLE 2-4 Potential Workforce in the Biomedical Sciences by Employment Status, 1991–2001

|  | 1991 | 1993 | 1995 | 1997 | 1999 | 2001 |
|---|---|---|---|---|---|---|
| Employed in S&E | 65,428 | 67,580 | 69,003 | 80,938 | 82,985 | 88,582 |
| Percentage | 84.1 | 80.4 | 75.9 | 77.1 | 77.6 | 78.2 |
| Employed out of S&E | 3,757 | 4,951 | 7,736 | 6,659 | 6,474 | 8,091 |
| Percentage | 4.8 | 5.9 | 8.5 | 6.3 | 6.1 | 7.1 |
| Unemployed, seeking work | 1,402 | 916 | 1,234 | 1,230 | 1,138 | 1,019 |
| Percentage | 1.8 | 1.1 | 1.4 | 1.2 | 1.1 | 0.9 |
| Unemployed, not seeking, not retired | 1,041 | 2,111 | 2,760 | 3,502 | 3,488 | 3,916 |
| Percentage | 1.3 | 2.5 | 3.0 | 3.3 | 3.3 | 3.5 |
| Postdocs | 6,182 | 8,474 | 10,194 | 12,587 | 12,825 | 11,680 |
| Percentage | 7.9 | 10.1 | 11.2 | 12.0 | 12.0 | 10.3 |
| Total | 77,810 | 84,032 | 90,927 | 104,916 | 106,910 | 113,288 |

SOURCE: National Science Foundation Survey of Doctorate Recipients.

compare their careers to four other groups of doctorates: MSTP-supported students who received only an M.D., Ph.D. recipients at MSTP institutions supported by NIH training grants, non-MSTP dual-degree graduates from an MSTP institution, and non-MSTP dual-degree graduates from a non-MSTP institution. The individuals in the study were divided into four 5-year cohorts from 1970 to 1995 to allow for changes over time in the educational characteristics and research environment. The cohorts and doctoral grouping were also compared on existing data from NIH files. The training and career paths of the MSTP graduates and the comparison groups were assessed from different perspectives, including time to degree, postdoctoral training, employment history, and research support and publication outcomes. By almost all measures, the MSTP-trained graduates fared better than the other groups. For example, they entered graduate training more quickly and took less time to complete the two degrees. Only the Ph.D. group applied for NIH postdoctoral fellowships at a higher rate, but the MSTP success rate was about the same as for the Ph.D. group. Depending on the cohort, between 60 and 70 percent of the MSTP graduates had a clinical fellowship and about 50 percent had both a clinical fellowship and postdoctoral training.

In terms of research activity, the NIH data showed that the MSTP graduates applied for research grant support from NIH at a greater rate and they were more successful in receiving support. The research productivity of the MSTP graduates across each of the cohorts as measured by published articles from the résumé data was about the same as that for the Ph.D. group and only slightly higher than the non-MSTP graduates from MSTP institutions. However, an examination of publications over the period from 1993 to 1995 showed that the earlier cohorts were more likely to be currently active than the Ph.D. graduates by publishing twice as many articles. The 1976–1980 non-MSTP cohorts, from MSTP institutions, also continued to be almost as active in publishing as the MSTP graduates.

The résumé analysis also provided insight into the professional and research activities of the different groups. About 83 percent of MSTP graduates in the study who were employed in 1995 had one or more academic appointments. This was higher than the M.D.- and Ph.D.-only groups and somewhat higher than the non-MSTP M.D./Ph.D.s group. Most of the dual-degree graduates in either group were in clinical departments and probably indicates some responsibility with regard to patient-oriented care. To better assess the type of research conducted by the different groups, the study classified the publications reported on the résumés into basic, clinical, and mixed type. Even though many of the dual-degree graduates are in clinical departments, they are still more likely to publish in basic journals, and this tendency is stronger in later cohorts.

The conclusions drawn from this analysis are that MSTP graduates appear to have been highly successful in establishing research careers, and their recent publication records suggest that members of all cohorts continue to be productive researchers. However, MSTP graduates appear most similar to non-MSTP M.D./Ph.D.s from the same institution; both groups are likely to be employed in academia with appointments in clinical or dual clinical and basic science departments, and both have similar publication patterns. This is not surprising, since non-MSTP-supported students at MSTP institutions follow the same program as their MSTP counterparts, complete the same degree requirements, and benefit from the MSTP-sponsored training efforts at those institutions.

## RESEARCH LABOR FORCE PROJECTIONS

The biomedical workforce with degrees from U.S. universities was estimated to be 100,262 in 2001. This included individuals in postdoctoral positions but did not count the 4,935 doctorates with degrees in biomedical fields who were unemployed or the 8,091 in positions not considered related to biomedical research (see Table 2-4). These three groups

TABLE 2-5 Projected Changes in U.S. and Foreign Doctorates Entering the Biomedical Workforce Between 2001 and 2011

| **Foreign Doctorates** | | |
|---|---|---|
| Scenarios | Estimated Number in 2001 | |
| Medium | 17,437 | |
| High | 24,787 | |
| Low | 17,437 | |
| | Total Projected Entrants Over the Period 2002–2011 | Increase in the Annual Number of Entrants from 2001 to 2011 |
| Medium | 11,435 | 280 |
| High | 20,375 | 502 |
| Low | 9,829 | 11 |
| **Doctorates from U.S. Universities** | | |
| Scenarios | Number in 2001 | |
| Actual | 5,386 | |
| Scenarios | Total Projected New Doctorates Over the Period 2002–2011 | Increase in the Annual Number of Doctorates from 2001 to 2011 |
| Medium | 60,846 | 1,055 |
| High | 67,204 | 2,047 |
| Low | 54,490 | 63 |

SOURCE: NRC analysis. See Appendix D Tables D-7 and D-8.

brought the potential workforce of U.S. doctorates to 113,288 (the only doctorates excluded were those who had retired). Table 2-4 also shows the change in this workforce over the past decade.

Note that in 2001 almost 80 percent of the potential workforce was employed in S&E and unemployment was less than 1 percent. Even with the inclusion of those unemployed and not seeking employment, only about 4.5 percent were unemployed.

The above figures represent only part of the total potential workforce, however, because foreign-trained doctorates also are employed in this country (and a few U.S. doctorates leave the country). Estimating this foreign component is difficult, given that no database describes the demographics of this group. Some data sources with information on foreign-trained doctorates exist, but they provide only a partial picture.[22] Based on these sources, it is estimated that about 15,500 such individuals are involved in biomedical research in the United States, though the size of this contingent could be as high as 25,000.

How the overall size of the S&E workforce might change over the next 10 years will be influenced by several factors: the number of doctorates who graduate each year, the unemployment levels in the field, the number of foreign-trained doctorates, and retirement rates. These factors can be accounted for by taking a multistate life-table approach, which models the workforce to estimate the numbers of researchers

who enter and exit the workforce at various stages. It is also important to know the age of the workforce and the age at which individuals enter it, as this information determines retirement rates. What follows in this section is a short summary of the findings from this model's analysis, with full details available in Appendix D (Demographic Projections of the Research Workforce).

The largest and most relevant source of new researchers is the set of graduates from U.S. doctoral programs. The size of this group grew significantly in the 1990s but has leveled off or declined in recent years. Making projections of the numbers of future graduates, therefore, depends on which years are used to develop the model (a quadratic regression). Rather than choose just one scenario, three different scenarios for Ph.D. growth were developed. The first was a regression from 1985 to obtain a high estimate; the second was a low estimate, based on the assumption of constant growth from the 2001 level; and the third was the average of the two to represent "moderate" growth. For the high estimate the annual number of Ph.D.s grows from 5,386 in 2001 to 7,433 in 2011, and the average of this number and the one resulting from no growth yields 6,441 in 2011 (see 10-year totals in Table 2-5).

A similar approach—with low, median, and high scenarios—was used for the inflow of foreign doctorates. However, because it is difficult to estimate the number of individuals in the current workforce with a foreign doctorate, the scenarios are based on estimates of the growth rate in the 1990s and the resulting population in 2001. Based on these estimates, it is possible to project the potential workforce in the biomedical sciences between 2001 and 2011. Using esti-

---

[22]Partial data are available from the Association of American Medical College's Faculty Roster and from the National Science Foundation, National Survey of College Graduates.

TABLE 2-6 Projected Workforce by Status for the Median Scenario, 2001–2011

| | 2001 | 2002 | 2003 | 2004 | 2005 | 2006 | 2007 | 2008 | 2009 | 2010 | 2011 |
|---|---|---|---|---|---|---|---|---|---|---|---|
| **U.S. Doctorates** | | | | | | | | | | | |
| Workforce | 113,289 | 117,175 | 120,953 | 124,661 | 128,335 | 131,992 | 135,590 | 139,135 | 142,632 | 146,082 | 149,482 |
| Employed in S&E | 100,262 | 103,148 | 105,851 | 108,544 | 111,305 | 114,147 | 117,010 | 119,875 | 122,730 | 125,564 | 128,361 |
| Out of science | 8,092 | 8,693 | 9,209 | 9,653 | 10,056 | 10,451 | 10,844 | 11,227 | 11,591 | 11,941 | 12,283 |
| Unemployed | 1,019 | 850 | 812 | 802 | 807 | 822 | 841 | 860 | 879 | 899 | 920 |
| Unemployed not seeking | 3,916 | 4,484 | 5,082 | 5,662 | 6,167 | 6,573 | 6,897 | 7,173 | 7,432 | 7,679 | 7,919 |
| Postdoc | 12,711 | 12,726 | 12,819 | 12,950 | 13,214 | 13,515 | 13,916 | 14,291 | 14,695 | 15,052 | 15,392 |
| **Foreign Doctorates** | | | | | | | | | | | |
| Workforce | 17,437 | 18,330 | 19,250 | 20,179 | 21,111 | 22,057 | 23,015 | 23,978 | 24,952 | 25,937 | 26,918 |
| Employed in S&E | 14,627 | 15,231 | 16,061 | 16,987 | 17,931 | 18,883 | 19,833 | 20,774 | 21,706 | 22,627 | 23,528 |
| Out of science | 1,231 | 1,240 | 1,216 | 1,166 | 1,096 | 1,011 | 921 | 837 | 765 | 709 | 671 |
| Unemployed | 106 | 110 | 113 | 114 | 116 | 118 | 122 | 128 | 134 | 139 | 142 |
| Unemployed not seeking | 1,473 | 1,749 | 1,859 | 1,910 | 1,967 | 2,043 | 2,136 | 2,239 | 2,347 | 2,461 | 2,576 |
| Postdoc | 2,079 | 2,037 | 2,164 | 2,342 | 2,522 | 2,696 | 2,848 | 2995 | 3,118 | 3,229 | 3,330 |
| **Total** | | | | | | | | | | | |
| Workforce | 130,726 | 135,505 | 140,203 | 144,840 | 149,446 | 154,049 | 158,605 | 163,113 | 167,584 | 172,019 | 176,400 |
| Employed in S&E | 114,889 | 118,379 | 121,912 | 125,531 | 129,236 | 133,030 | 136,843 | 140,649 | 144,436 | 148,191 | 151,889 |
| Out of science | 9,323 | 9,933 | 10,425 | 10,819 | 11,152 | 11,462 | 11,765 | 12,064 | 12,356 | 12,650 | 12,954 |
| Unemployed | 1,125 | 960 | 925 | 916 | 923 | 940 | 963 | 988 | 1,013 | 1,038 | 1,062 |
| Unemployed not seeking | 5,389 | 6,233 | 6,941 | 7,572 | 8,134 | 8,616 | 9,033 | 9,412 | 9,779 | 10,140 | 10,495 |
| Postdoc | 14,790 | 14,763 | 14,983 | 15,292 | 15,736 | 16,211 | 16,764 | 17,286 | 17,813 | 18,281 | 18,722 |

SOURCE: NRC analysis. See Appendix Tables D-9, D-11, and D-12.

mates of unemployment and the flow of doctorates in and out of the S&E workforce, the employed biomedical researcher population can also be estimated. Table 2-6 shows the results of the multistate life-table analysis under the medium scenario. These totals exhibit an annual growth rate in the biomedical workforce of 2 to 2.5 percent, which is comparable to the projected annual growth rate of the overall labor force.

Although these workforce projections are subject to many caveats, such as incomplete data and uncertainties in the economy and government spending, the balance between Ph.D. production and employment looks quite stable through 2011. Unemployment remains at about 1 percent, and the portion of the workforce remaining in science is about 80 percent. The committee believes this is a healthy percentage of trained people employed in science, but it has concerns about those unemployed and not seeking employment. The percentage of women in this category is significantly greater than their male counterparts, and there is a fear that some talented researchers may be lost because of the difficulty of balancing a career in science and raising a family. (This matter is considered further in Chapter 9, Career Progression.)

## CONCLUSION

The analysis in this chapter suggests that the number of researchers in basic biomedical research will remain stable for the next decade, as will employment opportunities, and the percentage of postdoctorals in holding patterns appears to be declining. Nevertheless, the committee's concern about the increased time to degree and the length of postdoctoral appointments should be noted—an infusion of young people into independent research positions, after all, is critical to the health of the research community. However, we also note that the increase in the average age of researchers parallels the aging of the general population.

"Success" is not easily quantified, but anecdotal evidence suggests that the NRSA program has successfully produced high-quality research personnel and has been important for the upgrading of research training in general. The MSTP program also merits special mention. It has been brilliantly successful at attracting outstanding physicians into basic biomedical research, much to the benefit of future health care. Given their special knowledge of human disease, physicians lend a unique perspective to such research.

The committee's recommendations for future training in the basic biomedical sciences are presented below, along with brief justifications based on the analysis described in this chapter.

## RECOMMENDATIONS

**Recommendation 2-1: This committee recommends that the total number of NRSA positions awarded in the biomedical sciences should remain at least at the 2003 level.**

**Furthermore, the committee recommends that training levels after 2003 be commensurate with the rise in the total extramural research funding in the biomedical, clinical, and behavioral and social sciences.**

Although manpower models have been developed in this report, they are not particularly useful in assessing the role of NRSA support in particular, as this represents only a small fraction of the total training support in the biomedical sciences. Available information, however, suggests that the system is in reasonable balance. Stipends clearly should rise over time, but this should be accomplished by the allocation of additional funds, not by decreasing the number of trainees. The relatively low unemployment among Ph.D.s in the biomedical sciences, an almost constant number of U.S.-trained doctorates from 2001 to 2003, and the fact that the pool of postdoctorates appears to be stabilizing or declining justify the suggested level, which should not fall below that of 2003.

The year 2001 is the last one for which reasonably accurate data were available for awards specific to the biomedical sciences. However, the total number of NRSA awards continued to rise (Figure 1-1) in 2002 and 2003, and it is assumed that the awards in the biomedical sciences have also increased. Using the percentage increase from 2001 to 2003 from Table 1-1 and the actual awards data for 2001 in Tables 2-2 and 2-3, the predoctoral and postdoctoral traineeships in the biomedical sciences in 2003 are estimated to be 5,390 and 1,740, respectively. Fellowship data for 2002 appear to be more complete and show that awards at the postdoctoral level are somewhat below those of 2001. Based on the totals for NRSA predoctoral and postdoctoral training in 2001 and 2003, the estimated levels for fellowships in 2003 for the biomedical sciences are 425 and 1,450, respectively.

The primary rationale for NRSA is to attract high-quality people into specific research areas and to set the training standards for major research fields. NRSAs should be a paragon for quality training and have served this role admirably. NRSA programs are an important investment in the future to ensure the health of the research enterprise and should be made by all NIH institutes and centers.

Beyond the monetary requirements of maintaining NRSA training numbers, this committee does not recommend that support be shifted from research grants to training grants (contrary to the recommendation of the previous committee). A balance is needed between research and training grants for the productive support of students and postdoctorates. Research grants offer an alternative training venue, and students and postdoctorates are essential for accomplishing the research specified in research grants. Moreover, a variety of support mechanisms for training is desirable. The NRSA provides multiple pipelines into the research endeavor, most notably for foreign students and postdoctorates. In certain technical areas, insufficient numbers of U.S. citizens are available to train in and carry out national research efforts in critical areas. The training of foreign scientists on research grants has also significantly enriched the talent pool in this country, as they often join the workforce for extended periods of time, including permanent residence.

Although two earlier National Academies committees[23,24] have recommended that some NIH research funding be shifted to training grants and fellowships, our committee has concluded—based on the uncertainty about the rate of future growth in employment opportunities in industry, and perhaps other sectors, and the considerations discussed above—that the number of graduate students supported on NRSA training grants should not increase any faster than NIH research funding, which is a principal determinant of employment demand. With regard to postdoctoral support, another National Academies committee[25] has recommended that foreign scientists be permitted to receive training grant and fellowship support—thereby increasing the size of the eligible pool—and that some research funds be transferred to training budgets. However, consideration of the current restriction on supporting foreign scientists on NRSA training was outside the scope of this study and was not discussed by our committee.

At the present time, the committee does not recommend a shift in the overall proportion of training dollars spent on NRSA versus other training vehicles but does suggest that the ratios of research dollars to fellows/students be maintained in approximate alignment for the different areas and that training efforts be supported by all NIH institutes and centers. Better coordination of training efforts across institutes is needed. The committee recognizes, however, that the balance may vary from field to field and will evolve over time.

**Recommendation 2-2: This committee recommends that the size of MSTP programs be expanded by at least 20 percent and that the scope be expanded to include the clinical, health services, and behavioral and social sciences.**

Available evidence suggests that it is increasingly difficult for physicians to move into research because of the high cost of medical training and graduates' enormous debt load. Nevertheless, the committee believes that it is very important to attract physicians into research and that MSTP programs have done so with remarkable success; the excellent record of these programs' M.D./Ph.D.s in obtaining research grants and remaining in research is well documented. This would increase the number of trainees from the 2003 level of 933 to about 1,120.

As has been the policy, MSTP grants should be confined to institutions where high-quality medical and research train-

---

[23]National Research Council. 2000a.
[24]National Research Council. 1998c. op. cit.
[25]National Research Council. 2005.

ing are both available. Expanding the range of disciplines should be helpful in attracting physicians into clinical and health services research but not at the expense of current MSTP support for basic biomedical training. Today's applicant pool for MSTP positions can easily accommodate a doubling of the size of the program without compromising its current quality. However, in recognition of the high cost of the MSTP program and budget constraints, the committee recommends a 20 percent increase as a significant and prudent investment.

# 3

# Behavioral and Social Sciences Research

The behavioral and social sciences cover a wide spectrum of health-relevant research areas. One end of the spectrum has a focus on the individual, including such areas as psychology, behavioral and cognitive neuroscience, and cognitive science. Here the focus is on the individual's behavior, with a direct relevance for mental health and mental disorders and a strong relevance for major health problems such as obesity; drug, alcohol, and tobacco abuse; and propensity for violent behavior and crime. The other end of the spectrum has a focus on interpersonal, group, and societal behavior, including sociology, economics, education, and political science. Research in these sciences has an equally important role in identifying key factors that underlie the complex health problems besetting our society.

The behavioral and social sciences are far more complex and variable than some of the natural sciences; not only is there an almost uncountable number of factors affecting individual and social behavior, but these factors combine and interact in extremely complex and mutable ways. Partly for this reason and partly for historical and cultural reasons, research support and research training in these areas lag well behind those in other sciences. While the behavioral and social sciences have addressed fundamental health care question for decades, methods and tools developed in recent years have provided useful and effective answers to some of the nation's most pressing health care problems.

At the same time that these sciences have been maturing, society has come to realize the absolute necessity of their research findings for the understanding, treatment, and prevention of its health problems. As a result, the behavioral and social sciences have been called on for advice to an ever-increasing degree by government agencies. This is evidenced by the number and range of government-commissioned committees, panels, and reports assigned to the Division of Behavioral and Social Sciences and Education (DBASSE) of the National Research Council. In the past 10 years, there have been over 300 publications resulting from DBASSE assignments that cover a wide range of areas directly or indirectly related to health concerns, including children and families; education, employment, and training; the environment; health and behavior; human performance; international studies; law and justice; national statistics; and population and urban studies. These studies range in scope from the level of the individual to the level of society and cover the entire range of social and behavioral sciences and extend to related fields (such as ecology and criminology).[1]

The social and behavioral sciences deal with many of the most complex and least predictable phenomena that affect people's health. Mental health, for example, is an important concern at the National Institutes of Health (NIH; particularly the National Institute of Mental Health, NIMH) as well as in the government and private sector generally. Yet mental health is only one part of a much larger picture because many of the most important health problems are determined and strongly affected by behavioral, social, and economic factors. At the level of the behavior of the individual, the behavioral and social sciences produce knowledge about health issues such as drug and alcohol abuse, obesity, violent behavior, smoking, maintenance of drug treatment regimens, stress management, ability to cope with illness, and health decision making. Moreover, there are many critical health issues that emerge at a larger scale. The economics of health

---

[1]A sample of reports directly relevant to health concerns include: *Educating Children with Autism* (National Research Council, 2001a); *Informing America's Policy on Illegal Drugs: What We Don't Know Keeps Hurting Us* (National Research Council, 2001b); *Preventing HIV Transmission: The Role of Sterile Needles and Bleach* (National Research Council and Institute of Medicine, 1995). *Preventing Reading Difficulties in Young Children* (National Research Council, 1998a); *Protecting Youth at Work: Health, Safety, and Development of Working Children and Adolescents in the United States* (National Research Council, 1998b); *Reducing Underage Drinking: A Collective Responsibility* (National Research Council, 2004b); *Understanding Risk: Informing Decisions in a Democratic Society* (National Research Council, 1996a); *Understanding Violence Against Women* (National Research Council, 1996b); *Work-Related Musculoskeletal Disorders: A Review of the Evidence* (National Research Council, 1999).

care and its delivery critically determines which diseases and problems are attacked, what research is carried out, and which treatments are given. The government has recognized these factors with multimillion dollar investments in surveys, such as the Health and Retirement Survey, the National Longitudinal Survey, and the National Survey of Families and Households. The behavioral and social sciences provide critical insights and knowledge. This knowledge covers a vast array of issues concerning our ability and willingness to deal with disability and our willingness to expend income and assets for health purposes, such as:

- promoting well-being;
- distributing health care geographically, sociologically, and economically;
- using and misusing health care institutions;
- monitoring health providers' behavior;
- studying the psychological and social effects of morbidity and mortality;
- tracking the social and psychological effects on treatment and recovery;
- transferring assets and beliefs across generations;
- documenting social support mechanisms;
- measuring the economics of alternative health care systems;
- verifying the effects of approaches to care and bereavement; and
- making health decisions.

Societal, behavioral, and economic factors work together to produce such problems as drug abuse, smoking, alcohol abuse, anorexia/bulimia, and obesity. Once-treatable diseases are making a comeback in more virulent forms because reliable methods cannot be found to ensure that curative drugs are taken as prescribed. Social and sexually transmitted diseases, such as HIV/AIDS, continue to be an increasing menace. Even crime and violence are rooted in elements that require the expertise of behavioral and social sciences research. It is now accepted that many diseases, historically considered mainly a matter for biomedical research, such as heart and lung disease, drug addiction, tuberculosis, and malaria, cannot be understood and treated without the benefit of behavioral and social research. When these far-reaching health implications of behavioral, social, and economic factors are added to the more direct implications of research for mental illnesses such as depression, schizophrenia, and various neurological illnesses, it is no surprise that the research demand in the behavioral and social sciences has grown rapidly in recent years.

Support for research in the behavioral and social sciences at NIH resides primarily in the NIMH, secondarily in the National Institute on Aging (NIA) and the National Institute of Child Health and Human Development (NICHHD), and is scattered in other institutes (with the present exception of the National Institute of General Medicine. It should be noted that the primary mission of NIMH is research into the prevention and treatment of mental disorders, and the mission of NIA and NICHHD is research into the health problems of young and aging populations. Consequently, neither institute directly supports research into key factors underlying societal health problems, such as smoking, alcohol and drug abuse, obesity, and the like. A case could be made that research in the behavioral and social sciences needs to be augmented significantly by other NIH institutes and centers. Most NIH institutes would benefit from scientists knowledgeable in the techniques, methods, and findings of the behavioral and social sciences. In particular, empirical design and quantitative and statistical methodology that have been so effectively refined in the social and behavioral sciences would be useful. Thus at institutes and centers that do not presently have a direct focus on research in the behavioral and social sciences, at least some training needs to be directed toward researchers with this focus. In addition, some of the training given to researchers with other primary foci needs to be informed by appropriate training in the social and behavioral sciences, a point that is taken up directly in Chapter 8.

## BEHAVIORAL AND SOCIAL SCIENCES RESEARCH WORKFORCE

The behavioral and social sciences workforce is as difficult to identify as the biomedical workforce but for different reasons. In particular, it is difficult to identify scientists who are doing basic health-related research, as opposed to those who are involved in clinical practice. Past studies of research training needs in the behavioral sciences generally defined the target workforce as Ph.D.s trained in anthropology, sociology, speech and hearing sciences, and psychology, with the exception of clinical, family, and school psychology. However, since professional organizations in psychology indicate that nonresearch-oriented doctorates are now receiving doctor of psychology (Psy.D.) degrees, the category of clinical psychology is included but not the other practice-oriented fields. Appendix C lists the fields included in the behavioral and social sciences. This inclusion is also supported by an experiment in which NIH was asked to identify whether the research topics for the theses of a sample of the Ph.D. population in the above-listed fields, including clinical psychology, would be considered for NIH funding. The results of this analysis showed that about 90 percent of the thesis topics could be funded and therefore a large portion of the clinical psychology Ph.D.s could pursue research careers. This may be an overestimate of the workforce, but it might provide a more accurate assessment. Whenever possible, the identification of those who do not participate in research will be addressed in the following analysis of the workforce. In particular, attempts were made to identify institutions with professional programs in clinical psychology and to exclude their doctorates from the analysis.

The critical role played by the behavioral and social sciences workforce is increasingly recognized as a key element in both the maintenance of good health and the treatment of disease. The research workforce that addresses the types of diseases and health problems described earlier in this chapter is much broader than the behavioral and social sciences as defined for this study. For example, even in the treatment of what are often considered biologically based diseases, behavior is a factor in getting patients to take their medicine or to participate in physical activities that would help or prevent their condition. These research areas have an interdisciplinary component with the life sciences, behavioral and social sciences, and even the physical sciences. Interdisciplinarity further complicates analysis of the workforce because people trained outside the medical field are doing research important to the medical community (e.g., an economist studying the public health system). However, it would be impossible to factor these researchers into the current workforce assessment.

Another complication is how students identify their research area when they receive their doctorates. The increasing tendency for some research areas in the biomedical and behavioral sciences to converge (neuroscience is the most notable example) may lead to the classification of some doctorates in the behavioral sciences as biomedical. This factor may lead to an undercount of doctorates in the behavioral sciences and an overcount in the biomedical sciences. These difficulties notwithstanding, an attempt has been made to identify doctoral fields for analysis and potential problems in the analyses. The behavioral and social sciences workforce will consist of Ph.D. graduates from universities in the United States in the fields listed in Appendix C and of foreign graduates seeking careers in science and engineering in this country. This definition of the behavioral and social sciences workforce will provide a general estimate of the number of investigators and an indication of the major trends affecting this workforce, such as changes in size, age, and composition.

## EDUCATIONAL TRENDS

The pool of college graduates in the behavioral and social sciences from which graduate programs would normally draw increased from about 74,000 in 1987 to almost 132,000 in 2001. In 1987 about 11 percent or 7,894 of these graduates matriculated to graduate programs in doctoral-granting institutions and in 2001 to about 6 percent or 8,305. The number of first-year graduate students was fairly constant during the late 1990s at about 8,500 and increased to 8,996 in 2002. This first-year enrollment resulted in a total full-time graduate enrollment of about 31,500 in 1987 and almost 40,000 in 2002. A portrait of the gender makeup of the graduate students (see Figure 3-1) shows a significant change from the late 1970s, when there were only a few more males than females, to 2002 when females outnumbered males by 2.5 to 1.

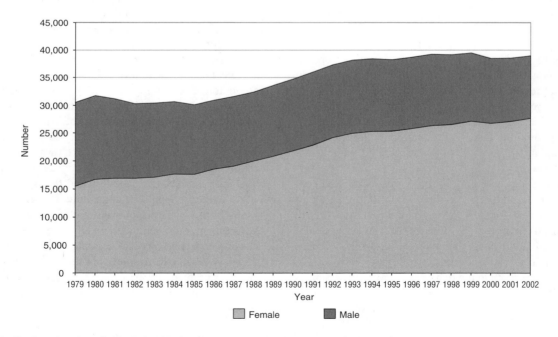

FIGURE 3-1 Graduate students in the behavioral and social sciences by gender, 1979–2002.
SOURCE: National Science Foundation Survey of Graduate Students and Postdoctorates in Science and Engineering.

The picture of support for graduate education at doctoral-granting institutions in the behavioral and social sciences is very different from that in the biomedical sciences (see Figure 3-2). Traditionally, about half of the graduate students are supported by their own funds or other sources, because external funding from traineeships is small and declining and teaching assistantships are the major source of support.

The fairly constant size of the graduate student population seen in Figure 3-1 is reflected in the number of doctoral degrees through 2000 (see Figure 3-3). However, over the period from 2000 to 2003, the number of doctorates declined by 368 or about 8.2 percent. From just a few hundred in 1970 the number of doctoral degrees granted to women grew to 2,908 in 2000 but declined slightly to 2,724 in 2003. The

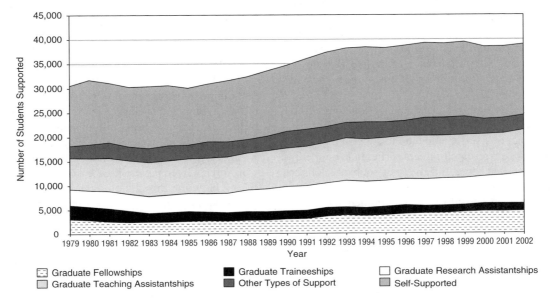

FIGURE 3-2 Graduate support in the behavioral and social sciences, 1979–2002.
SOURCE: National Science Foundation Survey of Graduate Students and Postdoctorates in Science and Engineering.

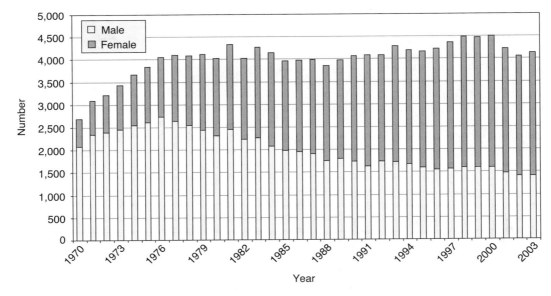

FIGURE 3-3 Doctorates granted in the behavioral and social sciences, 1970–2003.
SOURCE: National Science Foundation Survey of Earned Doctorates, 2001.

number of degrees granted to males dropped from a high of about 2,700 in the mid-1970s to a low of 1,411 in 2003. The decline in doctorates is a reflection of the graduate enrollment declines of the late 1990s, or the problem cited earlier with the classification of doctorates into closely related biomedical fields. On the one hand, the small increase in doctorates in 2003 may reflect the enrollment increases in the early 2000s and may predict a return to the degree production of the late 1990s in a few years. On the other hand, any increase may be temporary, since it may be a result of the national economic situation and will not continue into the future. Time to degree has increased by 3 years in total time and 2 years in registered time (see Appendix E). These increases have been greater than in the biomedical sciences by about a half a year. Similarly, the median age at time of degree has increased to almost 33 and is one of the highest in science and engineering.

Historically, behavioral and social sciences doctorates did not tend to go on to postdoctoral training, but this trend is changing. This fact by itself would tend to suggest that such doctorates could begin research careers earlier than biomedical doctorates, but such a trend is largely offset by the longer graduate training period. Recently, however, the fraction of doctorates planning on a postdoctoral appointment increased from about one-tenth in 1970 to more than one-third in 2003. Females are more likely to have additional research training since in recent years 15 percent of the females and 9.3 percent of the male doctorates have planned to pursue postdoctoral training. Another interesting aspect of the behavioral and social sciences doctoral population is the increased participation in postdoctoral training by individuals with degrees in clinical psychology (see Figure 3-4). This characteristic of clinical psychology doctorates also supports their inclusion in this assessment of personnel needs. For many years postdoctoral training was not considered essential, as was the case for other behavioral and social sciences fields, but in the early 1990s this changed and in recent years almost half of the behavioral and social sciences doctorates have planned to pursue postdoctoral training.

The large and increasing number of female doctorates seeking postdoctoral training suggests a special concern in the behavioral and social sciences. The traditional responsibilities of women to bear children and care for their families may lead to times when highly skilled researchers need to work in a less traditional format or even be absent from the workforce. Given the rapid pace of science, NIH might consider addressing this situation not only with retraining programs but also special postdoctoral research grants to keep

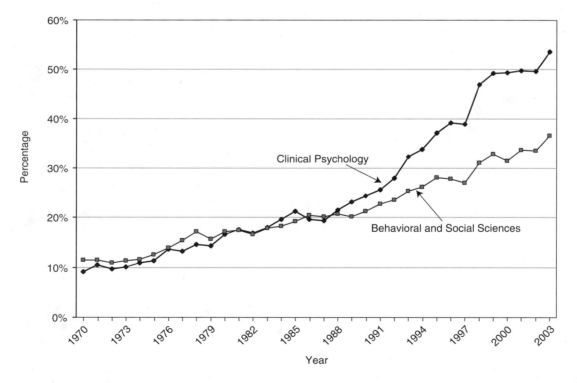

FIGURE 3-4  Doctorates planning postdoctoral training, 1970–2003.
SOURCE: National Science Foundation Survey of Earned Doctorates, 2001.

trained researchers in the workforce during periods in which personal priorities make it impossible to carry a full workload.

The proportion of doctorates facing potential immigration and visa difficulties is presently under 10 percent. An increasing proportion of doctorates in the biomedical sciences with temporary resident status and the problems that might occur if their residency status is jeopardized are not strongly seen in the behavioral and social sciences. Another positive development is the increase in minorities with doctorates. In the 1970s only 1 or 2 percent of the behavioral and social sciences doctorates went to minorities, but that has changed. In recent years, almost 15 percent of the doctorates have gone to minorities.

## EMPLOYMENT TRENDS

The behavioral and social sciences workforce grew steadily from 27,356 in 1973 to 99,145 in 2001. Most of the growth can be attributed to the increasing number of female doctorates (see Figure 3-5); while they are not a majority of the workforce, their numbers have increased at an average annual rate of 11 percent since the late 1980s. In this same time period, the growth in the number of male workers was only 2 percent. If the postdoctoral population is included in the workforce, the rates of growth have not changed since they comprise only a small part of the workforce. Figure 3-6 shows the number of postdoctoral appointments by employment sector and the rapid growth in appointments in recent years. However, the number of appointments declined from its high of 2,583 in 1997 to 2,093. This decline is similar to

that in the biomedical sciences and may be due to higher stipends imposed by NIH because interest on the part of new doctorates in postdoctoral training remains high, as seen by the data in Appendix E.

While the academic sector accounts for three-quarters of the appointments, as was the case for the biomedical sciences, there is stronger participation in the industrial sector. The other notable difference in postdoctoral training is the citizen/permanent resident and temporary resident ratio in academic institutions. In the biomedical sciences it is 1.4 to 1 with more temporary residents, compared to the behavioral and social sciences with a ratio of 3.6 to 1 with more citizens and permanent residents. It is possible that this difference reflects a divergence in technical training at virtually all levels of education between the U.S. and foreign systems. For example, the need for researchers with technical training (including laboratory training, instrumentation abilities, computational expertise, and mathematical and modeling skills) may have led to a large infusion of foreign researchers in the biomedical fields. If so, the increasing need for such types of training in the social and behavioral sciences may produce a tendency for a movement of the pattern seen in the social and behavioral sciences to that seen in the biomedical sciences.

The distribution of the nonpostdoctoral workforce in the behavioral and social sciences is very different from that in the biomedical sciences (see Figure 3-7). While academic employment is still the largest sector, industrial employment is growing at a rapid rate and almost equals that in educational institutions. The nonprofit sector is comparatively larger than in the biomedical sciences. By comparison, the

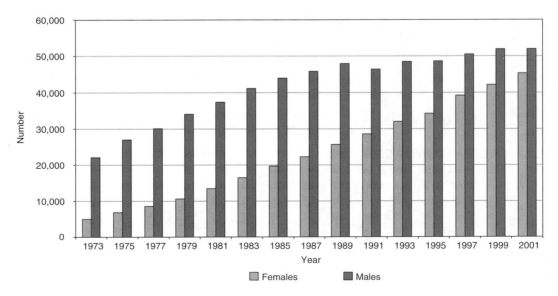

FIGURE 3-5 Behavioral and social sciences workforce (excluding postdoctorates) by gender, 1973–2001.
SOURCE: National Science Foundation Survey of Doctorate Recipients.

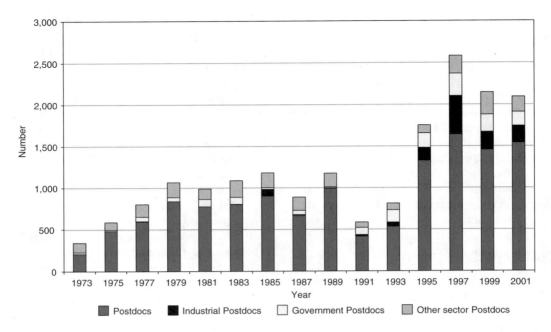

FIGURE 3-6 Trends in postdoctoral appointments by sector, 1973–2001.
SOURCE: National Science Foundation Survey of Doctorate Recipients.

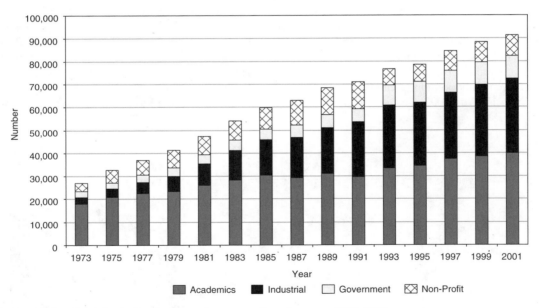

FIGURE 3-7 Behavioral and social sciences workforce by sector of employment, 1973–2001.
SOURCE: National Science Foundation Survey of Doctorate Recipients.

workforce in the behavioral and social sciences is almost as large as the biomedical sciences, with growth at about the same rate, 6.2 percent for the biomedical sciences and 5.4 percent for the behavioral and social sciences. The age distribution for the workforce, excluding postdoctoral appointees, for 1985 is similar for both the behavioral and the biomedical sciences but differs in that the median age in 2001 was 2.5 years older for the behavioral and social sciences workforce (see Table 3-1).

Another way to look at the aging of the behavioral and social sciences workforce is to compare the age distribution over time; note that there will be significant retirement in the next 10 years from the 55 to 65 age group (see Figure 3-8).

Academic employment in the behavioral and social sci-

TABLE 3-1 Median Age Cohort for the Biomedical Sciences and the Behavioral and Social Sciences

|  | Median Age 1985 | Median Age 2001 |
|---|---|---|
| Biomedical sciences | 40.7 Years | 46.2 Years |
| Behavioral and social sciences | 40.6 Years | 48.8 Years |

SOURCE: National Science Foundation Survey of Doctorate Recipients.

ences more than doubled from 1975 to 2001. Much of that growth was in nontenured positions and other academic categories, which together represent about one-third of the total academic staff in 2001. The size of the tenured and tenure-track staff has been almost constant since the late 1990s and grew by only 11 percent from 1989 to 1999 (see Figure 3-9).

Over the past 10 years two-thirds of the doctorates have been awarded to women. This is reflected in academic appointments, with about 60 percent of nontenured positions held by women (Figure 3-10). Those in tenured positions are far below their 47 percent representation in the workforce, but over time this should change as more women in tenure-track positions receive tenure.

The number of minorities in the behavioral and social sciences workforce increased dramatically from 520 in 1975 to 8,534 in 2001 (see Appendix E). While the number has grown in recent years by about 15 percent per year and is greater than the 5 percent growth of the total workforce, they still remain a small percentage of the overall workforce. In 2001, underrepresented minorities comprised 8.6 percent of behavioral and social scientists, compared to 1.9 percent in 1973. There are, however, twice as many in the behavioral and social sciences workforce compared to the biomedical sciences workforce, which is about the same size overall.

## RESEARCH TRAINING AND THE NATIONAL RESEARCH SERVICE AWARD PROGRAM

In general, the National Research Service Award (NRSA) program plays a smaller role in research training in the behavioral and social sciences than in the basic biomedical fields. Comparing the number of awards in Table 3-2 with a similar table in Chapter 2, the awards in the behavioral sciences are about one-tenth of those in the biomedical sciences. In terms of the percentage of students supported, less than 1 percent of the 40,000 graduate students in the behavioral and social sciences in 2002 had NRSA support. By comparison, about 9.3 percent of the biomedical sciences graduate students had NRSA support. It has been argued that much of the research in the behavioral and social sciences is not health related and that therefore, training in these research areas is not supportable under the NRSA program. The sample dissertation review, referred to at the beginning of this chapter, contradicts that reasoning because 90 percent of the reviewed dissertation abstracts were considered to be in areas fundable by NIH personnel.

NIH's basic mission is to support health-related research, and NIH has historically tended to consider such research to lie primarily in the physical structure of the body and hence

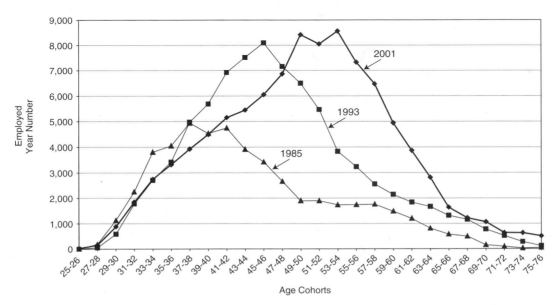

FIGURE 3-8 Age distribution of the behavioral and social sciences workforce, 1985, 1993, and 2001.
SOURCE: National Science Foundation Survey of Doctorate Recipients.

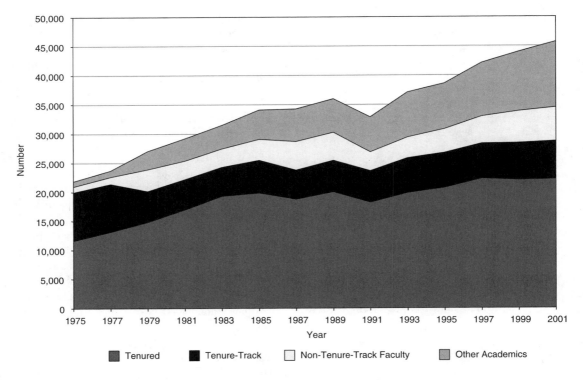

FIGURE 3-9 Academic employment in the behavioral and social sciences, 1973–2001.
SOURCE: National Science Foundation Survey of Doctorate Recipients.

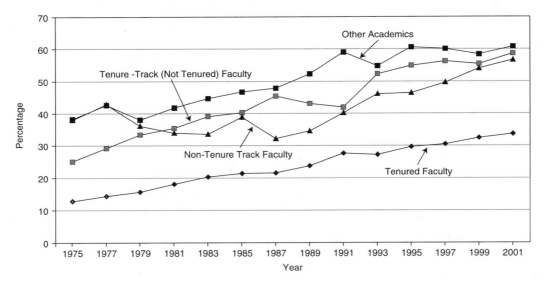

FIGURE 3-10 Percentage of women in academic positions, 1975–2001.
SOURCE: National Science Foundation Survey of Doctorate Recipients.

TABLE 3-2  National Research Service Award Predoctoral Trainee and Fellowship Support in the Behavioral and Social Sciences

|  | 1975 | 1980 | 1985 | 1990 | 1995 | 2000 | 2001 | 2002[a] |
|---|---|---|---|---|---|---|---|---|
| Traineeships (T32)[b] | 204 | 479 | 495 | 577 | 410 | 434 | 321 | 240 |
| Fellowships (F30, F31)[b] | 122 | 43 | 47 | 46 | 73 | 169 | 225 | 194 |

[a]For 2002 and possibly 2001, the data are incomplete for traineeships since educational institutions report on the number of students trained in certain fields and the information was last processed in February 2003

[b]See Appendix B for complete explanation of awards.

SOURCE: NIH IMPACII Database.

in biochemistry, genetics, and similar fields. Behavioral and social sciences research has traditionally been considered less relevant to the NIH mission. This may also be seen in the fact that NIH does not house an institute devoted to basic and applied research in the behavioral and social sciences. What research training there is in this area has tended to reside in NIMH, but NIMH has a mission to focus on mental disorders. Consequently, training in research-relevant areas for many other health problems with a social and behavioral component (such as smoking, obesity, drug abuse, violence, alcoholism) has lagged far behind society's needs. There may be added concerns for research training in the behavioral and social sciences by NIMH due to a recent decision by this institute to shift research funding to areas deemed to have more relevance to public health issues, such as neurological diseases and major mental disorders.[2]

Thus, research training in the behavioral and social sciences is not supported through a dedicated NIH institute or center but instead through the coordination of training and research by the Office of Behavioral and Social Science Research (OBSSR) in the Office of the Director. In recent years NIMH has supported a majority of the predoctoral trainees and fellows, followed by NICHHD, the NIA, the National Institute on Drug Abuse, the National Institute on Alcohol Abuse and Alcoholism, and the National Cancer Institute (NCI). A review of the 1,972 T32[3] training grants in 2002 showed that 98 were primarily in the behavioral and social sciences and about 150 others had some behavioral aspects to the training. Table 3-3 shows the distribution of the 98 awards across the NIH institutes and centers. Only 8 of the 21 institutes that could support T32 training made awards. NIMH far outnumbers the other institutes and centers for making these awards. If the institutes and centers with awards that contain behavioral aspects were included, this number would increase to 11 with the addition of the National Institute of Allergy and Infectious Diseases, the Na-

tional Institute on Deafness and Other Communication Disorders, and the National Institute of Neurological Disorders and Stroke.

The institutes and centers listed in Table 3-3 are the principal supporters of behavioral and social sciences research and training, with combined expenditures of $1.7 billion in 2001. Another 14 institutes and centers also provided $295 million in support in 2001. While NCI is a major supporter of behavioral and social sciences research, it provides little NRSA program training support in this area. NCI has used the R25T training mechanism to support training programs focusing on behavioral, prevention, control, and population sciences. In 2004, NCI made six awards under this mechanism to support behavioral science training.

A particularly notable omission from the list of institutes that support training in the behavioral and social sciences is the National Institute of General Medical Sciences (NIGMS). A few behavioral and social sciences doctoral students receive NIGMS training support, but only under institutional NRSA training grants that are focused on biomedical or clinical training. At one time NIGMS did support behavioral training but now claims that such training falls outside its mission. NIGMS has resisted calls from Congress to

TABLE 3-3  T32 Training Grants in the Behavioral and Social Sciences, 2002

| NIH Institutes | Number |
|---|---|
| National Institute on Alcohol Abuse and Alcoholism (NIAAA) | 4 |
| National Institute on Aging (NIA) | 6 |
| National Institute on Drug Abuse (NIDA) | 6 |
| National Institute of Diabetes and Digestive and Kidney Diseases (NIDDKD) | 2 |
| National Institute of Child Health and Human Development (NICHD) | 13 |
| National Institute of Mental Health (NIMH) | 46 |
| National Institute of Nursing Research (NINR) | 7 |
| National Heart, Lung, and Blood Institute (NHLBI) | 10 |

SOURCE: Tabulation from NIH IMPACII Database.

[2]Agres, T. 2002.
[3]See Appendix B for a complete explanation of awards.

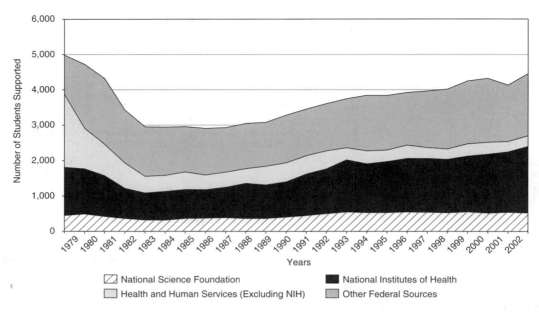

FIGURE 3-11 Funding sources for graduate education in the behavioral and social sciences, 1979–2002.
SOURCE: National Science Foundation Survey of Graduate Students and Postdoctorates in Science and Engineering.

develop collaborations with other institutes and centers at NIH to support behavioral research.[4]

Institutes and centers tend to support training in the behavioral and social sciences that is directed at particular subfields and often do not require interdisciplinary or multidisciplinary aspects generally found in training grants in the biomedical or clinical sciences. In order to encourage interdisciplinarity, it should not be forgotten that training support in the behavioral and social sciences promotes outreach and collaboration with other sciences.

The lack of support notwithstanding, efforts are being made by OBSSR to foster interdisciplinarity by highlighting research that joins the behavioral and social sciences with other health sciences. In July 2002, OBSSR held a workshop on interdisciplinary training in the behavioral, social, and biomedical sciences. It addressed a variety of issues, including the type and level of training, barriers that prevent investigators from doing interdisciplinary research, relevant fields for interdisciplinary training, and what fraction of the NIH training portfolio should support interdisciplinary training. More recently a working group for the NIH Advisory Council to the Director in a draft report recommended that OBSSR coordinate transinstitute basic research initiatives, and designate a home at NIH to foster basic behavioral and social

sciences research that is not linked to the mission of the categorical institutes and centers.[5]

The M.D./Ph.D. programs, particularly the Medical Scientist Training Program (MSTP) at NIGMS, foster interdisciplinarity. The MSTP was recently expanded to include Ph.D. study in the computer sciences, social and behavioral sciences, economics, epidemiology, public health, bioengineering, biostatistics, and bioethics. However, only a few institutions have students pursuing dual degrees with a Ph.D. in the behavioral and social sciences. The areas of computer science, biostatistics, and bioinformatics seem to be more attractive. Some institutions with well-established programs have expressed difficulty in developing a unified M.D./Ph.D. program with their behavioral and social sciences departments. Generally, the MSTP programs are housed in a biomedical sciences department or a medical school, and as such students are more likely to pursue biomedical research paths.

As shown in Figure 3-2, less than one-quarter of the graduate student population in doctoral-granting institutions in the behavioral and social sciences is supported by fellowships, traineeships, and research grants. While one of the missions of the National Science Foundation (NSF) is the support of the behavioral and social sciences, NSF support is only about one-tenth the total federal support and less than one-third of the support provided by NIH (see Figure 3-11).

It should be noted that total graduate support has declined since the 1970s and early 1980s, mainly due to reductions by

---

[4]Statement from the NIGMS justifying its 2003 budget request: "The Institute's research training programs mirror the areas of science that fall within the mission of the National Institute of General Medical Sciences. Except for a few fields of inquiry, behavioral studies largely fall outside of the Institute's research mission, and are instead deemed to be within the missions of other institutes at the National Institutes of Health." Also see *http://www.psychologicalscience.org/advocacy/issues/nigms_observer.cfm*.

[5]Draft Report of the Working Group of the NIH Advisory Committee to the Director on Research Opportunities in the Basic Behavioral and Social Sciences, *http://obssr.od.nih.gov/Activities/Basic%20Beh%20Report_ complete.pdf*, December 2, 2004.

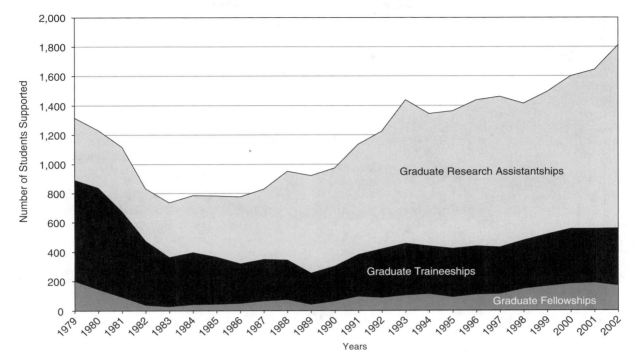

FIGURE 3-12  Graduate student support by NIH, 1979–2002.
SOURCE: National Science Foundation Survey of Graduate Students and Postdoctorates in Science and Engineering.

the non-NIH part of the U.S. Department of Health and Human Services. The current number of graduate students supported by NIH is about the same as in the 1970s. However, the proportion with NIH support has declined due to an increase in the total number of graduate students. In proportion to the total number of graduate students, NIH support has declined since the 1970s. The form of support has also changed over time. In the 1970s and early 1980s, NIH supported mainly graduate fellowships and traineeships, but by the 1990s its support shifted to research grants. Consequently, by 2001 over two-thirds of the support provided by NIH was in the form of research grants, and in 2002 it grew again by about 15 percent (see Figure 3-12).

As is the case at the predoctoral level, NRSA program support of postdoctoral training in the behavioral and social sciences is a fraction, between 10 and 15 percent, of that in the biomedical sciences (see Table 3-4). The decline in the number of postdoctoral positions supported by the NRSA program is similar to that in the biomedical sciences. This may be due to similar reasons: the higher stipend levels and the eligibility of individuals for NRSA support. There are no data on general postdoctoral support from NIH, but the picture for postdoctoral training support from all federal sources also shows growth in research grant support and the decline in trainee and fellowship support (see Figure 3-13). NIH's efforts to shift research training in the behavioral and social

TABLE 3-4  National Research Service Award Postdoctoral Trainee and Fellowship Support in the Behavioral and Social Sciences

|  | 1975 | 1980 | 1985 | 1990 | 1995 | 2000 | 2001 | 2002[a] |
|---|---|---|---|---|---|---|---|---|
| Traineeships (T32)[b] | 29 | 173 | 334 | 254 | 281 | 240 | 207 | 108 |
| Fellowships (F32)[b] | 131 | 99 | 83 | 76 | 94 | 102 | 109 | 111 |

[a]For 2002 and possibly 2001, the data are incomplete for traineeships since educational institutions report on the number of students trained in certain fields and the information was last processed in February 2003.

[b]See Appendix B for a complete explanation of awards.

SOURCE: NIH IMPACII Database.

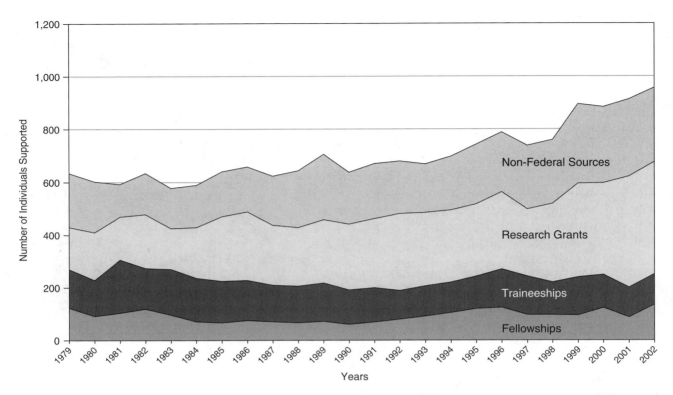

FIGURE 3-13  Academic postdoctoral support in the behavioral and social sciences, 1979–2002.
SOURCE: National Science Foundation Survey of Graduate Students and Postdoctorates in Science and Engineering.

sciences from the predoctoral to the postdoctoral level in the late 1970s and 1980s can be seen by comparing predoctoral support level in Figure 3-12 and postdoctoral support in Figure 3-13.

The discussion in Chapter 2 of an outcomes analysis for NRSA- and non-NRSA-supported researchers at the predoctoral and postdoctoral levels presented a case for reversing the trend toward more training on research grants. For the behavioral and social sciences, the same conclusions cannot be drawn. The most recent assessment of the career outcomes of NRSA predoctoral trainees and fellows in the behavioral and social sciences did not yield results that were clear-cut evidence. NRSA trainees and fellows, particularly those who received support at the start of graduate school, completed their Ph.D.s faster than other students, but there was no clear difference with regard to employment or research productivity. These findings should be interpreted with caution though since the number of trainees supported under the NRSA program is smaller in the behavioral and social sciences, and the sample used to assess the outcomes is also smaller and more prone to error.

## RESEARCH LABOR FORCE PROJECTIONS

As mentioned earlier in this chapter, individuals with doctorates in clinical psychology are considered part of the re-search workforce and as such may tend to overestimate the size of the actual workforce. Another uncertain component of the workforce are foreign-trained researchers now in the United States. Characterizing this component has proven problematic for the other two broad fields but is less so in the behavioral and social sciences since they appear to make up a small fraction of the population. The 1990 U.S. Census data estimate this group at about 3 percent of the workforce, and data from the U.S. Department of Education Survey of Postsecondary Faculty place the faculty percentage a little lower, at about 2 percent. In either case the numbers are small and will not have a significant effect on the projections. Table 3-5 shows the change in this workforce for U.S.-educated Ph.D.s over the past decade. A comparison of this workforce with that in the other broad fields shows a similar unemployment rate for those seeking employment and a rate for those not seeking employment similar to the biomedical sciences. As expected, the proportion of postdoctoral positions is lower than in the biomedical sciences and similar to that in the clinical sciences.

A life-table estimate of the science and engineering workforce in the behavioral and social sciences for the next 10 years is less problematic, since the variability introduced by the foreign doctorates is much less. The following is a short summary of the findings from the life-table analysis; full details can be found in the Appendix D.

TABLE 3-5 Potential Workforce in the Behavioral and Social Sciences by Employment Status, 1991–2001

|  | 1991 | 1993 | 1995 | 1997 | 1999 | 2001 |
|---|---|---|---|---|---|---|
| Employed in S&E | 74,814 | 80,327 | 82,674 | 89,570 | 93,796 | 97,010 |
| Percentage | 86.3 | 86.3 | 84.4 | 86.6 | 86.0 | 85.1 |
| Employed out of S&E | 8,424 | 8,576 | 10,513 | 7,807 | 8,914 | 10,644 |
| Percentage | 9.7 | 9.2 | 10.7 | 7.5 | 8.2 | 9.3 |
| Unemployed, seeking work | 1,396 | 1,098 | 573 | 672 | 972 | 789 |
| Percentage | 1.6 | 1.2 | 0.6 | 0.6 | 0.9 | 0.7 |
| Unemployed, not seeking, not retired | 1,439 | 2,296 | 2,342 | 2,784 | 3,204 | 3,418 |
| Percentage | 1.7 | 2.5 | 2.4 | 2.7 | 2.9 | 3.0 |
| Postdoctorates | 606 | 813 | 1,868 | 2,631 | 2,164 | 2,136 |
| Percentage | 0.7 | 0.9 | 1.9 | 2.5 | 2.0 | 1.9 |
| Total | 86,679 | 93,110 | 97,970 | 103,464 | 109,050 | 113,997 |

SOURCE: National Science Foundation Survey of Doctorate Recipients.

Graduates from U.S. Ph.D. programs will be the major contributor to the future workforce in the behavioral and social sciences, but since that population has shown little or no growth in the past, the projected growth and that of the workforce will be small. Table 3-6 shows the results of the multistate life-table analysis for the period from 2001 to 2011 under the median scenarios.

The projected median growth scenario for Ph.D. graduates increases from 4,221 in 2001 to only 4,619 in 2011, or about 0.5 percent per year. The inflow of foreign-trained Ph.D.s is only about 100 per year. Given this and the slow growth in the number of doctorates for U.S. institutions, the employed workforce is projected to grow from 102,193 in 2001 to 119,840 in 2011. This translates into about a 17 percent growth in the workforce and an annual growth rate of about 1.5 percent. This is the lowest growth rate of the three broad fields. The other segments of the workforce, except for postdoctoral appointments, are projected to decline over

TABLE 3-6 Projected Workforce by Status for the Median Scenario, 2001–2011

|  | 2001 | 2002 | 2003 | 2004 | 2005 | 2006 | 2007 | 2008 | 2009 | 2010 | 2011 |
|---|---|---|---|---|---|---|---|---|---|---|---|
| **U.S. Doctorates** | | | | | | | | | | | |
| Workforce | 113,997 | 116,267 | 118,368 | 120,408 | 122,375 | 124,247 | 125,960 | 127,497 | 128,868 | 130,101 | 131,154 |
| Employed in S&E | 99,146 | 101,902 | 104,256 | 106,418 | 108,416 | 110,281 | 111,957 | 113,432 | 114,729 | 115,887 | 116,874 |
| Out of science | 10,644 | 10,615 | 10,566 | 10,534 | 10,533 | 10,530 | 10,521 | 10,519 | 10,526 | 10,534 | 10,532 |
| Unemployed | 789 | 565 | 496 | 468 | 453 | 449 | 451 | 457 | 462 | 466 | 468 |
| Unemployed, not seeking | 3,418 | 3,185 | 3,050 | 2,989 | 2,974 | 2,988 | 3,031 | 3,089 | 3,151 | 3,215 | 3,281 |
| Postdoctorates | 2,391 | 2,527 | 2,651 | 2,746 | 2,842 | 2,905 | 2,968 | 3,021 | 3,072 | 3,109 | 3,144 |
| **Foreign Doctorates** | | | | | | | | | | | |
| Workforce | 3,469 | 3,470 | 3,465 | 3,454 | 3,438 | 3,423 | 3,411 | 3,395 | 3,376 | 3,349 | 3,312 |
| Employed in S&E | 3,047 | 3,049 | 3,046 | 3,046 | 3,041 | 3,038 | 3,036 | 3,030 | 3,018 | 2,997 | 2,966 |
| Out of science | 313 | 300 | 294 | 282 | 269 | 258 | 247 | 239 | 233 | 227 | 223 |
| Unemployed | 5 | 12 | 13 | 13 | 13 | 12 | 13 | 12 | 11 | 11 | 10 |
| Unemployed, not seeking | 104 | 108 | 111 | 112 | 113 | 113 | 114 | 113 | 114 | 113 | 112 |
| Postdoctorates | 69 | 69 | 69 | 70 | 71 | 73 | 73 | 74 | 75 | 74 | 74 |
| **Total** | | | | | | | | | | | |
| Workforce | 117,466 | 119,737 | 121,833 | 123,862 | 125,813 | 127,670 | 129,371 | 130,892 | 132,244 | 133,450 | 134,466 |
| Employed in S&E | 102,193 | 104,951 | 107,302 | 109,464 | 111,457 | 113,319 | 114,993 | 116,462 | 117,747 | 118,884 | 119,840 |
| Out of science | 10,957 | 10,915 | 10,860 | 10,816 | 10,802 | 10,788 | 10,768 | 10,758 | 10,759 | 10,761 | 10,755 |
| Unemployed | 794 | 577 | 509 | 481 | 466 | 461 | 464 | 469 | 473 | 477 | 478 |
| Unemployed, not seeking | 3,522 | 3,293 | 3,161 | 3,101 | 3,087 | 3,101 | 3,145 | 3,202 | 3,265 | 3,328 | 3,393 |
| Postdoctorates | 2,460 | 2,596 | 2,720 | 2,816 | 2,913 | 2,978 | 3,041 | 3,095 | 3,147 | 3,183 | 3,218 |

SOURCE: NRC Analysis, See Appendix Tables D-9, D-11, and D-12.

the same 10-year period. Postdoctoral appointments in the behavioral and social sciences have increased over the past decade, and this is projected to continue, with about one-third more doctorates in postdoctoral positions in 2011 than in 2001. Unemployment is projected to remain low and even decline to about 0.4 percent of the potential workforce in 2011.

## CONCLUSION

In assessing the overall picture for the behavioral and social sciences, the situation is similar to that for the biomedical sciences—namely, unemployment is low and the number of Ph.D.s entering the job market in the future is consonant with reasonable expectations about job availability. Appendix D discusses the uncertainties in the workforce model used to generate this conclusion. Based on this limited model, the status quo appears appropriate. However, all of these conclusions need to be placed in a broader context, which will be discussed in Chapter 10.

Finally, the NRSA program plays a special role in setting standards and attracting people to specific fields. This is vital for the health of the training system. A marked difference in training in the behavioral and social sciences relative to the biomedical sciences is in the concentration of support in a single institute, the NIMH. Because of the interdisciplinary nature of the subject matter and its general importance to the health of the nation, this does not seem desirable. A better distribution of training support across all NIH institutes and centers (including NIGMS) would be preferable. A specific recommendation in this regard is made in Chapter 5, but this issue also merits mention here.

## RECOMMENDATIONS

**Recommendation 3-1: This committee recommends that the total number of NRSA program positions in the behavioral and social sciences should remain at least at the 2003 level. Furthermore, the committee recommends that training levels after 2003 be commensurate with the rise in the total extramural research funding in the biomedical, clinical, and behavioral and social sciences.**

Data on the number of predoctoral and postdoctoral traineeships in the behavioral and social sciences are incomplete after 2000.[6] In 2000 there were 434 predoctoral trainees and 240 postdoctoral trainees. There was an 8.5 percent increase in the total number of predoctoral NRSA positions from 2000 to 2003 and an 8.4 percent increase in post-

---

[6]Data on the number of NRSA trainees in the behavioral and social sciences are incomplete after 2000 since educational institutions report on the number of students trained in a field. The information is returned to NIH as much as 2 years after training, and the information was last processed in February 2003.

doctoral NRSA training positions. Assuming these increases also held for the behavioral and social sciences, approximately 471 predoctoral and 260 postdoctoral NRSA training slots would have been filled in the behavioral and social sciences in 2003. Fellowship data are probably more current, since these awards are made to individuals in specific training areas, and the predoctoral and postdoctoral awards in 2002 were 194 and 111, respectively. This level of predoctoral support was probably also true for 2003, since there was little change in the total number of NRSA fellowships from 2002 to 2003. Therefore, the total number of individuals in the behavioral and social sciences supported by the NRSA mechanism in 2003 is about 665 at the predoctoral level. This is only a small fraction of the total support for graduate students. Much more comes from institutional support through teaching assistantships and self-support. Similarly, postdoctoral support is more likely to come from research grants and other forms of institutional support (see Figure 3-13).

The recommendation links the training level in the behavioral and social sciences to extramural research support across NIH, since all of the three broad fields for which NRSA training is available are becoming more interdisciplinary and training is needed to meet this trend. While NIH currently classifies research grants into a single area of research, it is also quick to recognize that the research may involve many fields and that expertise is needed in these fields to carry out the research.

The relatively low unemployment among Ph.D.s in the behavioral and social sciences suggests that having 2003 serve as a baseline for NRSA program support and having increases based on increases in extramural research support are both justified.

The discussion following Recommendation 2-1 with regard to the quality of the NRSA program and the relative balance of biomedical training to the workforce also applies to the behavioral and social sciences.

**Recommendation 3-2: This committee recommends that each NIH institute and center incorporate the behavioral and social sciences into its training portfolio, including institutes and centers that have not emphasized these disciplines in the past.**

The behavioral and social sciences are critical for the understanding, prevention, and treatment of most major health problems. For historical rather than rational reasons, most training has been centered in just a few NIH institutes and centers. In the case of NIGMS, Congress specifically instructed that the behavioral and social sciences be included, but this has not been done as of 2004. The result is that health decisions that arise in many institutes and centers are made without sufficient input from scientists and decision makers who have knowledge of and training in the techniques of the behavioral and social sciences.

# 4

# Clinical Sciences Research

The importance of clinical research is that it brings basic biomedical discoveries to the bedside to address patient care from the physical, behavioral, and social perspectives. It is also difficult to define the scope of this research. Perhaps the best definition of clinical research is the one developed in 1998 at the Graylyn Development Consensus Conference: *Clinical research is that component of medical and health research intended to produce knowledge valuable for understanding human disease, preventing and treating illness, and promoting health.*[1]

Clinical research embraces a continuum of studies involving interactions with patients, diagnostic clinical materials or data, or populations in any of the following categories: (1) disease mechanisms (etiopathogenesis); (2) bidirectional integrative (translational) research; (3) clinical knowledge, detection, diagnosis, and natural history of disease; (4) therapeutic interventions, including clinical trials of drugs, biologics, devices, and instruments; (5) prevention (primary and secondary) and health promotion; (6) behavioral research; (7) health services research, including outcomes, and cost effectiveness; (8) epidemiology; and (9) community-based trials.[2]

Clinical research and its translation into preventive and clinical care, in other words, are the primary means by which the nation's health care goals are fulfilled. It brings basic biomedical research to the bedside through the translation of increasingly remarkable basic research advances—such as the sequencing of the human genome—into human applications and into social, behavioral, and health care practice.

Nevertheless, these transformations do not happen in a vacuum. Health services research has become indispensable to understanding and informing the future of health care. Despite the promises of a newly competitive marketplace for health services, the costs of health care to all stakeholders have resumed their double-digit annual rise after a short hiatus in the late 1990s. Recent reports from the Institute of Medicine have highlighted the unacceptably poor status of the health care system as a whole[3] and the consequences of the continuing problem of the lack of insurance.[4] Others have described in great detail the impact of the organizational, administrative, financing, safety, access, and other deficits of the nation's cobbled-together health care "system" on individuals, communities, businesses, and the entire nation. These persistent challenges, along with the reemergent cost growth issue, make it increasingly important that clinical research not only deal with scientific advances per se but that it encompass the assessment of health outcomes, cost effectiveness, finance, access, and other research related to the deployment and utilization of the nation's health care services.

Despite its critical importance, the clinical research enterprise has for years been underdeveloped. Reasons include the extra time required for clinical research training; the difficulty in competing for sponsored research support; the inability to cross-subsidize clinical research from hospital and faculty practice income (as a result of major changes wrought in health care financing over the past 15 years); the debt burden that inclines many physicians in training to forgo opportunities for clinical research and focus instead on clinical care; and the unresolved status of clinical research within the culture of the academic health center, where basic science studies or clinical prowess are often valued more highly than clinical research.

This problem of clinical research underdevelopment has now been recognized as a critical issue to be addressed within funding programs—public, private, and philanthropic—and throughout the research community itself. For example, in FY 2001 the National Institutes of Health—the single largest public-sector source of funding for clinical research—awarded more than $6 billion in clinical research grants (con-

---

[1]Council on Scientific Affairs (I-99). 1998.
[2]Ibid.

[3]Institute of Medicine. 2001.
[4]Institute of Medicine. 2004.

stituting 37 percent of its total extramural research dollars). Among the successful innovations supported by these funds have been a nationwide network of general clinical research centers, where an estimated 9,000 researchers pursue a broad range of clinical research projects.[5] Nevertheless, the past two decades have been particularly challenging for the funding of all health professions, and especially for the support of research activities in the clinical environment that are not clearly tied to specified funding streams. Clinical research has yet to achieve the breadth and depth of currency (double entendre intended) it deserves.

Meanwhile, a key element in developing the nation's clinical research capacity is the building of a robust cadre of clinician-scientists able to realize the promise of 21st-century medicine. This objective depends, in turn, on continuing support, incentives, and educational and professional reforms throughout the existing clinical research workforce.

## DEFINING THE CLINICAL RESEARCH WORKFORCE

The clinical research workforce is as diverse as the definition of the field. It is composed of individuals with doctorates in the basic sciences, graduates of professional degree programs, graduates of health sciences and public health programs, and dual- or multiple-degree holders covering a wide range of health care research. Given the broad role these scientists play in providing the nation's health care—their research spans the spectrum from discovery to delivery—it is difficult to categorize them. For this report efforts will be made to identify individuals who fit the Graylyn definition. However, this definition is very broad. For example, it includes behavioral and social sciences research in the context of patient care, and it is difficult to separate this from the general area of health-related behavioral research that is addressed in Chapter 3. Many of them are involved in health services research (Chapter 7) and in other efforts that are increasingly interdisciplinary (Chapter 8). However, aspects of all these activities will be incorporated into the analysis of clinical research, as appropriate.

Apart from the problem of technically distinguishing the areas in which the clinical workforce conducts its research, it is also difficult to match these areas with workforce members' credentials—current databases focus on the specific degree and field of training for individuals and not on their research areas. This problem has hindered prior studies of the National Research Service Award (NRSA) program to the point where only partial descriptions of the workforce were given and no demographic projection of future workforce was made.

For this assessment's purposes, the basic workforce analysis will include Ph.D.s with degrees in the health fields listed in Appendix C, the fraction of the M.D. population in medical school clinical departments that conduct NIH-supported research, and doctorates with degrees from foreign institutions who are in some way identified as clinical researchers. This formula still does not capture the complete workforce, such as M.D.s in the non–medical school part of an academic institution or in industrial laboratories. Those doing clinical trials are also difficult to identify, as departments have different ways of allocating funds for clinical trials and of supporting associated researchers (from graduate students to postdoctorates to faculty). However, each of these groups will be included in the analysis when data are available. The nursing and dental workforces, as well as the health services researchers briefly mentioned above, will also be included in clinical research, but because each of these fields has its own special workforce issues, they will be examined separately in Chapters 5, 6, and 7.

## EDUCATIONAL BACKGROUND

The educational background of clinical researchers is difficult to assess in the same detail as that of biomedical and behavioral and social sciences since a small fraction of M.D. graduates enter the research workforce. However, data are available on the Ph.D. portion of this workforce, and these data can be analyzed. In particular, the graduate student population in the clinical departments of doctorate-granting institutions grew at an annual rate of 5 to 10 percent in the 1990s; it then leveled off until 2002, when there was growth of about 6 percent (see Figure 4-1). This growth pattern of the number of clinical research–oriented graduate students is much different than that of the biomedical sciences, whose population was virtually constant during the 1990s. Its growth in 2002, as in the other fields, may reflect a poor economy—where continued education is an alternative to the job market. It should also be noted that the growth was primarily caused by an increase in female graduate students and that nursing graduate students were excluded from the data (as most will not receive a doctorate).

The pattern of financial support for clinical science students is also quite different from that of the other fields (see Figure 4-2). Many more are self-supported, and research and teaching assistantships make up a smaller proportion. As is the case for the other broad fields, the number of graduate students supported on research grants has grown, while levels of assistantships, traineeships, and fellowships have been constant from the 1970s until now. The growth in self-support in 2002 is consistent with the general increase in graduate student populations and the limited forms of support available from external and institutional funds.

The growth in the graduate population is reflected by the number of doctorates in the clinical sciences, which increased by a factor of 5 from the early 1970s (see Figure 4-3). This increase is largely the result of growing participation by women. The proportion of male doctorates in the

---

[5]NIH competing and noncompeting research grants, fiscal years 1992–2002. Available at: *http://grants.nih.gov/grants/award/research/rgmech type9202.htm.*

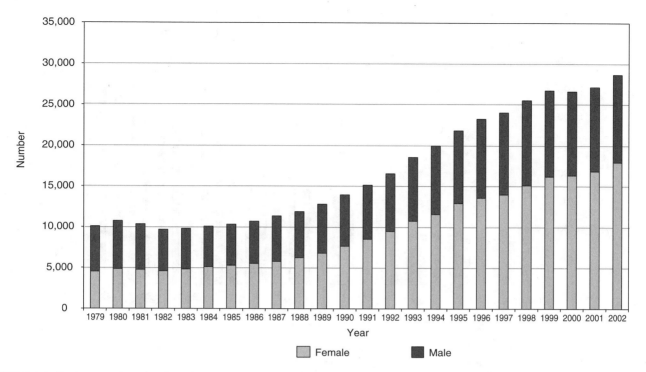

FIGURE 4-1 Graduate students in clinical departments by gender, 1979–2002 (does not include graduate students in nursing).
SOURCE: National Science Foundation Survey of Graduate Students and Postdoctorates in Science and Engineering.

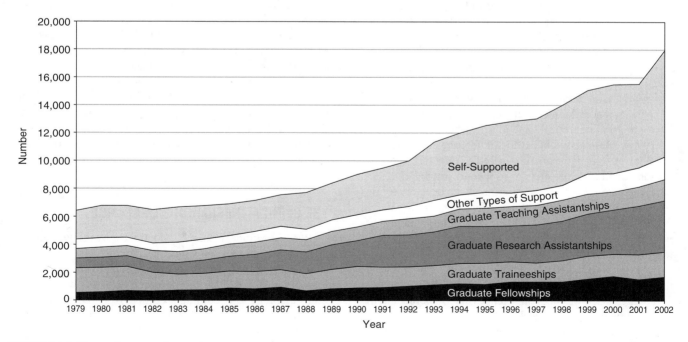

FIGURE 4-2 Type of support for graduate students in clinical sciences departments, 1979–2002 (does not include graduate students in nursing).
SOURCE: National Science Foundation Survey of Graduate Students and Postdoctorates in Science and Engineering.

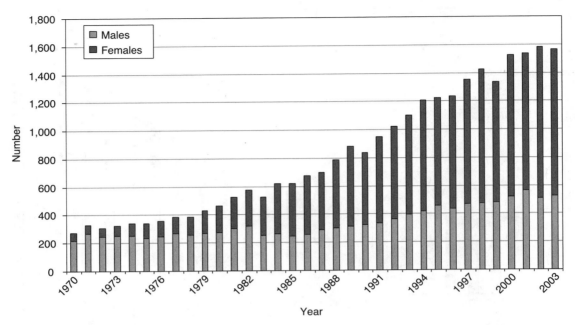

FIGURE 4-3  Doctorates in the clinical sciences by gender, 1970–2003.
SOURCE: National Science Foundation Survey of Earned Doctorates, 2001.

1990s was about 35 percent, but dropped below that level in 2002 and 2003, reflecting the decline in the male graduate student population in 2000 and 2001.

The citizenship pattern of clinical sciences doctorates, with only about 20 percent awarded to temporary residents and 5 percent to permanent residents, differs from that of the biomedical sciences. However, minority participation is similar to that of the biomedical sciences, accounting for only about 7 percent of the degrees in 2002 (see Appendix E).

In comparison to the biomedical as well as the behavioral and social sciences, clinical sciences differs significantly in time to doctoral degree and age at time of degree. Since the late 1990s, clinical sciences doctorate time to degree has been near or over 10 years, compared to about 7.5 years in the biomedical sciences and 8.5 to 9 years in the behavioral and social sciences. The age of clinical sciences doctorates at the time of receipt of their degrees averages 38 for clinical scientists, while doctorates in the other fields typically receive their degrees in their early thirties (see Appendix E). Moreover, of the three fields, clinical sciences doctorates are the least likely to have postdoctoral training. About 25 percent traditionally plan such training, in contrast to 70 percent of graduates in the biomedical sciences and 36 percent in the social and behavioral sciences.

It should be noted that these characteristics apply only to the U.S.-trained doctorates that will potentially make up the clinical research workforce. Some M.D.s and Ph.D.s with degrees from foreign institutions become part of this workforce as well, but data on this group are incomplete. Nevertheless, some indication of its contribution can be obtained from academic data. In 2002 of the 12,750 individual postdoctoral appointments in academic clinical departments, nearly 2,200 were U.S. citizens or permanent residents with M.D. degrees and 6,700 were temporary residents, a large proportion of whom were probably foreign educated with an M.D. or a Ph.D. degree. Given that the average postdoctoral appointment is 2 or 3 years and assuming that at least 50 percent of these doctorates will stay in the United States, some 2,000 researchers could be added each year to the country's clinical workforce. The above is only a partial estimate of the supply of clinical researchers, however, because M.D.s and foreign-educated doctorates could take postdoctoral training in the nonacademic sectors or have no postdoctoral training.

## THE CLINICAL RESEARCH WORKFORCE

Because clinical research is conducted by individuals with different degrees and no single data source comprehensively captures their activities, it is best to look at the clinical research workforce from the perspective of the different degrees that lead to becoming a clinical researcher. The basic workforce is the 17,180 doctorates with a Ph.D. in the clinical fields listed in Appendix C and as characterized in Appendix E, Table E-6. In addition, in 2001 the Association of American Medical Colleges (AAMC) roster of medical school faculty identified another 3,090 M.D.s with U.S. doctorates and R01 support as well as 750 individuals with Ph.D.s from foreign institutions and R01 support, for a total of about 21,000. A slightly different result is obtained from 2001 NIH data, which counted 4,563 M.D. principal investigators with R01 support, bringing the total for M.D.s and Ph.D.s to just under 22,500. However, neither of these counts captures the clinical researchers in the M.D. population who are not principal investigators on R01 grants; this could increase the M.D. research population by a factor of 2 or 3.

As was the case with the educational characteristics of clinical doctorates, data on their career progression and employment characteristics are only well known for Ph.D.s from U.S. institutions (Appendix E). This workforce has grown significantly over the past three decades, rising from about 2,500 in the early 1970s to about 17,000 in 2001 (see Figure 4-4). Much of this growth was in the academic sector, but the industrial sector also showed a significant increase. The growth in the academic sector in recent years has mainly resulted from the employment of non-tenure-track faculty and other academics (usually research associates; see Figure 4-5).

Tenured and tenure-track faculty still form the majority in academia, but their percentage fell from around 80 percent in the mid-1980s to 64 percent in 2001. This decline was not unexpected, given the tendency of many fields in recent years toward temporary or soft-money positions.

A major concern for the clinical research enterprise is the increase in the average age at which individuals receive their doctorates; this and other factors have contributed to the aging of the workforce. Between 1985 and 2001, the median age of the workforce increased from the 41- to 43-year cohort to the 49- to 50-year cohort (see Figure 4-6).

The Ph.D. workforce age distribution is greater by a few years on average than the age distribution for M.D. clinical researchers in medical schools. For example, the median age of Ph.D. clinicians is 50, while that of research clinical faculty in medical schools is a little under 47 (see Figure 4-7).

The declining interest of new doctorates in postdoctoral training is shown in Appendix E, Table E-5. Only a few hundred (about 2 percent) U.S.-trained clinical sciences doctorates held postdoctoral positions in recent years, and almost all of these positions were in academic institutions. However, the picture is somewhat different if the academic postdoctoral pool is examined on the basis of institutions' clinical departments. In 2002 there were almost 4,000 U.S. citizen or permanent resident Ph.D.s in these positions (see Figure 4-8). The number of temporary residents was about the same, but their percentage, like that of the biomedical sciences, was increasing. The difference between the data reported in Table E-6 and the data in Figure 4-8 is probably due to Ph.D.s with biomedical doctorates moving into clinical departments for training purposes.

Table E-6 shows that minorities represented 8.7 percent of the clinical research population in 2001, even though their numbers had grown from about 100 in 1973 to a little over 1,000 in 2001. This percentage is greater than in the bio-

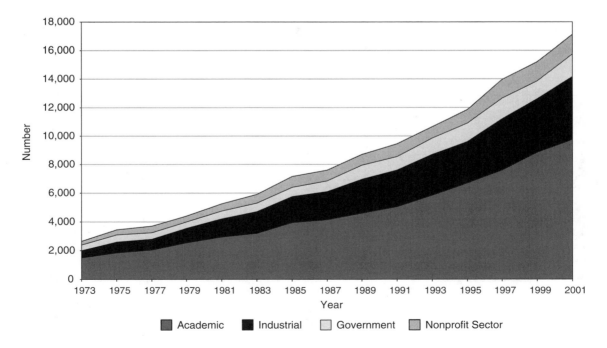

FIGURE 4-4 Employment sectors in the clinical sciences, 1973–2001.
SOURCE: National Science Foundation Survey of Doctorate Recipients.

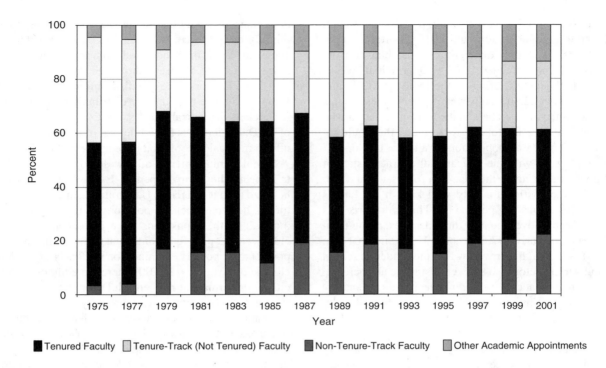

FIGURE 4-5  Academic appointments in the clinical sciences, 1975–2001.
SOURCE: National Science Foundation Survey of Doctorate Recipients.

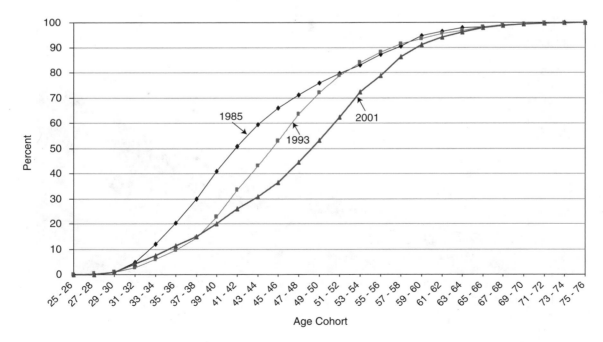

FIGURE 4-6  Cumulative age distribution of the clinical research workforce.
SOURCE: National Science Foundation Survey of Doctorate Recipients.

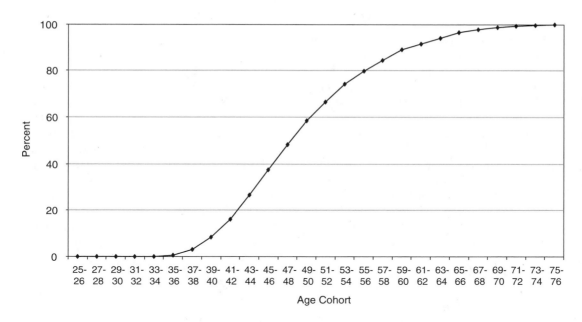

FIGURE 4-7  Age distribution of research clinical faculty in medical schools, 2002.
SOURCE: American Association of Medical Colleges Faculty Roster Database.

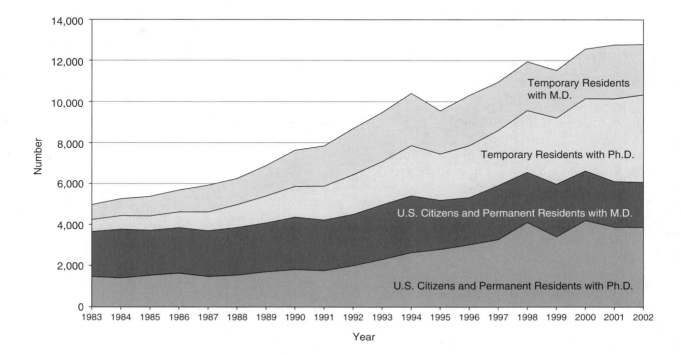

FIGURE 4-8  Postdoctoral appointments in clinical departments by citizenship and degree.
SOURCE: National Science Foundation Survey of Graduate Students and Postdoctorates in Science and Engineering.

medical sciences and about the same as that of the behavioral and social sciences. The data show, as in the other fields, a small number of temporary residents in the research population, but these are only individuals who were trained in U.S. institutions. There may actually be a larger percentage of temporary residents in the workforce when those with foreign doctorates are included.

The discussion until now has dealt only with part of the clinical sciences workforce (Ph.D.s), but medical doctors also participate in research. As seen in Figure 4-8, a number of M.D.s hold postdoctoral positions in clinical departments. In 2002 the number of postdoctoral positions occupied by U.S. citizens, permanent residents, and temporary residents was almost equally shared by M.D.s and Ph.D.s. However, the number of citizens/permanent residents, which was fairly constant in the late 1990s, is now declining, while the number of temporary residents in these positions is growing. This may also be a sign of the decreased postdoctoral participation noted in other fields by U.S. doctorates.

The number of domestic- and foreign-trained M.D. researchers on medical school faculties is estimated at 3,700. An additional 1,585 M.D./Ph.D.s received NIH support. About 40 percent of the M.D. grants were in clinical research areas, and 20 percent of the grants to M.D./Ph.D.s would be for clinical research. Therefore about 1,800 M.D. or M.D./Ph.D. researchers should be added to the 17,000 Ph.D.s educated in U.S. institutions in clinical fields. Although this brings the total to at least 18,800 clinical researchers, it is probably an underestimate, since a significant number of M.D.s work in industry to conduct or support clinical trials in the pharmaceutical and biotechnology companies, and the government employs M.D.s as researchers in its hospitals and laboratories. Also, about 15 percent of medical school faculties consist of researchers with foreign-earned doctorates; if this is typical, the above estimate should be increased again by 10 to 15 percent to at least 21,000.

While the exact number of M.D. clinical researchers is not known, it appears that individuals with Ph.D.s have dominated the field in recent years. There does not appear to be a change in the number of M.D.s in clinical research since the 1970s. While only 2,600 Ph.D.s made up the workforce and only a few hundred degrees were awarded each year in the 1970s, the Ph.D. workforce has since grown by a factor of 7. There may be several reasons for this change, but a logical one is the increased education debt incurred by medical school graduates. Most physicians and dentists today begin their professional careers with sizable education debts (though graduates of dual-degree—M.D.-Ph.D. or D.D.S.-Ph.D.—programs are the exception). From 1991 to 2001 the average medical school debt of M.D. graduates increased more than 50 percent, from almost $43,000 (in 2001 dollars) to just over $70,000. The level of educational debt for dental students is even higher—in 2001 it was over $75,000. This is primarily because dental students must purchase their dental instruments during their clinical training.

Although health care professionals are permitted to postpone payments on their student loans during NRSA or other authorized research training programs, this option may not be widely used. Even if it were, the fact is that additional training places its own financial and other burdens on young physicians. They must find time for research—an increasingly difficult challenge—particularly for those working in today's highly competitive health care market. Another obstacle for physician-investigators has been the limitation on salaries for NIH-funded investigators. It is now set at $175,000. While that is not an insignificant sum, it is below what many practicing clinicians or medical faculty can earn.

The M.D./Ph.D. programs were created as a way to bring more M.D.s into clinical research, but as noted earlier only about 20 percent of M.D./Ph.D.s pursue clinical research careers. Education debt does not appear to be the reason, as their debt averaged only about $15,000 in 2001. It is more likely that the research work they were exposed to during their Ph.D. program attracted them to a research career in the biomedical sciences instead.

Aside from the formal dual-degree programs, other mechanisms are being tried to encourage M.D.s to enter clinical research. Examples include master-level programs in special areas, such as Duke University's academic training in quantitative and methodological principles of medical genomics. Such programs appear to be very popular and may help redirect more physicians into clinical research.

## CLINICAL WORKFORCE ISSUES

For more than a decade now, concern has been expressed about the vitality of the clinical research enterprise. In 1997, Ahrens published a treatise that described the problems facing patient-oriented research and the economic and social factors that were driving the system.[6] He called for special training programs and greater cooperation between clinically trained M.D.s and technically trained Ph.D.s. Many other similar commentaries have been written, expressing the fear that because clinical investigators are not renewing themselves, many of the modern-day advances in biomedical research are not being translated into patient care.[7,8] For example, between 1983 and 1998 the number of physician-scientists decreased by 22 percent, from 18,535 to 14,479.[9] Another indication of the gap between basic research and the application of that research is the decline from 1995 to 2001 in the number of M.D.s applying for and receiving F32 postdoctoral fellowships.

In response to these concerns, NIH established in 1995 a Director's Panel on Clinical Research. A report issued in 1997, generally called the Nathan report (after its chairman,

---

[6]Ahrens, E. H. 1992.
[7]Arias, I. M. 2004.
[8]Gray, M. L. and J. Bonventre. 2002.
[9]Ley, T. J. and L. E. Rosenberg, 2002.

David G. Nathan), made recommendations concerning the need for more data on clinical research, the training of investigators, the expansion of clinical research centers, and the creation of partnerships. Shortly thereafter, in 2000, Congress passed the Clinical Research Enhancement Act, which called on NIH to implement many of the Nathan report's recommendations; and a 2003 Report Card later found that NIH had indeed implemented many of them.[10] In the area of training and career progression, three new K awards were established for clinicians. These included the K23, to support the career development of young investigators in patient-oriented research; the K24, to provide release time for midcareer clinicians to focus on research or mentor young researchers in patient-oriented research; and the K30, to allow for the development of clinical research training programs. Table 4-1 shows the growth in these awards since their establishment in 1998.

These programs appear to be fulfilling their mission, since 80 to 90 percent of the applicants are M.D.s, and they enjoy a higher acceptance rate than the Ph.D. applicants. The programs have also led the way for other organizations, such as the Doris Duke Charitable Foundation and the Howard Hughes Medical Institute, to establish similar programs.

In terms of training, NIH responded to the panel's report by encouraging internships at NIH for medical students and the establishment of a loan relief program that allows M.D.s to pay back their medical loans by making a 50 percent commitment to research for a period of 2 years. This program has been very successful in attracting physicians to research careers.

Other programs that appear to be successful at training clinical researchers come in the form of course work directed at physicians or Ph.D. students. For example, Duke University offers a master's level program for clinical fellows to develop quantitative and methodological principles of clinical research. The program offers formal courses in research design, research management, and statistical analysis. Another example is the joint Harvard/MIT Medical Engineering Medical Physics Ph.D. program that is aimed at training Ph.D. scientists in both their physical science or engineering specialty and the fundamentals of clinical medicine. Other forms of these programs range from a single course to a formal degree program, and there is some evidence to show that the graduates participating in these programs follow a clinical research path and join clinical departments in medical centers.[11,12]

## THE MEDICAL SCIENTIST TRAINING PROGRAM

Another effort aimed at addressing the shortage of individuals in translational research has been the establishment

TABLE 4-1 NIH Clinical Career Awards 1999–2002

| Year | K23 | K24 | K30 |
|------|-----|-----|-----|
| 1999 | 142 | 81 | 35 |
| 2000 | 327 | 158 | 57 |
| 2001 | 496 | 215 | 57 |
| 2002 | 664 | 261 | 59 |

SOURCE: NIH IMPACII Database.

of dual-degree programs, such as the Medical Scientist Training Program (MSTP) at the National Institute of General Medical Sciences (NIGMS). This program, which dates back to the 1960s, has produced several thousand M.D./ Ph.D.s who are highly qualified researchers. While the intent of the MSTP program is to develop translational research, it has not brought large numbers of individuals into patient-oriented research. Part of the problem might be the lure of bench science research, but there is also a long training period for these physician-scientists, which includes a postdoctoral appointment, internship, and residency. In the process, physicians may lose some of their medical skills in that they are not practicing medicine full time. The combination of the time commitment, loss of skills, and administrative challenges of research on human subjects may make basic research more attractive than patient-oriented research.[13,14]

Another career path for physician-scientists regards "late bloomers" who have an M.D. and for some reason decide to forgo private practice and pursue a research career. This path is generally longer than that of the M.D./Ph.D.s, as it includes medical school, a residency program, subspecialty fellowship training, and then a period of 3 to 6 years of research training. Prior to the medical scientist training programs, nearly all physician-scientists followed this path. Now the M.D./Ph.D.s make up about 30 percent of physician-scientists, according to NIH grant statistics, and at present only 2.5 percent of medical school graduates decide later to become researchers. While M.D./Ph.D. researchers leave medical school with relatively low debt, the debt of late bloomers stands at about $100,000 upon graduation and continues to grow through residency and fellowship training. If an individual elects a research career, it is almost impossible to begin bringing down this debt while on a $40,000 research training salary.

While increases in the number of individuals supported through the MSTP program would help alleviate the shortage of clinical researchers, ways to attract the late bloomers into research are also needed. For now the loan repayment program introduced a few years ago as part of the Public

[10]Nathan, D. G. and J. D. Wilson. 2003.
[11]Gray, M. L. and J. Bonventre. 2002. op. cit.
[12]Arias, I. M. 2004. op. cit.

[13]Nathan, D. G. 2002.
[14]Shulman, L. E. 1996.

Health Improvement Act has helped reduce the debt problem and possibly direct physicians into research careers. However, the program is small, with only about 250 trainees per year in authorized patient-oriented research programs receiving up to $35,000 each year for 2 years for repayment of their medical school debts and an additional 39 percent of the repayments to cover federal taxes, and possible reimbursement of state taxes that result from these payments. Also, there is a debate about whether the program should be expanded to allow repayment for M.D.s entering basic research training programs. While the addition of M.D.s to the bench science workforce may strengthen this research area, the added dollars for the program may be more effectively spent in attacking the shortage of clinical researchers.

## ROLE OF THE NATIONAL RESEARCH SERVICE AWARD PROGRAM

Earlier in this chapter, Figure 4-2 showed that clinical sciences graduate students' level of support from traineeships and fellowships was relatively constant—at about 3,500 students—and it also showed a decrease in the importance of these external support since the 1980s, as the number of research assistantships grew steadily to over 3,600 in 2002. This change in overall support is similar to the support from NIH, with an increase in clinical sciences research assistantships to the point where their number is a little greater than the level of trainee and fellowship support in 2002, though not to the level seen in the biological sciences (see Figure 4-9). It should also be noted that the National Science Foundation provides very little support for graduates, with about 100 awards equally divided between fellowships and research assistantships. However, another major source of support is the non-NIH part of the U.S. Department of Health and Human Services (DHHS), which in 2002 supported about 400 students on traineeships or fellowships.

The levels of graduate student support and Ph.D. production in the 1990s shown in Figure 4-2 are also reflected in the rapid growth in NRSA support of predoctoral trainees and fellows (see Table 4-2). Like the other two broad fields in this study, support was rather constant in the 1990s but declined in 2001, possibly because of higher stipend levels and the fixed NRSA budgets for the training programs. The differences between the numbers shown in Table 4-2 and

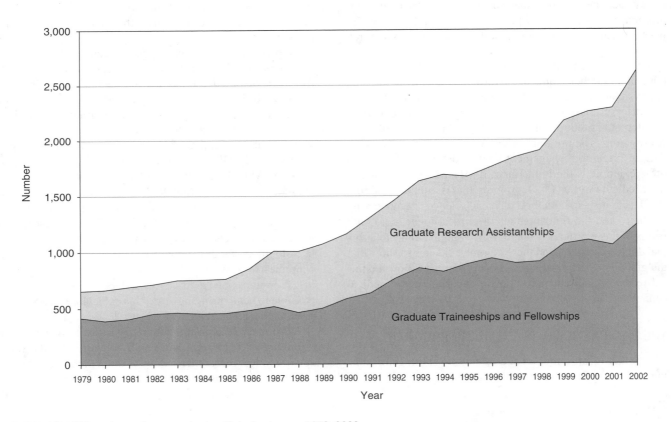

FIGURE 4-9  NIH predoctoral support in the clinical sciences, 1979–2002.
SOURCE: National Science Foundation Survey of Graduate Students and Postdoctorates in Science and Engineering.

TABLE 4-2 National Research Service Award Predoctoral Trainee and Fellowship Support in the Clinical Sciences

|  | 1975 | 1980 | 1985 | 1990 | 1995 | 2000 | 2001 | 2002[a] |
|---|---|---|---|---|---|---|---|---|
| Traineeships (T32)[b] | 83 | 609 | 559 | 641 | 1,334 | 1,395 | 1,577 | 875 |
| Fellowships (F30, F31)[b] | 4 | 129 | 44 | 151 | 108 | 126 | 143 | 151 |

[a]For 2002 and possibly 2001, the data are incomplete for traineeships since educational institutions report on the number of students trained in certain fields and the information was last processed in February 2003.

[b]See Appendix B for a complete explanation of awards.

SOURCE: NIH IMPACII Database.

Figure 4-9 are due to NRSA support through other DHHS agencies, such as the Agency for Healthcare Research and Quality.

Data on postdoctoral-level training support broken down by individual federal agency source are not collected, but information on the type of training—at least in academic institutions—is available (see Figure 4-10). The traineeships and fellowships portion of this support has been increasing at a slow rate, while the number of individuals on research grants has increased fivefold since the late 1970s.

The NRSA contribution to postdoctoral training support mirrors the general trend for fellows and trainees but at a lower level, given that support is available from sources other than NIH (see Table 4-3).

In addition to predoctoral and postdoctoral program support in the clinical sciences from the NRSA mechanism, dual-degree programs are another attractive option for health care professionals seeking clinical research training. Currently, NIH has three dual-degree training programs: (1) the MSTP, (2) the individual M.D./Ph.D. fellowships, and (3)

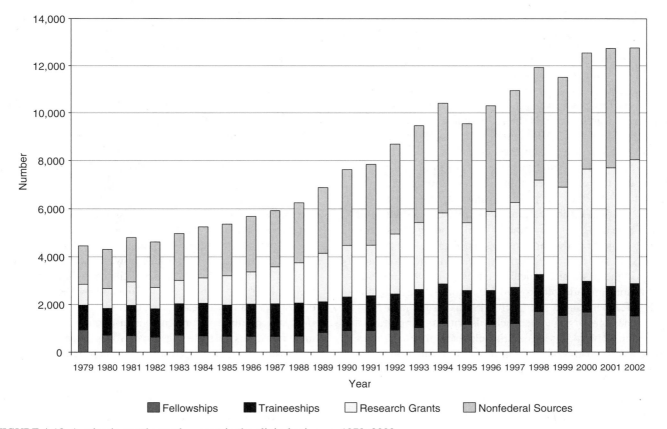

FIGURE 4-10 Academic postdoctoral support in the clinical sciences, 1979–2002.
SOURCE: National Science Foundation Survey of Doctorate Recipients.

TABLE 4-3 NRSA Postdoctoral Trainee and Fellowship Support in the Clinical Sciences

|                              | 1975 | 1980  | 1985  | 1990  | 1995  | 2000  | 2001  | 2002[a] |
|------------------------------|------|-------|-------|-------|-------|-------|-------|---------|
| Traineeships (T32)[b]        | 332  | 1,465 | 1,660 | 1,649 | 1,889 | 1,854 | 1,830 | 941     |
| Fellowships (F32)[b]         | 177  | 205   | 185   | 94    | 68    | 88    | 81    | 65      |

[a]For 2002 and possibly 2001, the data are incomplete for traineeships since educational institutions report on the number of students trained in certain fields and the information was last processed in February 2003.

[b]See Appendix B for a complete explanation of awards.

SOURCE: NIH IMPACII Database.

the Dental Scientist Training Program (DSTP). The MSTP is the largest and oldest program, dating back to 1964, and today is used to train about 1,000 students annually at 35 medical schools and universities. Fellowships for M.D./Ph.D. training, a more recent development, were instituted in 1989 by the National Institute of Mental Health, the National Institute on Alcohol Abuse and Alcoholism, and the National Institute on Drug Abuse to encourage dual-degree training in the areas of mental health, behavior, and neuroscience. This much smaller fellowship program supports about 40 students a year. The most recent dual-degree training program is the DSTP, which was created following recommendations from the 1994 study of the NRSA program. However, the DSTP is small and supports only a few students at three dental schools.

These dual-degree programs are very attractive to M.D. or D.D.S. students because they provide several career options and result in lower levels of education debt. However, relatively few participants receive much-needed training in clinical research methods. In 1996 an analysis of the fields of study chosen by MSTP participants found that nearly 60 percent of graduates from the late 1980s and early 1990s received their Ph.D.s in five basic science fields: biochemistry, neuroscience, molecular biology, cell biology, and pharmacology. Further, in their subsequent research careers, MSTP graduates focused almost entirely on laboratory-oriented research, and they sought NIH funding for such research projects at the same rate as did Ph.D.s.

MSTP students are generally directed toward doctoral study in the basic biomedical sciences simply because their institutions are oriented toward laboratory research in these fields. Recognizing a need, NIGMS has issued new MSTP guidelines that urge medical schools with training grants to extend their programs across disciplines to give M.D./Ph.D. students "a breadth of doctoral research training opportunities" in fields that include computer science, the social and behavioral sciences, economics, epidemiology, public health, bioengineering, biostatistics, and bioethics.

However, most M.D./Ph.D. programs have been slow to respond, as evidenced by little change in the descriptions of the programs. Finding mechanisms that will encourage stu-

dents in these dual-degree programs to conduct clinical research remains a challenge.

## RESEARCH LABOR FORCE PROJECTIONS

The lack of data for characterizing the clinical sciences workforce makes it extremely difficult to make accurate predictions of this workforce. Using the limited data from the Survey of Doctorate Recipients, the AAMC Faculty Roster, and 1990 U.S. Census data on immigrants, the 2001 potential clinical research population was estimated at 25,283. This included a combination of 19,105 U.S.-trained Ph.D.s and M.D.s, together with 6,178 individuals with doctorates from foreign institutions. This included individuals in postdoctoral positions but did not count the 563 doctorates with degrees in clinical fields who are unemployed or the 1,700 who are in positions that would not be considered scientific or related to clinical research. The employed workforce in the clinical sciences is 23,020. Table 4-4 shows the change in this workforce over the past decade for U.S.-educated Ph.D.s. However, this is only part of the total potential workforce in that there are foreign-trained doctorates who are employed and a few U.S. doctorates who leave the country and return at a later time. Estimating this foreign component is difficult, however, as no database describes the demographics of this group. The AAMC and 1990 U.S. Census data were used to provide the total workforce estimates given above, but no time series or characteristics were available.

It is also difficult to estimate how the science and engineering workforce in the clinical sciences will change over the next 10 years. Its size is influenced by the number of doctorates graduating each year, unemployment levels in the field, the number of foreign-trained doctorates, and retirement rates. It is possible to estimate some of these factors for U.S.-trained Ph.D.s, but only crude estimates have been made for the M.D. and foreign-earned degree holders.

The following is a short summary of the findings from the life table for clinical researchers. An analysis and the full details can be found in Appendix D. Graduates from U.S. Ph.D. programs are the largest and most relevant source of new researchers. The size of this group grew significantly in

TABLE 4-4  Potential Workforce in the Clinical Sciences by Employment Status, 1991–2001

| | 1991 | 1993 | 1995 | 1997 | 1999 | 2001 |
|---|---|---|---|---|---|---|
| Employed in S&E | 9,111 | 10,424 | 11,506 | 13,716 | 14,779 | 16,765 |
| Percentage | 89.9 | 87.1 | 83.7 | 88.1 | 86.6 | 87.8 |
| Employed Out of S&E | 654 | 815 | 1,315 | 785 | 1,328 | 1,394 |
| Percentage | 6.5 | 6.8 | 9.6 | 5.0 | 7.8 | 7.3 |
| Unemployed, Seeking Work | 149 | 163 | 171 | 170 | 203 | 127 |
| Percentage | 1.5 | 1.4 | 1.2 | 1.1 | 1.2 | 0.7 |
| Unemployed, Not Seeking, Not Retired | 79 | 327 | 266 | 388 | 333 | 404 |
| Percentage | 0.8 | 2.7 | 1.9 | 2.5 | 2.0 | 2.1 |
| Postdoctorates | 140 | 234 | 485 | 514 | 431 | 415 |
| Percentage | 1.4 | 2.0 | 3.5 | 3.3 | 2.5 | 2.2 |
| Total | 10,133 | 11,963 | 13,743 | 15,573 | 17,074 | 19,105 |

SOURCE: National Science Foundation Survey of Doctorate Recipients.

the 1990s, and unlike the pattern in the biomedical sciences, this growth continued into 2001. Since there appears to be continuing growth in the workforce, only median estimates are presented here for the inputs to the life-table model. A constant-supply scenario is unrealistic, and continued strong growth might not be sustained. The annual number of U.S. Ph.D.s grows from 1,551 in 2001 to 1,807 in 2011, and the inflow of foreign-degree holders increases from 504 in 2001 to 708 in 2011. This estimate of growth in the foreign population is problematic, however, because it is based on esti-

mates of the growth rate in the 1990s and the resulting population in 2001. Current immigration restrictions will have an impact on the number of foreign scientists who will be able to emigrate. Table 4-5 shows the results of the multistate life-table analysis for the period from 2001 to 2011, under the median scenarios. The 4 or 5 percent growth rate is much greater than in the biomedical sciences and in the 10-year period is projected to almost double.

Unemployment remains at 1 percent or less, and the portion of the workforce remaining in science is about 90 per-

TABLE 4-5  Projected Workforce by Status for the Median Scenario, 2001–2011

| | 2001 | 2002 | 2003 | 2004 | 2005 | 2006 | 2007 | 2008 | 2009 | 2010 | 2011 |
|---|---|---|---|---|---|---|---|---|---|---|---|
| **U.S. Doctorates** | | | | | | | | | | | |
| Workforce | 19104 | 20177 | 21273 | 22368 | 23454 | 24536 | 25621 | 26694 | 27744 | 28785 | 29818 |
| Employed in S&E | 17180 | 18281 | 19344 | 20405 | 21459 | 22504 | 23546 | 24563 | 25541 | 26498 | 27444 |
| Out of science | 1394 | 1389 | 1441 | 1482 | 1504 | 1529 | 1559 | 1597 | 1646 | 1703 | 1764 |
| Unemployed | 127 | 128 | 132 | 134 | 137 | 141 | 147 | 153 | 160 | 165 | 170 |
| Unemployed, Not Seeking | 404 | 380 | 356 | 347 | 354 | 361 | 369 | 381 | 396 | 410 | 426 |
| Postdoctorates | 507 | 546 | 585 | 620 | 659 | 705 | 750 | 785 | 813 | 834 | 859 |
| **Foreign Doctorates** | | | | | | | | | | | |
| Workforce | 6178 | 6661 | 7166 | 7691 | 8232 | 8796 | 9381 | 9985 | 10608 | 11246 | 11898 |
| Employed in S&E | 5840 | 6299 | 6781 | 7281 | 7791 | 8314 | 8853 | 9415 | 10001 | 10604 | 11218 |
| Out of science | 306 | 329 | 353 | 380 | 412 | 456 | 505 | 551 | 595 | 636 | 677 |
| Unemployed | 10 | 11 | 12 | 11 | 11 | 12 | 12 | 12 | 12 | 14 | 15 |
| Unemployed, Not Seeking | 22 | 22 | 19 | 19 | 17 | 15 | 12 | 5 | 1 | 0 | 0 |
| Postdoctorates | 320 | 343 | 366 | 390 | 414 | 440 | 464 | 486 | 508 | 531 | 552 |
| **Total** | | | | | | | | | | | |
| Workforce | 25282 | 26838 | 28439 | 30059 | 31686 | 33332 | 35002 | 36679 | 38352 | 40031 | 41716 |
| Employed in S&E | 23020 | 24580 | 26125 | 27686 | 29250 | 30818 | 32399 | 33978 | 35542 | 37102 | 38662 |
| Out of science | 1700 | 1718 | 1794 | 1862 | 1916 | 1985 | 2064 | 2148 | 2241 | 2339 | 2441 |
| Unemployed | 137 | 139 | 144 | 145 | 148 | 153 | 159 | 165 | 172 | 179 | 185 |
| Unemployed, Not Seeking | 426 | 402 | 375 | 366 | 371 | 376 | 381 | 386 | 397 | 410 | 426 |
| Postdoctorates | 827 | 889 | 951 | 1010 | 1073 | 1145 | 1214 | 1271 | 1321 | 1365 | 1411 |

SOURCE: NRC analysis. See Appendix Tables D-9, D-11, and D-12.

cent. The one thing this model does not account for is the possible growth in the physician-scientist workforce as the result of expansions in the M.D./Ph.D. programs—that is, the movement of more medically trained doctors into research careers.

## CONCLUSION

The importance of clinical research cannot be underestimated in today's health care system. Recent efforts to offset the growing shortage of clinical researchers, especially those initiatives aimed at attracting physician-scientists into patient-oriented research, have not been fully evaluated. One program that has been in existence for many years is the MSTP, but it has not brought researchers into patient-oriented research. The MSTP has produced a highly qualified workforce in the basic health sciences, but the potential remains for these scientists to become more involved in translational or patient-oriented research. The forces that constrain the clinical sciences workforce are beyond the control of training programs, as they involve national policies on health care and its delivery systems. Additionally, because many areas of clinical research require medical training, predoctoral support is not possible under a program like NRSA. Intervention must occur at a point beyond the doctorate, with postdoctoral and career development programs.

## RECOMMENDATIONS

**Recommendation 4-1: This committee recommends that the total number of NRSA positions awarded in the clinical sciences should remain at least at the 2003 level. Furthermore, the committee recommends that training levels after 2003 be commensurate with the rise in the total extramural research funding in the biomedical, clinical, and behavioral and social sciences.**

Data on the number of predoctoral and postdoctoral traineeships in 2001 appear to be consistent with earlier

years. In 2001 there were over 1,577 predoctoral NRSA training slots in the clinical sciences and 1,830 at the postdoctoral level. Projecting these numbers into 2003, on the basis of a 4.4 percent increase in total predoctoral training and a 5.6 percent increase in postdoctoral training, yields estimates of 1,665 and 1,910, respectively. The 2002 data on fellowships are probably more current at 151 predoctoral and 96 postdoctoral positions, and since there was little change in the level of fellowship support from 2002 to 2003, these levels could be applied to 2003. For both the traineeships and fellowships at the predoctoral and postdoctoral levels, NRSA support is only a small fraction of the total training support (see Figures 4-2 and 4-10). Much more comes from research grants and the retraining of physicians through the K23 and K24 programs or self-support at the predoctoral level.

The relatively low unemployment among Ph.D.s in the clinical sciences and the fact that the pool of postdoctorates appears to be stabilizing suggest that the NRSA training level should be maintained at least at the 2003 level and increase with extramural research funding.

The discussion following Recommendation 2-1 with regard to the quality of NRSA programs and relative balance of biomedical training to the workforce also applies to the behavioral and social sciences.

**Recommendation 4-2: This committee recommends that training grants be established for physicians to acquire the skills necessary for clinical investigation.**

Clinical research, such as clinical trials and outcome assessment, can be carried out by individuals in a variety of fields, but a shortage of well-trained people appears to exist. Attracting physicians into these areas is highly desirable. Training should include clinical trial design, statistics, and epidemiology. Training programs should be structured so that physicians can maintain other professional activities while pursuing this training and receiving degrees at the master's level.

# 5

# Oral Health Research

Although dentistry is often thought of in terms of professional practice, it is also a science that depends on researchers to develop new and better dental technologies and, through the training of dental practitioners, to bring those technologies to the general public. But the profession is now in jeopardy, since the need for dental school faculty to conduct research and to educate dental students is acute. Over the past decade, several hundred faculty positions in dental schools have gone unfilled each year. While not all of them would be filled by researchers, it is to the profession's advantage—as it is in other sciences—to have as many research-trained Ph.D.s or D.D.S./Ph.D.s as possible in these positions. The shortage of research staff in universities carries over to the industrial and governmental sectors as well, where a significant amount of dental research is conducted.

The reasons for this shortage are many. To cite just one, a culture exists within dental schools that values technical training and private practice over research, resulting in deficiencies in the support mechanisms for whoever does do research. The following sections describe the nature and scope of the problem.

## THE SHORTAGE OF DENTAL SCIENTISTS

In 2001 the American Dental Association issued a report, *Future of Dentistry*, which outlined many of the issues facing the dental profession including what is now called a crisis in dental education. This crisis may be more aptly termed a dental school faculty shortage that has become acute because few individuals choose academics and research as a career goal. In the late 1990s there were nearly 400 open faculty positions, but the estimate for 2002 was 373. This reduction in the number of unfilled positions has come mainly from the elimination of those positions (because of dental school budget cuts) rather than from faculty hires.

Figure 5-1 gives a 10-year history of vacant full-time faculty positions in U.S. dental schools. Given that the level has remained about constant over the past 5 or 6 years, the num-

ber is unlikely to decline in the near future. While the number of unfilled full-time positions is approximately 275, this should not be interpreted as the number of research faculty needed, as some of these positions are for clinical faculty. In Table 5-1, which shows the distribution of vacant positions by primary activity, 45 of them are in basic sciences and research. But in addition, some of the 194 clinical positions would be research oriented.

While the shortage is critical across all types of appointments, the job of filling research positions is particularly difficult because there is no pool of temporary or part-time employees—as is the case for the clinical positions, which can be filled by practicing dentists. Dental faculty are simply not trained to be researchers, and many of them may not have the interest or ability to explore new areas of knowledge. Clinicians who teach students to perform dental care are, without a doubt, critical to the mission of dental schools but are not discussed here.

This recruitment problem does not tell the whole story about the number of scientists needed in dental education for the next decade. A possibly more critical situation is the retention of current faculty. According to data from the American Dental Education Association's 2001–2002 Survey of Dental Schools, 1,011 faculty members, or 9 percent, vacated their positions in 2001–2002.[1] This level was about twice that of the previous academic year. In 2001–2002, 53 percent of faculty members left an academic position to go into private practice, an increase of 18 percent over the preceding year. Possible reasons for the shifts in 2001–2002 may be retirement, moving to other schools, and the downturn in the economy.

Institutional budgetary limitations are partly responsible for the recruitment and retention of dental faculty—in the past 10 years, faculty salaries have increased by about 25 to 30 percent, while income in private practice has gone up 78

---

[1]American Dental Association. 2001.

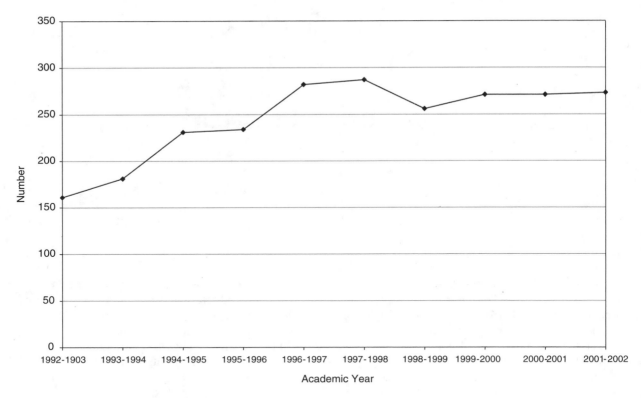

FIGURE 5-1 Unfilled full-time positions on dental school faculties, 1992–2002.
SOURCE: American Dental Education Association.

percent.[2] An important related financial issue is the debt incurred by dental students during their studies. Among students who entered dental school in 1998, about 60 percent had no education debt. Those who reported debt had an average burden of $25,300. Hence, a rationale might be that a pool of applicants with little or no education debt would be more at liberty to select a career path aimed at pursuing interests, rather than immediately generating income for debt service. However, of those graduating from dental school in 2002, 29 percent reported debt levels of $100,000 to $149,999.[3] Debt levels higher than $150,000 were reported by 29 percent of graduates. The average debt of all students upon graduation (from both public and private dental schools) was $107,500 (this average includes debt-free students). The average debt of those students who had at least some debt was $122,500. In general, their debt is higher than in any other profession, including medicine, because they are required to purchase instruments used in dental school. The impact of debt on career path is substantiated by the finding that nearly 24 percent of dental school seniors indicate debt as a factor influencing career plans. Further, as debt levels increase, a progressively higher percentage of

seniors with the higher debt levels opt to immediately enter private practice.

Perhaps the most significant factor driving the low interest in research among dentists is the prospect of a very lucrative career in private practice. General practitioners can expect an annual income of nearly $150,000, with specialists earning over $200,000, and there is no indication that these figures will decline in the future even with significant ad-

TABLE 5-1 Vacant Faculty Positions in Dental Schools, 2001–2002

| Primary Area of Appointment | Vacant Positions | | |
| --- | --- | --- | --- |
|  | Full-Time | Part-Time | Total |
| Clinical sciences | 194 | 63 | 257 |
| Basic sciences | 20 | 1 | 21 |
| Administration | 25 | 1 | 26 |
| Allied dental | 3 | 3 | 6 |
| Research | 25 | 2 | 27 |
| Other | 6 | 1 | 7 |
| Total | 273 | 71 | 344 |

SOURCE: American Dental Education Association.

[2]Haden, N. K., R. G. Weaver, and R. W. Valachovic. 2002.
[3]American Dental Education Association. 2001.

vances in oral health care. Thus many students who may be interested in research elect the higher-paid and, from their point of view, more secure careers in clinical practice.

The aging of the dental school faculty will only make the shortages of the past decade more of a problem in the future. The average age of faculty members in 2001 was 49.6 years, and 20 percent of the faculty were over the age of 60. Because there is little difference in the average age of the basic science/research faculty and the clinical faculty, the projections of about 1,000 retirements in the over-60 age group in the next 10 years would mean a reduction in the basic science and research faculty of about 200. The fact that few associate professors are following closely behind these senior faculty members means that the pipeline has many gaps and that an even greater need for researchers will exist over the next 10 years. The shortage of senior faculty will also create a period during which junior faculty have few mentors to assist them in the activities necessary for tenure and promotion.

In the context of the faculty shortage in dentistry, it is important to realize that not all research faculty in dental schools need be dentists. While clinicians trained as dentists are useful in answering clinical questions and are fundamental to clinical research, nondentist basic scientists trained to the highest standards are also an important part of the faculty mix. Although dental schools should have a mix of basic and clinical scientists to achieve the institutions' and the nation's research goals, few doctorates trained in the basic biomedical sciences have considered academic careers in a dental school. While some training may be necessary to make this adjustment in career goals, the benefit to the dental and biomedical professions would be significant. A complicating factor, however, is that some administrators in dental schools might not be willing to accept the qualifications of these basic scientists, even with the necessary training.

## POTENTIAL POOL OF DENTAL RESEARCHERS

The size and quality of the national applicant pool for U.S. dental schools merit scrutiny. Because this pool represents a large and relatively robust population of people who have an interest in oral health and are willing to further their formal education through an extensive training experience, a large proportion of the next generation of oral health researchers will likely be drawn from this group. Additional scientists may come from abroad or from among those practitioners who gravitate to oral health research as a consequence of their interest in its scientific challenges.

There are 56 dental schools in 34 states and Puerto Rico, enrolling 17,487 dental students and 5,266 dental residents in 2001. There were 4,448 first-year dental students, selected from a total applicant pool of 7,538.[4] The current ratio of applicants to first-year enrollment for dental school is 1 to 68. Among applicants to dental school in 2001–2002, 83.9 percent possessed baccalaureate degrees, 2.5 percent had master's degrees, and 0.1 percent had Ph.D. degrees, suggesting that preexisting research training or experience for this applicant pool is negligible. Clearly, if education in biomedical research is to be offered, it needs either to be a part of professional school study or provided as a postgraduate experience.

The predental grade point average for the year 2000 entering class was 3.35 overall and 3.25 in the sciences.[5] Dental Aptitude Test scores for the entering class of 2001–2002 were 18.65 (academic average) and 18.36 (science average), both on a 30-point standard scale.[6] Thus, given the number of slots available each year in U.S. dental schools, the applicant pool's academic quality, though above average, was not overwhelming.

A key question is whether a subset of individuals at the high end of the academic distribution can be drawn from the national pool and attracted to careers in biomedical research. Given both the size of this group and its mean GPA of 3.25 in the sciences, the existence of a sizable subset of academic high performers seems plausible, yet the percentage of graduates interested in teaching, research, or administration is small and declining. Few students entering dental school are aware of a career path that includes oral health research, and even fewer consider this option as they complete their training. Interest in research dropped from about 1.3 percent in 1980 to 0.5 percent in 2002.[7] This means that only about 20 of the nearly 4,000 dental school graduates each year consider a career in dental research.

The reasons for this low interest, as noted earlier, include the prospects of a high income in dental practice; the accumulated student debt; and a culture in many dental schools, especially among the clinical staff, that values the technical aspects of dentistry and often marginalizes research. The National Institutes of Health (NIH) has two grant programs that support the infrastructure in dental schools: the R24 for planning research facilities and infrastructure and the R25 for planning curriculum structure. It is generally believed that a higher percentage of students, although small, are interested in dental research earlier as opposed to later in their education; it might be possible to influence dental students later in their education by integrating research into professional training through the NIH grant programs. However, most dental school applicants are interested in becoming dentists, not biomedical researchers. This intention is presumably based on applicants' general understanding of what

---

[4]Weaver, R. G., K. Haden, and R. W. Valachovic. 2002.

[5]Center for Public Policy and Advocacy, American Dental Education Association (ADEA). 2003. *Dental Education At-A-Glance 2003*. Available at *http://www.adea.org/CPPA_Materials/default.htm*. Accessed on October 22, 2004.

[6]American Dental Association. 2001–2002.

[7]Ibid. 2:34.

dentists do. Inasmuch as 92.7 percent of professionally active dentists are engaged in private practice, with 92.1 percent of that number holding an equity share in a practice,[8] it seems reasonable that most dental school applicants aspire to a career as a small-business person rather than as a biomedical scientist. Yet it is still from such a pool that the future biomedical research scientists in this field are likely to come. In other words, biomedical researchers in the oral health sciences start out wanting to be practicing dentists; but they apparently undergo a significant shift in career plans and professional identity sometime during either dental school or specialty training, usually under the influence of a mentor or because of some other significant academic experience. What dental schools can do to foster such a shift is an important question.

Each year competition is great for the highest academic performers graduating from dental school. The most effective at siphoning off the best are the nine specialties in dentistry: oral and maxillofacial surgery, orthodontics, periodontics, endodontics, pediatric dentistry, prosthodontics, oral and maxillofacial pathology, oral and maxillofacial radiology, and public health dentistry. For 2001–2002, 1,264 students enrolled in these specialty programs. Although the number of applications for these positions is reported as 43,612, this figure is misleading because "applications" refers to the cumulative number of applicants to all programs and represents a duplicated count.[9] Because of the inordinate length of some specialty training programs—anywhere from 2 to 7 years after dental school—some residents may exclude themselves from the additional training needed to become a biomedical scientist. On the other hand, departmentally based dental schools are, arguably, run by research-oriented dental specialists. Thus, while there are positions for general dentists in dental schools, leadership positions are often held by research-oriented specialists. The preferred model for training biomedical research scientists in the oral health sciences is to have dental specialists go on to research training, usually by studying for a Ph.D. Hence, the approximately 1,200 specialty students can be seen as the potential pool for the recruitment of future scientists—though a relatively small percentage of this number are actually attracted by the prospect of actually doing so. In recognition of this possibility, the National Institute of Dental and Craniofacial Research (NIDCR) has tried several programs leading to advanced research training (usually through the vehicle of a Ph.D.) in combination with either the dental school curriculum or clinical specialty training.

One initiative that was instituted by NIDCR, in response to a recommendation from the National Research Council's study of the National Research Service Award (NRSA) program, was a Dental Scientist Training Program (DSTP)—a dual-degree program leading to a D.D.S. and a Ph.D. In 2001–2002, 11 institutions had NIH-supported DSTPs, with a total of about 30 students. There were another 10 institutions with D.D.S./Ph.D. programs that did not have NIH support. The applicant pool for the DSTPs is very strong, and more students could be accepted into them if funding were available. The curriculum sequence for the DSTP at many institutions is similar to that of the Medical Scientist Training Program (MSTP)—the first 2 years are spent in dental training, the next 2 to 3 years are devoted to research training for the Ph.D., and then students return to dental school for 2 or more years to complete their dental degrees.

One serious drawback to the DSTP is its funding mechanism. The MSTP students may receive support for up to 6 years under the NRSA requirements, and MSTP policy requires that every student be supported with stipends and total tuition for the entire period of dual degree. However, the DSTP student may only receive 5 years of support with the possibility of a sixth year under the T32 mechanism, and no full support requirement exists. This support usually applies during the Ph.D. portion of students' training and part of their dental training, but other sources must be found to support their studies for the rest of the program. Some institutions have used the K award mechanism to secure the needed funding. Consequently, students can complete the DSTP and still have debt. This program is new—only a few students have completed it—but graduates appear to be dedicated to research careers and are now in postdoctoral training.

Some insight comes from studying other training programs funded by NIDCR, given that this single institute funds the overwhelming majority of research training for oral health researchers. In fact, about 8.5 percent of the NIDCR budget in FY 2002 was spent on research training and career development[10]—approximately $20.4 million (total of both direct and indirect costs).[11] In 2002 NIDCR supported at least a dozen separate categories of research training and career development awards, including 157 NRSA grants and research career development awards. Further, for FY 2003, 50.6 percent of training grant proposals reviewed by NIDCR were funded (averaged over the individual awards). Though useful, these data do not in themselves provide much information concerning the actual number of persons currently in training through these various vehicles since some represent awards to individuals while others represent awards to institutions—each of the institutional awards providing funding for multiple individuals (and differing numbers of indi-

---

[8]Weaver, R. G., K. Haden, and R. W. Valachovic. 2002. op. cit.

[9]American Dental Association. 1999.

[10]American Dental Association. 2002.

[11]Gordon, S. July 16, 2003. Presentation to the Committee to Monitor the Changing Needs for Biomedical and Behavioral Research Personnel Oral Health Panel. New York, NY. Note: Personal Communication. Director. National Institute of Dental and Craniofacial Research. Note: Success rate averages must be regarded with some caution inasmuch as applicants often apply more than once prior to award and often a single applicant may straddle fiscal years. Success rate also varies by type of mechanism.

viduals per training program). Further, they provide even less information about the number of applicants to each program. Were such data available—such as the number of applicants for each training slot—they would be useful as a gauge of interest in training programs, and they would inform projections concerning the potential shortfall of biomedical research personnel relative to the nation's needs. Also they would help determine whether, from a national perspective, the number of applicants exceeds, matches, or falls short of the number of training slots available. A one-to-one match of applicants to available positions or, even more alarming, unfilled research training slots would not bode well either for the number of persons in the pipeline or, perhaps more significantly, for their quality.

In any case, although the number of individual awards may give one indication of the demand for training through institutional awards, this effect has never been quantified— in part because NIH grants are attributed to the principal investigator, not the individual trainee.

## RESOURCES FOR RESEARCH TRAINING

There is a need to systematically identify sources of collaborative funding for research training across government agencies and within the private sector. The goal of this effort is to facilitate communication and thereby expand the pool of funds that could be used for research training in fields related to oral health.

Although it provides the largest single source of all dental research training funds, the research training budget of NIDCR is limited and under financial pressure in the current economic climate. For example, in 2002 there were 31 NRSA grants, 70 research career development awards, and 48 K12 and K16 awards, for a total of 149 research training awards across the nation. The level of support in NIDCR for NRSA T32 and T35 grants was about 2.9 percent of its total budget, and for NRSA F31 grants the support was at 0.4 percent. This was about average for these awards across the NIH institutes. When considering the relatively large amount of research training support within other agencies of the government and the private sector, it becomes apparent that the possibility of augmenting NIDCR research training funds with other governmental and private-sector funds could markedly increase the total research training capacity for dental research in the United States.

Inspection of Tables 5-2 and 5-3 suggests that the research areas of concentration for FY 2002 could be linked to scientific research areas that are funded by other disciplines. For example, there are many research training programs across NIH and in other agencies of the government that fund the same or similar research disciplines being targeted by the NIDCR, such as microbiology, microbial pathogenesis, immunology, biotechnology, mammalian genetics, epithelial cell regulation, physiology, pharmacogenetics, molecular and cellular neurobiology, clinical trials and patient-oriented

TABLE 5-2 Research Areas of Research Career Development Awardees, Fiscal Year 2002[a]

| Research Area | Total |
|---|---|
| Microbiology and microbial pathogenesis | 6 |
| Immunology and immunotherapy | 4 |
| AIDS | 2 |
| Biotechnology and biomaterials | 4 |
| Developmental biology and mammalian genetics | 17 |
| Epithelial cell regulation and transformation | 7 |
| Physiology, pharmacogenetics, and injury | 6 |
| Molecular and cellular neurobiology | 2 |
| Clinical trials and patient-oriented research | 14 |
| Behavioral research | 3 |
| Population sciences | 4 |
| Health disparities | 1 |
| Total | 70 |

[a]Research areas defined by primary NIDCR project code are self-reported; programs have more than one research area.

SOURCE: NIH/NIDCR tabulation.

research, behavioral research, and population sciences. Dental researchers being trained in any of these NIDCR-funded research training programs could be co-funded or co-supported by other research training funds that are similarly targeted toward these research disciplines.

An NIH policy could facilitate and encourage co-funding of research trainees. Also, a barrier that needs lifting is the tendency to discourage dentist scholars from applying for research training funds within these disciplines. If applicants other than physicians are eligible, dentists should also be

TABLE 5-3 Research Areas of Institutional National Research Service Award T32 Programs, Fiscal Year 2002[a]

| Research Area | Total |
|---|---|
| Microbiology and microbial pathogenesis | 14 |
| Immunology and immunotherapy | 14 |
| AIDS | 0 |
| Biotechnology and biomaterials | 9 |
| Developmental biology and mammalian genetics | 7 |
| Epithelial cell regulation and transformation | 6 |
| Physiology, pharmacogenetics, and injury | 6 |
| Molecular and cellular neurobiology | 7 |
| Clinical trials and patient-oriented research | 6 |
| Behavioral research | 2 |
| Population sciences | 7 |
| Health disparities | 0 |
| Total | 78 |

[a]Research areas defined by primary NIDCR project code are self-reported; programs have more than one research area.

SOURCE: NIH/NIDCR tabulation.

eligible, while funds targeted specifically for physician research training would stay limited to physician applicants. With this broadening of the spectrum of research training sources to which dentist-researchers could apply, the opportunity for collaborative funding for research training in fields related to oral health would expand. Sources of research training funds could include various government agencies, foundations, universities, industrial organizations, and foreign governments.

Aside from the funding method used for the DSTP program, there are serious problems with the way NIH programs are now being administered. For example, there is a need for more dental-oriented clinical researchers, especially those involved in translational research; clinical studies, such as Phase II or case-control studies; randomized controlled trials, including hypothesis-driven NIH Phase III type trials and Food and Drug Administration Phase II- and III-type trials; and Phase IV studies of side effects and interactions with co-therapies. Researchers with the ability to participate in all of these types of clinical investigations are needed. Clinical researchers who can participate in high-level development and applications research, such as the engineering of products, also are needed. The K30 institutional grants are designed to do just this. However, most of these applications appear to come from medical schools and nondental institutions, and the emphasis is not on training dental researchers.

Finally, training in interdisciplinary and emerging fields is not now traditionally thought of as being within the dental research training profile. Dental research relies on or crosses other disciplinary areas (see the next section), but little support is given for training in these areas. This problem is partly one at NIH, where the tendency is not to support such training; but the educational institutions are also responsible, since they do not apply for T32 awards in interdisciplinary or emerging fields.

## NATIONAL RESEARCH SERVICE AWARD PROGRAM AND OTHER NATIONAL INSTITUTES OF HEALTH PROGRAMS

In 2002, NIDCR funded 31 new, continuing, or non-competing T32 training grants. These grants supported a total of 81 predoctoral students and 86 postdoctoral appointees. In addition, they provided support for 27 short-term projects under the T35 mechanism. Of the 31 funded T32 awards, 20 provided support for students in Ph.D. programs and the other 11 were for support of the DSTP. The 20 non-DSTPs supported about 50 students at the predoctoral level, and based on the statistics on vacant research positions in dental schools, these programs could eliminate any shortage in a few years. But many of the trainees do not view dental school and dental-oriented research as a career option. In terms of individual fellowship awards, there are 16 F30 awards for support of predoctoral students in dual D.D.S./Ph.D. and D.M.D./Ph.D. programs, one F31 award for predoctoral support in a Ph.D. program, and nine post-doctoral fellowships. While the F30 award is designed to support training in an established dual-degree program for students who intend to be researchers, it is no guarantee that students will not pursue professional careers.

Individuals in the dental community have made extensive use of the K award program, securing 70 awards in 2002. A little over half of these awards were for clinical training through the K02, K08, K23, and K24 mechanisms. There are 30 awards that could be considered transitional training, and 20 are the new K22 awards. This level of participation in the K22 is unusually high, since there were only 93 K22 awards across all NIH institutes. Of all the fields of study the K awards seem to work well for the dental profession, since the mission-oriented research of the profession fits with the rigid structure of these awards.

One program at NIH that has not been widely used by dental professionals is loan repayment. In 2002 only six individuals with a D.D.S. participated in the clinical research loan repayment program, and no one with this degree applied to the program under the health disparity or disadvantaged-background features of the program. Considering the high level of debt that dentists have when they graduate from dental school, it seems this program would be attractive.

Even though many committees and working groups have addressed the issue of clinical research training, there remains a critical shortage of clinical scientists in dentistry, particularly to perform Phase II- and III-type trials. There are a few oral health scientists trained in epidemiology who could carry out these clinical trials, but epidemiology or public health training often does not include the skills needed to conduct clinical trials. The recommendation in the clinical sciences chapter of this report that addresses the need for physician training in this area should apply equally to the training of dental clinicians.

The issue of minority researcher training, and of the training of researchers in general to address the health of minorities, is as important in dentistry as it is in other fields. African Americans, Hispanic Americans, and Native Americans make up only about 10 percent of all students enrolled in dental schools, reflecting a steady 10-year downward trend that could have a major impact on the dental health of minority populations. After a slight increase in enrollment through the mid-1990s, only 810 African Americans, 913 Hispanic Americans, and 99 Native Americans were enrolled in dental schools during the 1999–2000 academic year. Minorities are also underrepresented in private practices, with African Americans making up 2.2 percent of dentists, Hispanic Americans accounting for 2.8 percent, and Native Americans representing 0.2 percent. The second aspect of minority research is the training of investigators who have competence and commitment to investigate health care disparities among populations. A broad array of investigators is needed—people with skills in molecular epidemiology, clinical trials, and field studies and who have knowledge and interest in diseases that occur in populations that suffer from health care disparities.

While many programs exist at NIH to address the shortage of minority researchers, the success of these programs is unclear. And in light of the general shortage of dental school faculty, it is unlikely that any changes will take place without strong programs that are specifically targeted in this area.

## CONCLUSION

The need for augmented research in oral health clearly exists. However, equally clear is the shortage of faculty to carry out the training and act in the interest of dental trainees in research. For this situation to improve, dental schools must place a higher priority on research and ensure that exposure to research is part of the curriculum. Unfortunately, recommendations in this regard are beyond the scope of this committee. However, some positive steps can be taken in existing programs to provide incentives to prospective trainees.

## RECOMMENDATIONS

**Recommendation 5-1: This committee recommends that NIDCR fund all required years of the D.D.S./Ph.D. program.**

The current program is not sufficient to attract high-quality students. As with the highly successful MSTP, full support must be provided as an incentive for students to enter research. The partial support currently provided is not a good test as to whether a D.D.S./Ph.D. program is viable. The program should be closely monitored to assess the quality of applicants, the training of applicants, and the research success of applicants.

**Recommendation 5-2: This committee recommends that the NIDCR loan forgiveness program require documentation of time spent in research and scholarly success.**

Loan forgiveness should not be viewed as a means of providing general support for dental faculty but should instead be regarded as a means of promoting high-quality research in dentistry. Faculty members who receive loan forgiveness should provide evidence they have performed productive research, as judged by grant support and publications.

**Recommendation 5-3: This committee recommends that NIDCR should design and implement programs intended to increase the number and quality of dental school applicants who are committed to careers in oral health research.**

The creation of a cadre of high-quality oral health researchers has been severely hampered by the culture in dental schools, where the clinical faculty are often drawn from private practice and students enter with the intention of pursuing such careers. Dental schools associated with research universities can draw on colleagues in the basic sciences to supervise doctoral training for D.D.S./Ph.D. trainees, but D.D.S./Ph.D. programs in those schools will have trouble finding qualified applicants until a more suitable cadre of research-oriented students are attracted to dental schools. Innovative programs will likely involve the promotion of D.D.S./Ph.D. programs to undergraduates considering biomedical research careers. The dental school research culture will evolve slowly, but a necessary step toward the resolution of current problems may be the creation of well-trained D.D.S./Ph.D. graduates who can assume faculty positions and serve as role models in the future.

# 6

# Nursing Research

Research training in nursing prepares investigators who are a part of the larger health sciences workforce. Study questions are raised from the nursing perspective but contribute to knowledge in general. For scientists in the discipline of nursing, the ultimate intent of the knowledge generated through research is to provide information for guiding nursing practice; assessing the health care environment, enhancing patient, family, and community outcomes; and shaping health policy.

The science of nursing is characterized by three themes of inquiry that relate to the function of intact humans: (1) principles and laws that govern life processes, well-being, and optimum function during illness and health; (2) patterns of human behavior in interaction with the environment in critical life situations; and (3) processes by which positive changes in health status are affected.[1] Thus, within the health sciences, nursing studies integrate biobehavioral responses of humans. The science of nursing can also be classified as translational research because it advances clinical knowledge and has the directional aims of improved health care and human health status.[2] As stated in a classic policy paper, research for nursing focuses on ameliorating the consequences of disease, managing the symptoms of illnesses and treatments of disease, facilitating individuals and families coping or adapting to their disease, and dealing in large part with promoting healthy lifestyles for individuals of all ages and under different backgrounds and disease conditions.[3] In addition, nursing research focuses on enhancing or redesigning the environment in which health care occurs in terms of the factors that influence patient, family, and community outcomes.

Focusing on ameliorating the consequences of illnesses or their treatment is the intent of many research programs conducted in nursing. For example, a new protocol for en-

dotracheal suctioning has been tested and implemented in a number of hospital critical care units. Endotracheal suctioning is a frequently performed procedure that can have serious consequences if not done correctly. Another example in the area of symptom management is understanding the factors that influence common problems such as pain. In one study that focused on developing a longer-acting pain medication, investigators found that gender is a major factor in whether drugs are effective, with women responding well to seldom-used kappa-opioid drugs while men have little benefit from such drugs.

Another major area for research in nursing is facilitating individuals and families as they cope or adapt to long-term chronic disease. An excellent example of this area of study is a self-help program developed for Spanish-speaking people with arthritis. For many years, Hispanics with arthritis did not have many educational resources for how to cope with or adapt to their illness. Two investigators at Stanford University's medical center have now developed and tested for effectiveness a self-management program with accompanying exercise and relaxation tapes. This self-help program is being considered for nationwide dissemination by the National Arthritis Foundation.

Research in nursing also has a strong focus on health promotion and risk reduction. The intent is to promote healthy lifestyles for individuals of all ages and backgrounds and with various disease conditions. One example is a school-based program now adapted by most North Carolina schools that is a tested health promotion program in exercise and diet for young children at risk for cardiovascular disease. The research results from this school-based intervention program are impressive; the young people's total cholesterol levels and measurements of body fat were significantly reduced following the education and exercise interventions, and their fitness levels, physical activity, and knowledge about cardiovascular disease risk factors improved.[4]

[1]Donaldson, S. K. and D. M. Crowley. 1978.
[2]Sung, N. S., et al. 2003.
[3]American Nurses Association. 1985.

[4]National Institute for Nursing Research. 2003.

Together, influencing, redesigning, and shaping the environment for patients, families, and communities is another major area of study in nursing. For example, over 80 studies have shown the influence of nursing surveillance and presence on positive patient outcomes.[5] The shortage of nurses, a critical factor, in a health care environment has been demonstrated to increase patient mortality and morbidity.[6] Other studies show the benefit of home visits by nurses in improving the health and quality of life of low-income mothers and children.[7]

Research in nursing is often referred to as "nursing science" or "nursing research," which has led some to confuse it with the nursing profession. This terminology exists at the National Institutes of Health (NIH) in the name of the National Institute for Nursing Research (NINR); however, the funding from NINR supports scientific research relevant to the science of nursing, and the investigators may be nurses or nonnurses. Nursing science is a knowledge structure that is separate from the profession and clinical practice of nursing.[8] Furthermore, the term "nurse-scientist" is not reserved for graduates of Ph.D. programs in nursing; it refers to any scientist conducting research in the disciplinary field of nursing. For example, highly trained nurses under the supervision of a principal investigator could conduct the bulk of the work in a clinical trial.

Research training for nurses, as for other biomedical and behavioral researchers, needs to occur within strong research-intensive universities and schools of nursing. Important characteristics of these training environments include an interdisciplinary cadre of researchers and a strong group of nursing research colleagues who are senior scientists in the sense of consistent extramural review and funding of their investigative programs and obvious productivity in terms of publications and presentations. These elements are essential to the environment required for excellence in research training.

The NINR has traditionally placed a greater emphasis on research training in relationship to the relative size of the institute's budget than is evident with NIH in general. This is due to the current stage of development of nursing research and the need for greater numbers both as investigators and academic faculty. At least 8 percent of NINR funds go to research training, which is roughly twice the percentage invested by other institutes.[9] This commitment has been consistent for a number of years. This committee's Nursing Research Panel members commend the wisdom of this tradition and encourage its continuation.

This chapter focuses on the following two areas that are of major concern to the discipline: (1) changing the career trajectory of research training for nurse-scientists to include earlier and more rapid progression through the educational programs to and through doctoral and postdoctoral study as well as increasing the number of individuals seeking doctoral education and faculty roles, and (2) enhancing postdoctoral and career development opportunities in creative ways.

## CHANGING THE CAREER TRAJECTORY FOR NURSE-SCIENTISTS

The following three major factors motivate the critical need to change the career trajectory for nurse-researchers: (1) enhancing the productivity of nurse-researchers to build strong, sustained research programs generating knowledge for nursing and health practice as well as shaping health policy; (2) responding to the shortage of nursing faculty and the advancing age of current nurse-investigators, and (3) emphasizing the need for strong research training of nurse-investigators in research-extensive and research-intensive universities with equally strong interdisciplinary research opportunities.

## ENHANCING SUSTAINED PRODUCTIVITY FOR NURSE-SCIENTISTS

Nurse-scientists play a critical role in the conduct of research and the generation of new knowledge that can serve as the evidence base for practice and improvement of patient health outcomes. However, nurses delay entering Ph.D. programs. There is particular concern because of inherent limitations in the number of years of potential scientific productivity. Starting assistant professors in other scientific fields typically have a research career trajectory of 30 to 40 years in duration. The average age of an assistant professor in nursing is 50.2 years. Hinshaw reasons that for a faculty member who enters the nursing academic workforce at the age of 50 and retires at 65, this productive period will be only 15 years for developing research programs and contributing to science for nursing and health practice in general.[10] Thus, nurse-investigators tend to have a short career span. This limitation severely constrains the growth of nursing research and thus knowledge for nursing practice.

The median time elapsed between entry into a master's program to completion of a doctorate in nursing is approximately 15.9 years compared to 8.5 years in other disciplines.[11] In addition to having a long period of graduate training, the time has increased by 3 years since 1990, and there are no signs of the trend being reversed. Because there are many factors that reinforce the late entry of nurses into Ph.D. programs, there is a need to create incentives to change the career path. The challenge of promoting earlier entry into

[5]Ibid.

[6]Aiken, L. H., et al. 2002.

[7]National Institute of Nursing Research. 2003. op. cit.

[8]Donaldson and Crowley. 1978. op. cit.

[9]Grady, P. A. 2003.

[10]Hinshaw, A. S. 2001.

[11]National Opinion Research Center. 2001.

science careers was discussed by this panel. Of several proposals considered, there was strong support for one that would encourage and support education trajectories with fewer interruptions. To facilitate this, there needs to be greater awareness of nursing as a scientific discipline. Once students enter undergraduate programs in nursing, those students with interests in science should be identified early and encouraged to consider doctoral education. Exposure to nurse-scientists during the undergraduate program would also entice students to consider research as a primary focus in nursing. A few programs of this type exist, such as the Early-Entry Option in the school of nursing at the University of Wisconsin, Madison. In this program highly talented undergraduates are moved directly into the Ph.D. program.

A "fast tracking" of undergraduates into doctoral programs also necessitates dispelling myths related to the need for clinical practice prior to graduate school entry. There is a need to evaluate the requirement of the master's degree for individuals interested in an academic career with an emphasis on research. The lengthening of most master's programs due to certification requirements for advanced-practice roles has resulted in two plus years for master's program completion, which further delays entry into doctoral education.

In addition, the average number of years registered in a doctoral program is longer for nursing than for other fields. On average, it takes 8.3 years for nursing Ph.D. students to complete their degrees compared to 6.8 years for all research program doctoral students.[12] This is due in part to the fact that the majority of doctoral nursing students are part-time students. As of 2002, there were 81 research-focused doctoral programs in nursing with a total of 3,168 enrollees; 55 percent of enrollees were part-time students. This accounts for the low percentage of graduates; 12.8 percent of enrollees graduate each year.[13]

Nursing developed both its Ph.D. and its D.N.Sc.[14] programs to build on the master's degree in nursing as well as to accommodate breaks between degrees for clinical practice. Early reliance on the master's degree is understandable in that it was nursing's highest degree for many years before the establishment of a significant number of research doctoral programs. As doctoral programs were developed, they built on the master's content, which at the time was predominantly research and theory focused. Over time the master's programs have changed to become primarily preparation for advanced clinical practice, yet nursing continues to require the master's degree for entry into doctoral study in most programs. Currently, very few doctoral programs in nursing admit baccalaureate graduates directly into the program, and for those that do, the master's degree is usually required as a progression step. This requirement for entry into the Ph.D. program makes the group of advanced nurse-practitioners, rather than baccalaureate students, the major pool from which applicants are recruited into research. This is problematic in that this practitioner pool has the same demographic characteristics as the profession and thus is older in average age and more limited in diversity compared to applicants for science Ph.D. programs in general. Incorporation of the clinical/professional content from the master's degree as foundational to the Ph.D. in nursing also encourages faculty to recruit and teach only nurses. Currently there are only a few doctorate programs in nursing that admit nonnurses.

Even though there are other fields that require a master's degree as a requirement for earning the professional research doctorate, such as the M.P.H. for the Dr.P.H., the master's degree has a completely different meaning relative to the science Ph.D. degree. The master's degree is usually awarded as a "consolation prize" for students who are unable to complete the requirements for the science Ph.D. By making the master's degree a requirement for its Ph.D. program, nursing has created confusion as to the meaning of the degree outside the nursing profession.

In considering strategies for increasing the number and length of productive research years for scientists in nursing, it is important to distinguish between the educational needs and goals of nursing as a practice profession that requires practitioners with clinical expertise from nursing as an academic discipline and science that requires independent researchers and scientists to build the body of knowledge.[15] To improve the productivity and research focus of the Ph.D. in nursing, doctoral programs need to be reengineered to admit directly from baccalaureate programs, to admit nonnurses, to decrease the number of years from high school to Ph.D. graduation, and to expand the interdisciplinary scope of the program and the research. The need for doctorally prepared practitioners and clinical faculty would be met if nursing could develop a new nonresearch clinical doctorate, similar to the M.D. and Pharm.D. in medicine and pharmacy, respectively. The concept of a nonresearch clinical doctorate in nursing is controversial, but some programs of this type exist.

Nursing should be encouraged to reengineer some of its doctorate programs to exclusively meet the goal of producing scientists and researchers who are the most capable in terms of skills and projected career life, to meet the needs of nursing as a science and for the development of its research-based disciplinary knowledge. Doctorate programs currently require core coursework in theoretical systems, philosophy of science, qualitative and quantitative methods, and statistical/data analysis techniques. What is different from other science degrees is the amount of advanced practice usually required prior to the doctoral program. Some educational

[12]American Association of Colleges of Nursing. 2003b.
[13]American Association of Colleges of Nursing. 2003a.
[14]McEwen, M., and G. Bechtel. 2000.

[15]Donaldson and Crowley. 1973. op. cit.

depth in a clinical area or in practice is important for the study of clinical questions, but how much is the issue.

There is no clear research career trajectory evident among scientists in nursing today. The common thread is that they entered their doctoral programs later than most other scientists and have not benefited from postdoctoral education. This is because most nurses enter doctoral programs following receipt of the clinical master's degree, also often with many years of clinical experience, and their primary socialization has been as practitioners. As such, they bring with them rich experiences that may help shape the focus of their inquiry. However, they also carry with them enormous burdens relating to their readiness for entering rigorous science training, their interest in continuing training following their predoctoral experience, and their long-term capacity for developing a research career. In addition, when nurses complete their doctoral training, most move directly into an academic career. There they frequently encounter settings in which the demands for teaching and lack of pervasive research programs, socialization, and further mentoring make continuing progress as a scientist difficult.

There is evidence to suggest that a successful career in science is the result of a number of key factors across the life span. These factors include inspiration and "connection" to science and the field; involvement in the enterprise of discovery and science; knowledge, skill, and leadership development; opportunities for coaching, role modeling, and mentoring; a scientific community with peer engagement, assessment, support, and critique; an intensive research environment; and adequate support for research in all of its phases. With these factors in mind, each stage of nursing from precollege, undergraduate, predoctoral, and postdoctoral to the career scientist can build strategies to enhance the career path.

The development of future scientists begins very early in the educational experiences of young people. These include education in school but also beyond. This begins with exposing students interested in nursing at the precollege level to both the profession and nursing science. Undergraduate development of scientists moves individuals from a more general interest in and connection to science to actually beginning to embark on a career in science. The context should be designed to support both the acquisition of a solid academic foundation for further study, a clear notion of pathways for becoming a scientist, and educational experiences that move the student into actual conduct of research. Predoctoral training should begin before the doctoral student starts a course of study. The student's program should assure a very strong match between the research interests of the student and the capacity of the program and faculty. Programs should be fundamentally grounded in a commitment to and processes that support the development of scientists. The postdoctoral phase is the point at which one's own science career should begin to take hold and the intrinsic rewards of science and discovery drive the work of the postdoctoral fellow. Ultimately, the career scientist is at the stage of developing and maintaining his/her program of research. For academic scientists this is the point at which mentoree becomes mentor and teacher, based on the program of research. It is also the point at which the scientist should become an active member of the academic community.

## RESPONDING TO THE SHORTAGE OF NURSE-INVESTIGATORS

It has been well established that there is both a current shortage and a projected continued shortage of nursing faculty, especially those who are scientists and researchers. At this time, approximately 50 percent of faculty that teach in nursing baccalaureate programs are doctorally prepared. This represents a marked increase from the late 1970s, when only 15 percent were. This 50 percent level was achieved in 1999 but has not increased since then despite a large increase in the number of doctoral degree programs available to nurses during the same time period (e.g., in 2002 there were 81 research-focused programs). Two factors that likely contribute to this stalemate are (1) the relatively constant number of doctoral degrees earned each year, despite the increase in the number of programs, as shown in Table 6-1, and (2) the older age of graduates, as evidenced by an increase in the average age of assistant professors from 45 to 49.6 years for the period 1996 to 1999. In 2002 the average age of doctorally prepared faculty was 53.3, compared to 50.2 in 1999 and 2000.[16] These statistics suggest that the doctorally prepared faculty is aging, and because the percentage of faculty members with doctorates is not increasing, it does not appear that younger replacements are being put in place. Thus, this older group of doctorally prepared faculty members in nursing is likely to retire from the academic workforce over the next few years, leaving nursing programs with too few faculty members to conduct research and educate the next generation of scientists.

The need to dramatically increase, even double, the number of nurse-scientists is acute, especially at earlier points in their careers. A recent Special Survey of Vacant Faculty Positions conducted by the American Association of Colleges of Nursing indicated that 59.8 percent of the vacancies require an earned doctoral degree.[17] Training opportunities are available, including predoctoral and postdoctoral fellowship programs offered primarily by the NINR. The number of applicants for these awards has remained relatively stable over time, consistent with the flat doctoral graduation rate for nursing. It is important to provide research training incentives that increase the number of nurses selecting a research career and at a much earlier point in their professional development.

---

[16]American Association on Colleges of Nursing. 2004.
[17]Grady. 2003. op. cit.

TABLE 6-1 Nursing Doctorates from U.S. Institutions, 1991–2003

| | 1990 | 1991 | 1992 | 1993 | 1994 | 1995 | 1996 | 1997 | 1998 | 1999 | 2000 | 2001 | 2002 | 2003 |
|---|---|---|---|---|---|---|---|---|---|---|---|---|---|---|
| **Number of doctorates** | 261 | 325 | 338 | 373 | 336 | 354 | 354 | 420 | 399 | 353 | 414 | 363 | 437 | 411 |
| Number of males | 10 | 12 | 12 | 15 | 20 | 14 | 12 | 13 | 17 | 14 | 15 | 24 | 23 | 34 |
| Number of females | 251 | 313 | 326 | 358 | 316 | 340 | 342 | 406 | 380 | 337 | 399 | 335 | 414 | 377 |
| **Minorities** | 9 | 10 | 13 | 23 | 15 | 21 | 19 | 24 | 22 | 29 | 21 | 31 | 30 | 38 |
| **Citizenship** | | | | | | | | | | | | | | |
| U.S. citizen | 244 | 300 | 313 | 344 | 301 | 307 | 307 | 356 | 336 | 296 | 344 | 290 | 350 | 336 |
| Permanent resident | 2 | 3 | 6 | 5 | 5 | 5 | 9 | 11 | 11 | 8 | 9 | 10 | 7 | 7 |
| Temporary resident | 12 | 17 | 9 | 17 | 27 | 36 | 33 | 40 | 33 | 36 | 45 | 48 | 49 | 49 |
| Unknown status | 3 | 5 | 10 | 7 | 3 | 6 | 5 | 13 | 19 | 13 | 16 | 13 | 2 | 19 |
| **Postdoctoral plans** | | | | | | | | | | | | | | |
| Postdoctoral fellow | 18 | 15 | 24 | 20 | 27 | 21 | 15 | 23 | 25 | 18 | 30 | 35 | 45 | 34 |
| Postdoctoral research | 9 | 5 | 4 | 5 | 3 | 4 | 5 | 6 | 7 | 9 | 10 | 12 | 12 | 14 |
| Postdoctoral trainee | 0 | 0 | 1 | 0 | 0 | 1 | 0 | 0 | 0 | 1 | 1 | 0 | 2 | 3 |
| Other study | 2 | 3 | 5 | 4 | 2 | 3 | 9 | 1 | 3 | 9 | 8 | 6 | 4 | 6 |
| Employment | 209 | 284 | 280 | 323 | 287 | 300 | 298 | 342 | 303 | 285 | 330 | 274 | 314 | 312 |
| Other plans | 5 | 4 | 5 | 5 | 2 | 8 | 9 | 9 | 16 | 7 | 16 | 8 | 14 | 14 |
| Unknown plans | 18 | 14 | 19 | 16 | 15 | 17 | 18 | 39 | 45 | 24 | 19 | 26 | 46 | 28 |

SOURCE: National Science Foundation Survey of Earned Doctorates, 2003.

## EMPHASIZING RESEARCH-INTENSIVE TRAINING ENVIRONMENTS

Strong, research-intensive environments are critical in both the general universities and the schools of nursing for doctoral, postdoctoral, and career development preparation. Such environments provide the experience of being immersed in scientific inquiry with mentors and the intellectual cohort of investigators required for the preparation of nurse-researchers. Research-intensive environments also promote crucial interdisciplinary research opportunities. Nursing research confronts complex questions. Thus it needs to involve multiple perspectives and bodies of interdisciplinary expertise.

To date, scientific training for nurses and others committed to nursing research has utilized a variety of National Research Service Awards (NRSAs) and Career Development K awards. These research training awards are funded by the NINR. The individual predoctoral awards (F31) have been slowly increasing, with very limited numbers of individual postdoctoral awards (F32) evident. The NRSA institutional awards (T32) have grown considerably over time, with 43 such awards made between 1986 and 2002 and 27 operational in 2003. Within the T32s, 65 postdoctoral trainees and 93 predoctoral awards were anticipated for 2003. For the individual NRSA awards there were five postdoctoral awards (F32) and 100 predoctoral awards (F31) for 2003 (see Figure 6-1).

The level of scientific productivity differs among the NRSA mechanisms for the individuals and institutions funded by the NINR. Analysis of the funding record for successfully acquiring either research (R) or career (K) development awards later in the career shows a pattern similar to that of the total NIH research training programs. NINR trainees and fellows funded on individual NRSAs are more apt to successfully acquire R and K awards (see Table 6-2) at a later date.

The difference is sizable, with predoctoral awards being 17 percent of the individual awards (F31) and 5 percent of the T32 predoctoral positions. The pattern is similar with a greater difference for the postdoctoral fellows—38 percent for the F32 and 18 percent of the T32 positions. However, productivity in terms of publications shows the opposite pattern (see Figure 6-2).

The 2 years 1997 and 1999 illustrate a consistent pattern of higher publications for trainees and fellows on the T32 awards. In 1997 and 1999, 158 and 154 publications resulted from trainees and fellows on the institutional T32 awards versus 66 and 23, respectively, for doctoral students holding the individual F awards.

Both institutional and individual research training awards under the NRSA program should continue. The individual awards build strong scientific capability and independence when working with a research-active mentor. With the T32 institutional awards, the cadre of strong senior researchers

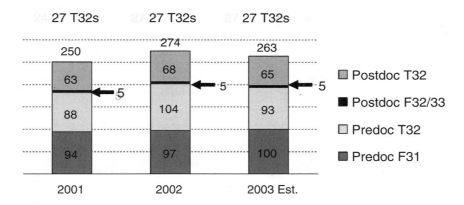

FIGURE 6-1 Training positions at the postdoctoral and predoctoral levels.
SOURCE: National Institute for Nursing Research Budget Office.

TABLE 6-2 Analysis of Pre- and Postdoctoral Fellows with Subsequent Funding

| n | % | |
|---|---|---|
| 116 | 17 | F31 awardees receiving subsequent K or R series funding (N = 696) |
| 23 | 38 | F32 awardees receiving subsequent R series funding (N = 61) |
| 22 | 5 | Predocs on T32s receiving subsequent K or R series funding (N = 439) |
| 44 | 18 | Postdocs on T32s receiving subsequent K or R series funding (N = 245) |

SOURCE: NIH IMPACII Database.

forming a scientific community is valuable in terms of mentoring and publications. The individual predoctoral awards (F31) can be used for a variable length of study. The NINR/NIH is encouraged to allocate three to four years per award in order to support full-time, consistent progression for research training.

The lower productivity of trainers and fellows, who have been funded on the institutional NRSAs (T32) and later obtain R01 and K awards, is of concern. The research training offered through T32 mechanisms needs to be strengthened in the following manner:

• T32 awards should be placed in research-intensive universities with strong interdisciplinary opportunities and

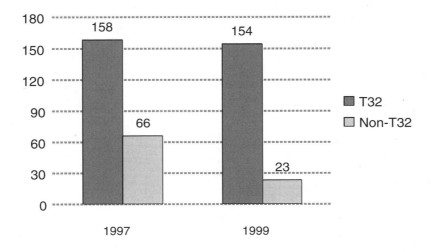

FIGURE 6-2 Publications, T32 versus non-T32.
SOURCE: Outcome analysis by National Institute for Nursing Research at NIH.

research funding, and research interdisciplinary activities should be a critical aspect of the initial NRSA application and annual reports.

• The T32 awards should be allocated only to schools with research-intensive environments, including a cadre of senior investigators with extramurally funded research or research track records and research infrastructures that support research and research training.

• The application process for T32 positions as predoctoral trainees or postdoctoral fellows should be more formalized, with specific proposals submitted in relationship to their research and the match with faculty at the institution made explicit.

• Trainees and fellows on a T32 award position should provide evidence of the interdisciplinary strength that is part of their program of study.

• Criteria for selection of T32 fellows and trainees should be based on a consistent, full-time plan for research training and long-term potential for contribution to science and nursing.

• The monitoring and tracking of trainees and fellows should be formalized, with changes in research plans or mentor(s) filed as part of the annual report.

A small but growing cadre of nurse-investigators is supported in their research development by K awards. In addition to the awards from NINR, other institutes and centers also support nursing research through the K mechanisms, since elements of nursing research are intrinsic to other fields. These awards are usually awarded to nurse-scientists in their early or midcareer stages when they are shifting the substantive or methodological focus of their research. NINR has primarily used the following four types of career awards: K01, Mentored Research Scientist Development Award; Minority K01, Mentored Research Scientist Development Award for Minority Investigators; K22, Career Transition Award, and K23, Mentored Patient-Oriented Research Career Development Award; and K24, Mid-Career Investigator Award in Patient-Oriented Research.[18]

These awards could be important in advancing both career development and science development. Unfortunately, there is limited information regarding the outcomes of these awards, including successful research grants and publications by awardees.

## CONCLUSION

In summary, three major factors influence the recommendation to change the research training career trajectory pattern for nurse-scientists: the need to enhance the productivity of each investigator's study for nursing practice and for shaping health policy; increasing the numbers of nurse-investigators to respond to the investigator and faculty shortage; and emphasizing the need for research training within strong research-intensive environments.

## RECOMMENDATION

**Recommendation 6-1: The committee recommends that a new T32 program be established that focuses on rapid progression into research careers. Criteria might include predoctoral trainees who are within 8 years of high school graduation, not requiring a master's degree before commencing with a Ph.D., and postdoctoral trainees who are within 2 years of their Ph.D.**

This new program would produce strong research personnel and lengthen the research careers of the trainees. These grants should be placed in research-intensive universities with strong interdisciplinary opportunities and research funding, including a cadre of well-established senior investigators.

---

[18]See Appendix B for a complete explanation of awards.

# 7

# Health Services Research

Health services research provides the information needed to understand the strengths and weaknesses of our health care delivery system.[1] Health services research has documented inadequate access to health care for uninsured, rural, and inner-city populations; failures of patient safety practices that kill as many as 98,000 Americans in hospitals each year;[2] and poor-quality care for chronic diseases.[3] Health services researchers have studied factors contributing to rising health care costs and clarified the contribution of new technologies and lack of incentives for efficiency.[4] In general, the goal of health services research is to contribute to the health and well-being of individuals and populations. This requires health services researchers to go beyond disease outcomes and examine health status and health-related quality-of-life outcomes, as well as focus attention on prevention and health promotion services.

The contributions of health services research to policy, management, and clinical care have been diverse. Planners and policy makers, for example, look for ways to generalize findings from efficacy studies: persons recruited to randomized control trials testing new treatments typically are not representative of the larger population expected to benefit from the treatment. Thus, it is up to health services research to fill this information gap by assessing the impact of diagnostic and treatment technologies on patient outcomes and costs across practice settings and populations.

Health service interventions are inherently complex and usually involve multiple system levels, including patients, providers, health care organizations, financing, and community context (e.g., health resources, population sociodemographic and risk factors). The design, conduct, and analysis of complex interventions require the input of many disciplines, as well as advances in multilevel longitudinal statistical methods. The Agency for Healthcare Research and Quality together with the National Institutes of Health (NIH) and the Centers for Disease Control and Prevention (CDC) recently convened a conference on "Research Designs for Complex, Multi-level Health Interventions and Programs"[5] to explore the design, implementation, and analysis of complex service interventions.

Translational research recently emerged as another important dimension of health services research design and analysis. Americans receive treatments consistent with the best scientific evidence only half of the time, which has raised questions as to what should be done to accelerate the adoption of "best practices."[6] This is a small but growing area of health services research and is likely to become a much larger and more important area in the future. Meeting the challenge of translational research can be expected to require additional disciplinary breadth, drawing on areas of marketing research, adult learning, and real-time decision support technologies.

Central to advances in any scientific field are measurement tools, and for health services research measurement tools span payment and financing, appropriateness of utilization, quality of care, and patient outcomes of care. In the past these tools have provided measurement systems to support financing innovations to increase hospital efficiency and to adjust capitation payments and in the future research will need to extend payment methodologies to provide incentives for quality performance, as well as efficiency and equity.

---

[1]Note: Many definitions of this multidisciplinary field are available in the literature, including those developed by previous NRC committees on personnel needs in the biomedical and behavioral sciences. For example, see National Research Council, 1977, 1983, 1989, and 1995. Other authors include the Institute of Medicine, 1995. A recent definition circulated within the community was developed by Kathleen N. Lohr and Donald M. Steinwachs (Lohr and Steinwachs, 2002).

[2]Institute of Medicine. 1999

[3]McGlynn, E. A., et al. 2003.

[4]Although spending more than other nations on health care, the United States has failed to achieve population health indicators equal to countries that spend substantially less (Reinhardt, 2002); furthermore, our quality-of-care indicators are not consistently higher (Hussey et al., 2004).

---

[5]NIH, Bethesda, MD, May 4–5, 2004.
[6]McGlynn. 2003. op. cit.

A goal for health care access is the timely receipt of appropriate care, and criteria for evaluating the appropriateness of service use have been developed and are widely applied for utilization review. With fee-for-service financial incentives and comprehensive insurance coverage having the potential to encourage overuse of services, the measurement of appropriateness has been applied to identify unnecessary admissions and days of inpatient care. In contrast, those without health insurance are likely not to seek needed services or to delay doing so until severely ill, and methods have been applied to assess the consequences of inadequate access to primary care. Future work will need to provide better metrics of timeliness and appropriateness, and from a patient's perspective, measuring appropriateness needs to take into account desired outcomes and social context.

From another perspective, advances in measuring quality of care have provided tools to evaluate the processes of care and patient outcomes. Clinical research provides the foundation for establishing diagnostic and treatment criteria based on scientific evidence. In the absence of strong consistent evidence, clinical expert consensus has been used to set quality standards. One largely unanswered question is whether process standards can be expected to apply to 90 percent of patients, 80 percent, or less. Research is needed to improve our capability to match treatments to patients and minimize the need to try multiple treatments before achieving desired outcomes.

## FEDERAL SUPPORT OF HEALTH SERVICES RESEARCH

In 1968 Congress recognized the emerging role of health services research for improved health care delivery in the United States and created the National Center for Health Services Research and Development (NCHSRD) in the U.S. Department of Health, Education, and Welfare. During those years, NCHSRD sought to develop research on issues of access, cost, and quality and to develop data systems to support research on utilization and cost of care.[7] However, in the years that followed, the budget for NCHSRD declined and the future of the NCHSRD and its funding were uncertain. Private foundations played a critical role in sustaining the health services research field.[8]

In 1989 health services research once again found strong support in Congress, and a new vision for health services research was created in the authorization for the Agency for Health Care Policy and Research. Congress directed the agency, subsequently renamed the Agency for Healthcare Research and Quality (AHRQ), to undertake research on patient outcomes, develop practice guidelines, and disseminate research to change the practice of medicine.[9] The agency placed greater emphasis than previously on the examination of clinical practices, decision making, and comparing the cost effectiveness of alternative approaches to diagnosis and treatment.

While the National Research Service Award (NRSA) program included support for health services research from its inception (see, for example, NRC, 1977), Congress specified in 1989 that one-half of 1 percent of the NRSA budget for training be allocated for training health services researchers through AHRQ, subsequently expanding that allocation to 1 percent of NRSA funding in 1993. By August 2003, AHRQ had provided support for research training through the NRSA program to nearly 800 individuals in the form of predoctoral/postdoctoral traineeships and to another 80 individuals in the form of individual fellowship awards.[10]

It should be noted that in the early 1990s Congress authorized a 15 percent set-aside for NRSA training in service-related research supported by the National Institute of Mental Health (NIMH), the National Institute of Drug Abuse (NIDA), and the National Institute of Alcohol Abuse and Alcoholism (NIAAA) as part of the reorganization of the former Alcohol, Drug Abuse, and Mental Health Administration into the NIH. Nonetheless, AHRQ is seen as the lead agency in the area of health services insofar as NIH funding for health services research focuses on questions related to the delivery of health care related to NIH-specific diseases and disorders.

## CURRENT MARKET FOR HEALTH SERVICES RESEARCHERS

Health services researchers work in a variety of settings, including academic health centers, the policy and planning offices of the federal and many state and local governments, throughout the health care delivery sector, and in the phar-

---

[7]The center initiated large-scale demonstrations, including the Experimental Medical Care Review Organization (EMCRO) to develop tools for quality measurement and their evaluation. The EMCRO demonstrations provided the Medicare program with the methodologies it needed in the Professional Standards Review Organization (PSRO) to evaluate hospital use. The NCHSRD also competitively funded health services research centers in academic institutions and for Kaiser Permanente.

[8]See the NIH/NLM-sponsored database, "HSRProj," for details regarding health services research projects supported by various sectors: *http:// www.nlm.nih.gov/hsrproj*. It should be noted that health services research

in focused areas like mental health services, alcohol and drug abuse treatment services, and veterans' health care continued throughout this time. Health services research funding also comes from the Centers for Medicare and Medicaid Services, the Centers for Disease Control and Prevention, the Department of Defense, and other NIH institutes.

[9]In 2001 the reauthorization of Agency for Health Care Policy and Research led to a name change to the Agency for Healthcare Research and Quality (AHRQ). The word *policy* was dropped from the title and *quality* was added to reinforce the quality-of-care research mission of this agency.

[10]These counts are based on the number of individuals who completed a minimum of 6 months of NRSA training, beginning their training sometime after August 1986 and completing their training by August 2003. P. Flattau, personal communication, September 2004.

maceutical and health insurance industries.[11] Unfortunately, no national statistical system reports on the size and composition of the health services research workforce, since national workforce statistics usually capture information about these scientists in terms of their primary discipline of training or employment and fail to identify the field of scientific inquiry as "health services research."[12] In other words, many scientists who work on health services research problems may do so while conducting research in other areas, such as social, biological, or health research. Furthermore, many health services researchers conduct research as part of their primary employment in nonacademic settings, such as those working in government policy and planning offices or those employed in the pharmaceutical or insurance industries. Therefore, this "part-time" involvement in health services research only further exacerbates efforts to estimate the size and composition of this workforce.

Despite the absence of a national database, a number of studies over the years have yielded important insights into the nature and composition of this group of specialists.[13] For example, the field of health services research draws talent several ways. In the early years of the field's development in the 1960s and 1970s, clinicians and other health scientists simply redirected the focus of their research on the matter of improving health care delivery.[14,15] Today, individuals enrolled in more traditional fields of science and engineering have the opportunity to focus their studies at the doctoral level specifically on problems related to health care services and delivery. They may do so as doctoral candidates in public health or health policy; in the social sciences, including health economics; in other health sciences such as epidemiology or biostatistics; or in health services research itself. Indeed, the NRSA program has made it possible for many individuals interested in receiving formal training in health services research at the predoctoral level to do so.[16]

Postdoctoral research training is another mechanism that has emerged over the past 20 years to foster the growth of a skilled health services research workforce.[17,18] The AHRQ T32 NRSA program has proven to be an especially effective mechanism for attracting clinicians into a health services research career. Of the nearly 200 individuals who received postdoctoral NRSA support through AHRQ between 1986 and 1997, two-thirds had earned a doctorate in one of the clinical professions prior to NRSA training, primarily in internal medicine.[19] Among those individuals holding a research doctorate and pursuing postdoctoral training, half had earned a doctoral degree in the social sciences.[20]

The best data available on the actual size of the health services research workforce comes from the membership roles of the professional organization, AcademyHealth. AcademyHealth draws its members from both health services research and health care policy and includes student memberships. While this database more than likely underestimates the total size of the workforce, it does provide some insights into its composition.

The total AcademyHealth membership in 2004 was 3,745, and 1,688 members (45 percent) reported having a Ph.D., Sc.D., or other doctoral-level training in science. There were another 710 (19 percent) reporting an M.D. and only 15 with a D.D.S. The primary locus of employment for doctoral degree holders who are members of AcademyHealth is the academic sector. Table 7-1 shows the distribution of these individuals across all sectors.

AcademyHealth membership includes roughly equal gender representation, females (51 percent) and males (45 percent), while student membership has greater female representation (64 percent) than male (30 percent). The ethnic mix of members is 13 percent from minority ethnic backgrounds, including Asian/Pacific Islanders (7 percent), African Americans (3 percent), and Hispanics/Latinos (1 percent); 24 percent are "unknown." The remainder (63 percent) are Caucasians. Student membership shows greater diversity—24 percent coming from minority ethnic backgrounds, including 14 percent Asian/Pacific Islanders, 6 percent African Americans, and 2 percent Hispanics/Latinos, plus 54 percent Caucasians and 22 percent unknown.

Table 7-2 shows the primary fields of interest of AcademyHealth members. Most members classify themselves into health services research, and only 15 to 20 percent, depending on their degree, list health policy. The exceptions are those with J.D. degrees, who are strongly oriented toward policy.

---

[11]Based on data collected by the Agency for Healthcare Research and Quality, 2000.

[12]As NIH moves more toward transdisciplinary research, the problem of lacking multiple classifications for both "discipline" and "field of application" may be faced by basic science and clinical researchers, as well as those working in health services research.

[13]Institute of Medicine. 1995.

[14]National Research Council. 1978.

[15]Ebert-Flattau, P. 1981.

[16]An AHRQ-funded review of the curricula vitae (CV) provided by former AHRQ trainees and fellows revealed that 73 percent of the AHRQ T32 predoctoral trainees had earned a doctoral degree by 1998, and the remaining 27 percent was either in training or ABD. Of those who earned a doctorate by 1998, about three-quarters had earned them in a health science field, including health services research, a related multidisciplinary health field such as health policy, health administration, or public health or in one of the other health sciences. Over three-quarters of the T32 predoctoral trainees had earned their baccalaureate degrees in one of the sciences, with 38 percent in the social sciences, 19 percent in the health sciences, and 22 percent in other scientific fields, including the physical and mathematical sciences.

[17]In addition to federal programs of support, private foundations such as the Pew Charitable Trust have played a significant role in promoting training in health policy and health services research. See Institute of Medicine, 1997.

[18]Institute of Medicine. 1997.

[19]Other clinical postdoctoral T32 trainees had specialized in pediatrics (16 percent) or family practice (8 percent).

[20]Ibid.

TABLE 7-1  AcademyHealth Ph.D. and Professional Degree Members' Employment Sector, 2004

| Employer | Total | % | Ph.D. | % | M.D. | % | D.D.S. | % | Pharm.D. | % | J.D. | % |
|---|---|---|---|---|---|---|---|---|---|---|---|---|
| Total | 3,748 | 100 | 1,524 | 100 | 713 | 100 | 15 | 100 | 23 | 100 | 91 | 100 |
| University | 2,023 | 54 | 951 | 62 | 427 | 60 | 14 | 93 | 18 | 78 | 43 | 47 |
| Research/policy center | 444 | 12 | 182 | 12 | 90 | 13 | 0 | *a* | 1 | 4 | 6 | 7 |
| Corporation | 355 | 9 | 92 | 6 | 63 | 9 | 1 | 7 | 3 | 13 | 12 | 13 |
| Government agency | 292 | 8 | 118 | 8 | 54 | 8 | 0 | *a* | 0 | 0 | 6 | 7 |
| Association | 164 | 4 | 41 | 3 | 7 | 1 | 0 | *a* | 0 | 0 | 10 | 11 |
| Consulting firm | 148 | 4 | 44 | 3 | 11 | 2 | 0 | *a* | 0 | 0 | 6 | 7 |
| Foundation | 131 | 3 | 41 | 3 | 15 | 2 | 0 | *a* | 0 | 0 | 3 | 3 |
| International agency | 15 | *a* | 5 | *a* | 4 | 1 | 0 | *a* | 0 | 0 | 0 | 0 |
| Unknown | 176 | 5 | 50 | 3 | 42 | 6 | 0 | *a* | 1 | 4 | 5 | 5 |

*a*Less than 0.5 percent.

SOURCE: AcademyHealth Membership Survey.

The employment opportunities and careers in health services research vary widely. Academic careers may be in schools of medicine, nursing, public health, and other health professional schools, as well as engineering and traditional arts and sciences departments (e.g., sociology, psychology, economics, political science). To effectively manage interdisciplinary research, academic institutions usually have organizational structures such as centers or institutes for health services research. At some institutions there are multiple centers reflecting different areas of specialization and the availability of funding for specialized centers from federal and private sources.

Private-sector health services research careers are available in many areas. Federal contract work evaluating major public policy initiatives is primarily done by private research firms. These organizations include RAND, Mathematica, Abt Associates, Westat, and others. These organizations are organized to do large-scale studies that are not as easily managed in most academic settings.

Other private-sector health services research careers are in research organizations sponsored by health maintenance organizations and health plans, hospital systems, pharmaceutical firms, insurers, and other major stakeholders in health care. Health services research positions may involve directing research, translating research into practice and products, and management evaluation of health care operations.

Associations for professional groups, manufacturers, and advocacy groups recruit people trained in health services research to strengthen their capacity to use information coming from health services research for their members. As efforts to translate science into practice accelerate, the demand for individuals skilled in health services research and communication to users is likely to grow.

Government agencies recruit substantial numbers of health services research professionals to lead and manage research programs, to support policy analysis and development, and to work with managers and providers in the Veterans Administration (VA) and Department of Defense (DOD) health care delivery systems.

New career paths for health services research professionals may emerge as research into effective translation of knowledge into practice grows. For example, the recently passed Medicare prescription drug legislation mandates comparative effectiveness studies of health care services, including prescription drugs, increasing the need for health services researchers trained in pharmaco-economics. The development of tools and techniques to support translation is

TABLE 7-2  Primary Field of AcademyHealth Members by Ph.D. and Professional Degree, 2004

| Primary Field | Total | % | Ph.D. | % | M.D. | % | D.D.S. | % | Pharm.D. | % | J.D. | % |
|---|---|---|---|---|---|---|---|---|---|---|---|---|
| Total | 3,748 | 100 | 1,524 | 100 | 713 | 100 | 15 | 100 | 23 | 100 | 91 | 100 |
| Health services research | 1,457 | 39 | 764 | 50 | 322 | 45 | 6 | 40 | 13 | 57 | 4 | 4 |
| Health policy | 709 | 19 | 177 | 12 | 102 | 14 | 3 | 20 | 2 | 9 | 42 | 46 |
| Both | 1,203 | 32 | 517 | 34 | 202 | 28 | 4 | 27 | 4 | 17 | 27 | 30 |
| Unknown | 376 | 10 | 66 | 4 | 87 | 12 | 2 | 13 | 4 | 17 | 18 | 20 |

SOURCE: Academy Health Membership Survey.

likely to become an industry that will require research skills in the design, evaluation, and testing of new technologies. Translation of knowledge for clinicians may be the initial priority, but priorities will likely expand to include managers, patients, and the public. The demand for well-trained health services researchers is currently strong and likely to continue to expand in the future.

## DEGREE PRODUCTION AND EMPLOYMENT

Ideally, it would be useful to document the flow of individuals into the health services research market. However, graduate programs in health services research are not separately accredited and since the graduates could come from doctoral programs reflecting a wide variety of specialties, there is no accurate tally of doctoral students earning degrees in health services research. In 2004 AcademyHealth published a directory of health services research programs based on "self-identification," which included 81 programs offering master's or doctorate degrees. (Doctoral programs are mainly Ph.D. programs, including both disciplinary [e.g., health economics, medical sociology] and general training in health services research.)

One source of information that reveals the complex educational history of the contemporary health services researcher workforce is an AHRQ-supported study of former NRSA trainees and fellows who received NRSA support from AHRQ between 1986 and 1997 and their employment situation as of December 1998.[21,22] That study showed that these former trainees and fellows actively pursued research careers through a variety of employment paths. Most T32 predoctoral trainees who had completed their doctorates by 1998 did not pursue formal postdoctoral research training. Only 20 of the 102 individuals providing curricula vitae (CVs) reported pursuing postdoctoral research training following receipt of their doctorate. However, a majority (11 of 20, or 55 percent) had NRSA postdoctoral support. Employment information is available for 93 of the 102 individuals having received AHRQ T32 predoctoral support, and just over half (51 percent) accepted a position in an academic setting, another 29 percent took a first job in business/industry, and another 17 percent went to work in government following NRSA training.

Of the 181 individuals who received AHRQ T32 postdoctoral research training support and provided CVs, 62 held research doctorates, and more than three-fourths only re-

ceived AHRQ NRSA training support. By 1998, 58 of the former AHRQ T32 postdoctoral trainees with research doctorates were employed. The vast majority had accepted a first employment position in academia (44 of 58, or 76 percent), and the fraction grew slightly higher when their sector of employment in 1998 was analyzed (46 of 58, or 79 percent). A proportionately larger share of women held academic employment, 30 of 36 (83 percent) in 1998 than men, 16 of 22 (73 percent). On the other hand, of the 181 individuals who received T32 postdoctoral research training through AHRQ between 1986 and 1997 and provided CVs, 119 held clinical doctorates. Of these, two-thirds (78) relied solely on AHRQ for postdoctoral research training support. By 1998, 112 individuals had completed their postdoctoral research training. The first employment positions of these clinicians were chiefly in academia: 95 of 112, or 85 percent. However, it is interesting to note that another 10 percent took a first job in government (12 of 112). In 1998 the fraction working in government settings had grown to 20 percent (22 of 112) as had the fraction in industry/business (21 of 112, or 19 percent). Proportionately fewer individuals reported academic employment in 1998 (86 of 112, or 77 percent). Women holding clinical doctorates and having received AHRQ T32 postdoctoral training support were as likely (31 of 41, or 76 percent) as men (55 of 71, or 77 percent) to be working in academia. For AHRQ F32 fellows, 56 of the 57 trainees had been employed. The vast majority (42 of 56, or 75 percent) were employed in academia in 1998 regardless of degree type: 24 of 30 clinical doctorates (80 percent) and 18 of 26 research doctorates (69 percent).

Over one-third of the T32 predoctoral trainees who were employed in 1998 reported having received grant/contract support (34 of 93, or 37 percent). Most of those with support reported having obtained it from private foundations (18 of 34, or 53 percent), although a number received support from NIH (14), AHRQ (9), or other U.S. Department of Health and Human Services (DHHS) agencies (13).

By contrast, 60 percent of the postdoctoral Ph.D. T32 trainees who were employed by 1998 reported having had research grant/contract support (34 of 58). Besides having received support for research from private foundations (62 percent), some had received support from NIH (15 of 34), AHRQ (4 of 34), or other DHHS agencies (9 of 34). Similarly, 60 percent of the former T32 postdoctoral trainees with clinical doctorates who were employed in 1998 reported having received research grant/contract support (65 of 112). Most received support from private foundations (49 of 65). Other sources of research support included NIH (26 of 65), AHRQ (26 of 65), and/or DHHS (22 of 65). Of the AHRQ NRSA F32 fellows who were employed by 1998, over 70 percent received research grant and contract support (40 of 56). The majority of these grants and contracts were privately funded, as reported by 27 of 40 fellows. Of federal sources, most reported having received support from NIH (19 of 40), AHRQ (12 of 40), and other DHHS agencies (14

---

[21]The AHRQ-funded study involved the collection of CVs from former NRSA trainees and fellows, the extraction of information about their educational and employment histories, and the analysis of career outcomes, including publication patterns. Information was summarized in *The AHRQ Research Training and Career Development Databook: 1986 to 1998,* (Agency for Healthcare Research and Quality, 2001).

[22]*The AHRQ Research Training and Career Development Databook: 1986 to 1998,* 2000. Rockville, MD: Agency for Healthcare Research and Quality.

of 40). In summary, the majority of these former NRSA trainees and fellows were actively engaged in health services research careers.

## OUTLOOK FOR HEALTH SERVICES RESEARCH FUNDING

The broad relevance of health services research has contributed to federal funding through multiple agencies, unlike the funding of most other areas of health research. AHRQ research is expected to address cross-cutting access, quality, and cost issues that are faced by the entire American health care system. Other funding sources seek to fund health services research in support of their organizational missions. The VA and DOD focus on their delivery systems, the Center for Medicare and Medicaid Services (CMS) on financing Medicare and Medicaid, CDC on prevention, and NIH on delivery of services for specific diseases. These funding sources are complemented by private sources, including major foundations (e.g., Robert Wood Johnson Foundation, Commonwealth Fund, MacArthur Foundation, Kellogg Foundation, Kaiser Family Foundation, California Wellness Foundation) and private corporations. The following discussion will be limited to federal funding of health services research.

In 2001 the Coalition for Health Services Research, the advocacy affiliate of AcademyHealth, began an initiative to document health services research funding levels across the federal government. The first report was completed in 2003, and now there are annual updates. The 2004 report found:

> From information provided to us by the following federal agencies, we estimate that $1.5 billion was expended for health services research and related activities by the federal government in Fiscal Year 2003. This total is distributed to the following agencies:
> ○ Agency for Healthcare Research and Quality (AHRQ)
> —$309 million;
> ○ Centers for Disease Control and Prevention (CDC):
> —National Center for Health Statistics (NCHS)
> —$126 million;
> —Extramural Prevention Research Program
> —$14 million;
> ○ Centers for Medicare and Medicaid Services (CMS)
> —$74 million;[23]
> ○ National Institutes of Health (NIH) (All Institutes)
> —$873 million;
> ○ Veterans Health Administration (VHA)
> —$52 million; and
> ○ The Department of Defense (DOD)
> —$15 million.

Given that these agencies do not use a standard definition or uniform categories to report their expenditures, questions

remain about what is included in these totals. From the data reported by AHRQ, CMS and NCHS we know that a total of $191 million was spent to support data systems used in health services and health policy research. We also know that the NIH expenditures include both health services research and dissemination activities.

The health services funding of $1.5 billion when compared to total federal health research funding of $34.3 billion in 2003 shows that approximately 5 percent is being devoted to health services research, based on classifications used in each agency and institute.

AHRQ allocates its funding by major programmatic areas (see Table 7-3, which shows the distribution of funding for fiscal year 2004). The largest categories in the budget are data development and informatics. Informatics is primarily in support of patient safety and the evaluation of electronic health records systems. Adding informatics, quality/safety, pharmaceutical outcomes, and chronic disease management together represents over 45 percent of the research portfolio addressing quality-of-care concerns. Data development funds include the cost of data collection and analysis of the Medical Expenditure Panel Survey, the primary source of data on medical expenditure patterns in the United States. AHRQ's budget covers other major areas of health services research, including prevention, socioeconomics of health care, long-term care, and bioterrorism.

TABLE 7-3 Health Services Research Funding by Major Programmatic Area, Agency for Healthcare Research and Quality, Fiscal Year 2004

| AHRQ Portfolios as a % of the Total Fiscal Year 2004 Budget | |
| --- | --- |
| Budget Line/Portfolio | % of Total Budget |
| Quality/safety of patient care[a] | 10.5 |
| Infomatics[a] | 21.0 |
| Data development[b] | 22.3 |
| Chronic care management | 9.7 |
| Prevention | 9.5 |
| Bioterrorism[c] | 0 |
| Socioeconomics of health care | 12.9 |
| Pharmaceutical outcomes | 4.8 |
| Training | 2.6 |
| Long-term care | 5.6 |
| Organizational support | 0.9 |
| Total | 100 |

[a]There is a significant link between the quality/safety of patient care and the informatics portfolios. This budget is primarily the patient safety earmark.

[b]18.2 percent of the data development portfolio is devoted to the Medical Expenditure Panel Survey.

[c]AHRQ's bioterrorism research is funded through support from the Office of Public Health Emergency Preparedness. This funding is reimbursable and is therefore not part of the agency's appropriated budget.

SOURCE: Agency for Healthcare Research and Quality.

---

[23]Most of the funding in CMS's research budget actually represents congressional earmarks for activities that are only remotely related to CMS's research and demonstration interests.

NIH institutes report funding health services research as shown in Table 7-4. NIMH, NIDA, and the National Cancer Institute have the largest programmatic commitments, ranging from 17 to 23 percent of their budgets. Other institutes report smaller budget commitments to health services research.

Overall, AHRQ provides 20 percent of all health services research funding as reported by federal agencies. Other federal agencies support more focused program-specific and disease-specific health services research. Private funding of health services research is substantial, but no comprehensive source of information is available on nonfederal sources.

## THE NATIONAL RESEARCH SERVICE AWARD PROGRAM IN HEALTH SERVICES RESEARCH: THE AGENCY FOR HEALTHCARE RESEARCH AND QUALITY

The NRSA program provides support for training in health services research. AHRQ receives funding equal to 1 percent of all NRSA funds for NIH. In 2003, AHRQ supplemented NRSA funding with $500,000 to fund a total of 82 predoctoral candidates and 69 postdoctoral fellows, plus six pre- and postdoctoral minority positions. In terms of success rates for training grant applications, the agency in recent years was able to fund only about 55 percent of the requested training positions. This is very similar to the rate for all NIH training awards. In addition, several NIH institutes provide

NRSA awards in health services research, including NIMH, NIAAA, and NIDA and probably others. Overall, the total number of trainees is likely less than 2 percent of all NRSA training positions. No data are available on graduates of doctoral programs who plan to pursue health services research careers and are not funded by NRSA. It would be expected that these numbers far exceed NRSA recipients, as they do in other health research fields.

While there is incomplete information on all individuals with training in health services research and those supported by NIH, since they are part of a larger training activity within several institutes, there is some information on NRSA trainees supported by AHRQ. In particular, the AHRQ-commissioned outcome study cited earlier[24] documented AHRQ-supported 383 predoctoral and postdoctoral trainees through 24 university-based or university-affiliated T32 training sites. Of these, 160 represented T32 predoctoral institutional trainees and another 223 T32 postdoctoral institutional trainees. Another 67 AHRQ F32 individual NRSA fellowships were awarded, for a total of 450 trainees. The majority of AHRQ-supported NRSA trainees and fellows between 1986 and 1997 were female (265 out of 450, or 59 percent), a difference especially evident among T32 predoctoral trainees (115 of 160, or 72 percent) and F32 fellows (41 of 67, or 61 percent). There were slightly more males (114) than females (109) among T32 postdoctoral trainees during this period. No data are currently available on the characteristics of trainees since 1997, but it is known that about 450 have been supported by AHRQ through individual awards and 27 institutional training grants.

Information on the trainees before 1997, which came from this review of current CVs, revealed that 377 (or 84 percent) of the 450 trainees provided their CVs and that 139 had T32 predoctoral support, 181 had T32 postdoctoral support, and 57 had F32 fellowships. By 1998, 102 (or 73 percent) of the AHRQ T32 predoctoral trainees had earned a doctoral degree, and the remaining 37 were still in training. Of those who earned a doctorate by 1998, about three-quarters (74) earned them in a health science field, including health services research (23 of 102, or 23 percent); related multidisciplinary health fields such as health policy, health administration, or public health (30, or 29 percent); or in one of the other health sciences (21, or 21 percent). Over three-quarters of the T32 predoctoral trainees had earned their baccalaureate degrees in one of the sciences, with 38 percent in the social sciences, 19 percent in the health sciences, and 22 percent in other scientific fields, including the physical and mathematical sciences.

At the postdoctoral level, T32 training has proven to be a mechanism that attracts clinicians into a research career. Of the 181 AHRQ postdoctoral trainees providing CVs, two-

TABLE 7-4 NIH 2004 Health Services Research Budget Estimate (Dollars in Thousands)

| Institute | Health Services Research Budget | | |
|---|---|---|---|
| | Total | % of Total Institute Budget | % of NIH's Total |
| National Institute of Mental Health | $208,543 | 15.10 | 23.20 |
| National Institute on Drug Abuse | $153,572 | 15.50 | 17.10 |
| National Cancer Institute | $151,094 | 3.20 | 16.90 |
| National Institute on Aging | $74,800 | 7.30 | 8.40 |
| National Institute of Diabetes and Digestive and Kidney Diseases | $70,936 | 3.90 | 7.90 |
| National Institute on Alcohol Abuse and Alcoholism | $65,000 | 15.20 | 7.30 |
| National Heart, Lung, and Blood Institute | $53,940 | 1.90 | 6.00 |
| National Library of Medicine | $23,606 | 7.60 | 2.60 |
| Other National Institute of Health Services Research | $94,442 | 30.30 | 10.50 |
| Total | $895,933 | | |

SOURCE: Coalition for Health Services Research (2004). *Federal Funding for Health Services Research*, Washington, D.C.

---

[24]AHRQ, 2000. op. cit.

TABLE 7-5  Field of Research Doctorate for Agency for Healthcare Research and Quality T32 Postdoctoral Trainees by Cohort

| Cohort (Start Year) | N | Social Sciences | Health Sciences | Other Research Doctorates |
|---|---|---|---|---|
| 1986–1989 | 11 | 6 | 3 | 2 |
| 1990–1993 | 24 | 13 | 8 | 3 |
| 1994–1997 | 27 | 17 | 8 | 2 |

SOURCE: Tabulation for the Agency for Healthcare Research and Quality.

thirds (119, or 66 percent) had earned a doctorate in one of the clinical professions prior to NRSA training, the majority of which were in internal medicine (62, or 52 percent). Other clinical postdoctoral T32 trainees specialized in pediatrics (16 percent) or family practice (8 percent). Among the 62 research doctorates pursuing postdoctoral research training through AHRQ NRSA T32 awards, half earned a doctoral degree in the social sciences. Furthermore, it appears that AHRQ T32 postdoctoral research training has increasingly attracted individuals from the social sciences since 1986 (see Table 7-5).

The AHRQ NRSA F32 fellowships attracted individuals from both the clinical professions and the sciences into careers in health services research. Nearly half (26, or 46 percent) held a doctorate in a research field such as epidemiology, health policy, sociology, or psychology. The remainder (24, or 42 percent) earned a clinical doctorate in such fields as internal medicine or pediatrics and held both an M.D. and a Ph.D. degree prior to pursuing AHRQ fellowship training (7, or 12 percent). The majority (two-thirds) of individuals holding AHRQ F32 fellowships between 1986 and 1997 worked prior to receiving NRSA support. More than half (55 percent) had been employed in academia prior to F32 training, especially those with research doctorates.

## CONCLUSION

Health services research relies on the knowledge and understanding of a broad spectrum of research fields, and the field is growing as both public and private research funding increase and as the breadth of research expands to include greater emphasis on intervention and translational research. Data show an increasing demand for researchers in this area and the need for increased training to meet the demand, both for students in doctoral programs and health professionals who bring specialized skills to the field. This training should include the knowledge and skills needed to function effectively as a member of an interdisciplinary team, and the NRSA program is the appropriate vehicle for this training.

## RECOMMENDATIONS

**Recommendation 7-1: Health services research training should be expanded and strengthened within each NIH institute and center.**

Biomedical research has created a growing gap between research advances in biomedical science and the ability to apply them effectively to improve the health of the public. Thus, there is a need for more effective health care delivery practices to ensure effective and evidence-based care and to reduce waste and unnecessary risk to patients. These issues are not particular to just a few NIH institutes and centers where training support for health services research is now focused, and the health services research would be better served if training occurred more broadly across NIH.

**Recommendation 7-2: AHRQ training programs should be expanded, commensurate with the growth in total spending on health services research.**

Recognition of the rising costs of care, together with concerns about quality and consistency, has driven increases in health services research. Health services research has established an important evidence base to enable patients and health care organizations to evaluate the benefits and risks of diagnostic and therapeutic intervention and to compare relative values of older and newer approaches as choices proliferate. This field can also evaluate different approaches to health care delivery and financing, which will allow the nation to benefit optimally from the dramatic advances in biomedical science. Training programs should grow proportionately with the need for individuals who have a wide range of disciplinary skills to conduct this research effectively.

# 8

# Emerging Fields and Interdisciplinary Studies

Thus far we have conveniently classified training areas as basic biomedical, behavioral, and clinical. This is obviously an oversimplification. There are many disciplines within each of these areas and significant overlap in and between these three major groupings. In point of fact, some of the most significant research occurs at the interfaces between traditional research areas. This is even more likely to be true in the future because the solution to complex biological and health care problems will require experts and expertise in many different disciplines—and increasingly expertise in more than one field. Consequently, it is important to encourage such research. If this research is to be successful, individuals must be broadly trained so that they can understand and contribute to research that overlaps different fields.[1] In considering these issues, it is important to remember that today's interdisciplinary research often ends up as tomorrow's "traditional" discipline. A few examples are discussed below.

## INTERDISCIPLINARY/MULTIDISCIPLINARY RESEARCH

Enzymology began as a field primarily of interest to biologists who wanted information about metabolic cycles and the proteins catalyzing physiological reactions. However, as soon as relatively pure enzymes were available, organic chemists joined the fun, trying to delineate mechanisms through organic synthesis and physical chemistry principles. They were quickly joined by physical chemists and physicists, bringing in the strength of kinetics, spectroscopy, and structural biology. The advent of cloning and site-specific mutagenesis has sparked further advances in the field. Drug development based on detailed knowledge of enzymology began very early on and continues to be an important area. Enzymology was once considered a demonstration of the strength of interdisciplinary research. However, today single individuals are simultaneously carrying out research in all of the fields mentioned above, and any modern biochemistry/molecular biology department should have all of these skills represented on its faculty.

Who would have guessed that the discovery in 1946 that nuclei can be oriented in a magnetic field would lead to modern nuclear magnetic resonance and magnetic resonance imaging? Yet this fundamental observation by physicists was rapidly developed by physical chemists and biologists into instrumentation that is indispensable for modern research in chemistry, biology, neuroscience, and psychology and that is likewise indispensable for diagnostic work in clinics. Several Nobel prizes have been awarded in this area of research.

Physicians recognized very early that deficiencies in certain substances could lead to severe health problems. Early examples included vitamins and hormones. Physiologists, biochemists, and cell biologists soon found that specific proteins mediated the mechanism of action of these substances, and this led to the field of receptor biology. Physicians, biochemists, cell biologists, and physical scientists have all contributed to the elucidation of receptor biology for such diverse substances as insulin, cholesterol, and adrenaline. Moreover, the medical implications have been very significant.

A more recent example is the sequencing of the human genome. The techniques required for this impressive accomplishment involved the collective efforts of many traditional fields, including physics, chemistry, biology, and computer science. Understanding the health implications of the sequences that have been obtained will be even more difficult and surely will involve areas such as mathematics, computer science, and bioinformatics. The identification of specific genes associated with a specific disease is an obvious health implication of this work.

Cognitive science began as an attempt to broaden the traditional accounts of behavior to account for high-level cognition such as language by reaching out to concepts and ap-

---

[1]National Research Council. 2004a.

proaches from fields such as linguistics and anthropology. Soon cognitive science moved in another direction and attempted to explain behavior with neural networks, reaching out to another emerging field, neuroscience. Among other outcomes, this juxtaposition led to language models couched in neural terms. Neural net models in turn led to general algorithms for machine learning and machine classification, combining the emerging field with newly emerging trends in statistics, computer science, information science, and informatics. Applications of this synergy are now found everywhere in society.

Another good example, overlapping with the previous one, concerns the emerging fields of cognitive neuroscience and behavioral neuroscience, which represent a blend of neuroscience, functional anatomy, psychology, and physiology. These developments occurred hand in hand with the emergence of new brain imaging techniques such as positron emission spectroscopy and functional magnetic resonance imaging. The result has been an enormous growth in the understanding of mental illness and cognitive abnormalities.

When new theory building is pertinent at the intersections among disciplines, coupled with long-term programmatic changes such as those that characterize the linkages between the health and social sciences, some observers have argued for the recognition of a notion called *transdisciplinary research*,[2] contrasting it with interdisciplinary and multidisciplinary research. The notion is to provide a systematic, comprehensive framework for the definition and analysis of social, economic, political, environmental, and institutional factors that influence human health and well-being. The implications are challenging for training a new generation of individuals with a broad, integrative view of the health and social sciences.

Many major health problems faced by society are extremely complex and inherently require research from many areas of science. Examples include obesity, drug abuse, smoking, alcohol abuse, and even violent behavior. In these and other cases, inter-, multi-, and transdisciplinary research is a necessity rather than an option. It is to be noted in this regard that training in the behavioral and social sciences is only one component, but nonetheless an essential component, of the training required to deal with these health issues. At present such training largely resides in the National Institute of Mental Health. This policy places many obstacles in the way of the interdisciplinary research training that the committee regards as an essential part of the research package required for such health problems. Therefore a specific recommendation that much larger efforts be made to integrate research training in the behavioral and social sciences with research training in other fields in all the relevant institutes of the National Institutes of Health (NIH) has been included.

---

[2]Rosenfield, P. L. 1992.

## EMERGING FIELDS

As a result of the advancing edges of research, new fields are constantly emerging. Some come and go, whereas others develop into new, well-recognized entities. Some recent examples, in addition to those previously mentioned, are cited below.

Probably the best-recognized examples are the fields of genomics and proteomics. Both are an outgrowth of the vast number of genome sequences becoming available. Genomics is usually considered the study of DNA itself, whereas proteomics is broadly construed to represent the study of proteins expressed by genes. In both cases, regulation of genetic processes is an important factor. Work in these fields, as noted previously, requires quantitative skills in mathematics and computer sciences, along with a thorough knowledge of the associated biology.

Nanotechnology, including nanomedicine, is a closely coupled wave of the future. Already nanodevices such as DNA/RNA chips have been used to make important advances in basic research and diagnostics.

The study of biological molecules has reached the stage where single molecules can be visualized. The new techniques include fluorescence correlation spectroscopy, single-molecule fluorescence microscopy, and cryo-electron microscopy. Recent advances in nuclear magnetic resonance and X-ray crystallography have bolstered the level of information that can be obtained. This area of research will permit a new level of understanding to be reached with regard to the function and mechanism of action of biological molecules.

Impressive progress has been made in understanding the physiology of organisms by isolating the major components, such as enzymes and nucleic acids. The time is now ripe for the development of systems biology. This requires integration of the entire biological framework of an organism, starting with bacteria and ending with humans. This effort will require broad training in the basic sciences and medicine, from biology to mathematics.

Modern biological research has become nearly impossible without the use of computers. Recognition of this new reality has led in part to the emergence of a burgeoning discipline at the intersection of biology and computer science: *bioinformatics*. Closely related to computational biology, bioinformatics takes a computer science perspective in developing new methods and techniques pertinent to analysis of the vast amounts of data being produced by biology researchers and especially in the fields of genomics and proteomics. Bioinformatics draws heavily on methods developed by the slightly older field of clinical (medical) informatics; however, a new breed of scientist is being produced by academic programs in the evolving field of biomedical informatics (which subsumes both clinical and biological applications of informatics principles and methods).

An interdisciplinary field concerned with decision making has emerged in recent years. It is represented, for example, by the Society for Judgment and Decision Making and a related organization with a health care focus, the Society for Medical Decision Making. Scientists in this developing field come from economics, social psychology, business, law, artificial intelligence, statistics, epidemiology, anthropology, and cognitive psychology and are concerned with all aspects of decision making in the real world, both normative (what decisions are optimal) and actual (what people do). There is often a large gap between the two, and resolving the difference is of vital importance for society and health care.

Another relatively new interdisciplinary field in the social sciences combines political science, sociology, public and environmental affairs, economics, international business investment, and psychology and is concerned with rational decision making and resource management at the level of societies. This field has been supported in part by a variety of recent National Science Foundation initiatives in global change. It includes subfields such as ecological economics, environmental science, urban and rural affairs, international resource management, and much more of a similar nature.

Sometimes an interdisciplinary field is in such early stages that it has no name and there remains uncertainty about whether it will in fact emerge. Yet one cannot withhold support from such fields at early stages because support would arrive too late to do any good during the critical formative stages. One current example is in the intersection of robotics, computational models, machine learning, and developmental psychology and is concerned with behaving organisms and devices learning to operate in a real-world environment.

Currently, U.S. population demography clearly indicates a shift to older people. Hence, the study of aging will be of increasing importance. This includes not only the biology but also the psychology and sociology of life stresses, chronic medical problems, and mental health. This has already been recognized, for example, by the award in 2002 of a $26 million grant to the University of Wisconsin Institute on Aging from the National Institute of Aging. The purpose of the grant is to carry forward a project initiated in 1995 by a multidisciplinary team interested in the behavioral, psychological, and social factors of how people age. The Mind-Body Center, created at the University of Wisconsin in 1999 and funded by the National Institute of Mental Health, investigates the age profiles of physical and mental health in humans and animal models. Integrated study of aging phenomena is an important target for the future.

## TRAINING IMPLICATIONS

Clearly, research in emerging areas and interdisciplinary/multidisciplinary research are important for making major breakthroughs in health-related research. Therefore, it is important that research training be broadly based. This has been well recognized at many universities and funding agencies with the creation of programs bridging multiple departments and institutions. The Burroughs Wellcome Fund, for example, provides specific grants for the purpose of bringing students with backgrounds in the physical, computational or mathematical sciences into research in the biological sciences. Ten such programs have been funded since 1996. The National Research Service Awards (NRSAs) have long promoted broad training. The National Library of Medicine has supported training at the intersection of biomedicine and computer science for over 20 years. Training grants typically span multiple departments. In fact, this is often a requirement for a training grant.

The term "broadly based training" is not to be taken too literally. The fundamental problem with much of present-day training is caused by the increasing depth of understanding of increasingly narrow fields. However, these factors make it difficult to train any scientist truly broadly, other than in a superficial fashion. Thus, a balance should be struck in which sufficient training is provided in a discipline to allow deeper scientific progress in an established field with sufficient breadth in relevant alternative fields to allow new progress outside established boundaries. Given the impossibility of training in every field, means must be found to identify other relevant fields through which a field can be transmuted and enriched and then to encourage sufficient numbers of scientists to achieve sufficient mastery of those fields so identified. The difficulty of this task is easy to underestimate. One solution is to create "bridge" people who have sufficient breadth and understanding of two disciplines that they can help meld and catalyze communication among members of larger teams drawn from the discipline themselves. It should also be recognized that interdisciplinary training is time consuming since there is more to learn on the part of the trainees and a need for greater coordination of the trainees' research projects on the part of the mentors.

A further distinction helps delineate the concept of "broad training." There are some skills that are so fundamental to all scientific fields and to scientific progress that all trainees must learn them; these include mathematics, quantitative approaches, statistics, computation, writing, speaking, and communication. This may seem a tautology, but all of us have seen examples of scientists who have not received reasonable training in one or more of these essential skills, and in fact there are some fields where one or another of these skills is routinely overlooked. The first and foremost recommendation is that policies be implemented that ensure all trainees receive intensive training in such areas, noting the special need for quantitative and computational training, while recognizing that potentially good science too often goes unnoticed if the researchers are unable to describe their work effectively in talks and journal articles.

The second concept of "broad training" is field-specific training that allows new concepts and approaches to develop through synergy with new areas. Examples of such synergy were provided in the introduction to this section. Identifying such areas is an ongoing enterprise that requires creativity and insight, but some general procedures and approaches can help ease the difficulties. Research supervision by mentors from more than one department should be encouraged. Emerging areas need to be quickly recognized and supported, a process that can and should occur within individual funding agencies but also can be furthered by outside groups (such as this committee) instructed to help in this enterprise. Establishing training grants in emerging areas is important, but it is a lengthy process and may be too slow to encourage the appropriate training. Individual awards, however, can respond rapidly to immediate needs, so the committees making such awards should be especially sensitive to the need to provide awards for research training proposals that move beyond traditional field boundaries. Further, the instructions to those applying for such awards should emphasize the importance of this criterion.

## RECOMMENDATIONS

**Recommendation 8-1: The standing committee created to monitor the continuing needs of the biomedical research community should also be charged to provide recommendations to NIH as to the identity of emerging research fields.**

The need to react quickly to recognize important new research developments and to support the training of appropriate personnel is of obvious importance to the health sciences. To track the evolution of existing fields, the changes in relations among existing fields, and the emergence of new fields, both NIH and the standing committee should make use of techniques that analyze electronic databases to map existing scientific structures and their changes over time.

It is extremely difficult for individuals, no matter how knowledgeable, to grasp the structure of science and the way this structure evolves. Fields overlap in confusing ways, and existing mechanisms (funding and otherwise) often are rooted in old scientific divisions and classifications that have

become partly irrelevant and hinder scientific progress. Perceiving the evolving structure of science is critical for NIH to make good decisions. Computational techniques are available now that produce "knowledge maps." These maps can provide important information about the future of research.

**Recommendation 8-2: The NIH should target individual NRSAs in emerging fields, interdisciplinary areas, and specific fields of interest. Such applications should be given priority in the awards process, and special review panels should be used as needed.**

This approach will encourage scientists in the various fields to contribute to the task of identifying new areas. Individual awards can respond most rapidly to new initiatives. In addition they can be easily adjusted as fields mature or evolve in unanticipated directions. Moreover, a small number of awards can be very effective in attracting people to new fields and establishing standards. These awards should be made at both the predoctoral and postdoctoral levels.

The committee recognizes that such efforts are ongoing, but these efforts should be integrated across the institutes, including a formal structure to ensure a long-term vision.

**Recommendation 8-3: Quantitative subject matter should be integrated into and required for training programs in all areas. Quantitative subjects include statistics, mathematics, physics, physical chemistry, computer science, and informatics.**

The need for quantitative training is stressed throughout this report. With the overwhelming amount of new data becoming available, it is essential that scientists understand how to analyze and critically interpret the information. In all areas of biology and medicine, understanding biological processes and health issues on a quantitative basis will be of increasing importance. Although quantitative training is already prescribed in many cases, it is a necessity for all areas of biomedical, behavioral, and clinical research.

# 9

# Career Progression

The continued strength of this nation's health research enterprise will depend on the quality of doctoral programs in U.S. educational institutions, the continuing education and training of researchers after the doctorate, the utilization of an international pool of scientists, and the establishment of a diverse workforce. How careers progress is important in establishing this research enterprise. It depends on the efficient progression of individuals from student to independent researcher, the ability to attract and retain talented foreign-educated scientists, and the engagement of minorities in science at all education levels. The discussion in this chapter concerns research careers in all three major fields: biomedical, clinical, and behavioral/social sciences.

Professional education begins with graduate education, continues and matures with specialized training, and ends when full status as an independent researcher is obtained. It is long and arduous, with graduate school being the place where individuals are initially exposed to research tools and specialized knowledge and are required to carry out an original research project. This is typically followed by a period of postdoctoral training to learn additional skills and develop in-depth knowledge in a particular area. However, this part of the career path is not as well defined as it is for a medical degree with an internship and residency appointments of fixed duration. The career path varies widely across fields. The biomedical sciences often include multiple or extended postdoctoral appointments. The clinical fields, at present, are not usually followed by additional postdoctoral training. The behavioral and social sciences traditionally did not have much postdoctoral training but recently are becoming more like the biomedical sciences. In particular, the increasing interdisciplinary nature of research will require more training. The advancement of science continues to require more knowledge and skills on the part of new entries into the research workforce, and this can be obtained through postdoctoral training. It is, additionally, a time when individuals can refine research interests and begin to establish research careers.

For decades the United States served as the training ground for scientists from all parts of the world. The structure of the research enterprise in educational institutions, government, and industry, on the one hand, has provided foreign-born scientists with an environment that promotes research careers and, on the other hand, has helped meet the increasing demand for highly skilled researchers. In the biomedical and clinical sciences a significant proportion of the doctorates are temporary residents at the time of their degree and many stay in this country for postdoctoral study or permanent employment. There are also a large number of foreign-educated doctorates who come to this country for postdoctoral study and many gain permanent resident status. Of the foreign students who come to the United States for an education, some stay and become part of the workforce, and some return to foreign countries. In either case they are an essential part of the research community in all research fields in the biomedical and behavioral sciences. Changes in immigration policy in this country that make it more difficult for foreign researchers to enter the country, or stay once they have arrived, will increase the attraction of research opportunities in other countries, will reduce the number and quality of researchers in this country, and will almost certainly affect the nation's ability to carry out its research agenda.

In regard to domestic research training, the under-representation of minorities continues to be an issue. In fields that require the most technical and quantitative training, the proportion of underrepresented minorities is vanishingly small.[1] It is well documented that this problem will not be rectified by programs aimed solely at doctoral and postdoctoral training levels. One reason for the low level of participation of minorities is the failure of the education system to provide an adequate background.[2,3] Predicted demo-

---

[1]May, G. S., and D. E. Chubin. 2003.
[2]Babco, E. L. 2003.
[3]May and Chubin. 2003. op. cit.

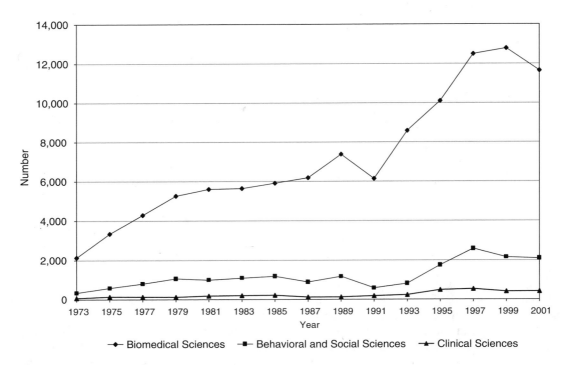

FIGURE 9-1  Postdoctoral appointments in the three broad fields, 1973–2001.
SOURCE: National Science Foundation Survey of Doctorate Recipients.

graphics for the next 20 years warrant a more aggressive approach to providing opportunities for minority students to develop their interests in science research, and it is essential that such programs are aimed at all levels of education. Mentorship and faculty involvement during the graduate years play a significant role in nurturing students to continue their progression.[4] Doctoral and postdoctoral training programs that target minorities are being examined by another National Research Council (NRC) committee to determine their effectiveness on increasing the participation of minorities in research careers.

## POSTDOCTORAL TRAINING

Postdoctoral training is not a new phenomenon in the biomedical sciences, but it has become increasingly important over the past decades. It has grown in importance to the point where about 70 percent of the doctorates in recent years have elected additional training compared to about 50 percent in 1970. Although not as prevalent, the proportion of behavioral and social sciences doctorates in postdoctoral training increased from about 10 percent in 1970 to 30 percent in 2001. In the clinical sciences, postdoctoral training has been between 15 and 20 percent over the recent 30-year period. The lower level of training in the clinical sciences applies

only to Ph.D.s since there are other mechanisms by which M.D.s receive research training. While some M.D.s enter the traditional postdoctoral appointment, many are trained instead on career development awards, which will be discussed in the next section. Figure 9-1 compares the number of postdoctoral trainees in the three broad fields and shows the differences in the level of postdoctoral training.

While postdoctoral training is traditionally defined as a period during which researchers increase knowledge and sharpen research skills, it is also the case that it is a period of employment. For those supported by principal investigators' (PIs) research grants, employment generally is in a laboratory in which the director sets the work agenda, and the postdoctorate trainee's work is dedicated to that grant. In such cases, scientific and professional mentoring of the postdoctoral trainees is thoroughly mixed with the grant goals and, as a result, may be an implicit but marginal component of the director's responsibilities.[5] Institutions do not keep track of the positions for postdoctorates paid out of research grants and hired into laboratories and typically do not even know how many people are on postdoctoral appointments. As a result, postdoctorate trainees may not be included in the support structure that includes health and other insurance benefits available to students and university personnel. These conditions have prompted the formation of

---

[4]Tsapogas, J. 2001.

[5]National Research Council. 2000b.

organizations within institutions to serve as postdoctoral trainee representatives. These local-level organizations spawned the National Postdoctoral Association (NPA) in order to draw attention to their concerns.[6] Consequently, some institutions have started to become responsive by establishing offices to oversee postdoctoral appointments and by setting policies to address working condition issues.

In a 2000 report the National Academies recommended increasing stipend levels for predoctoral and postdoctoral trainees on the National Service Research Award (NRSA) program.[7] The National Institutes of Health (NIH) responded to this recommendation by setting $45,000 as a target stipend level for first-year postdoctoral appointments, with plans to reach that level through annual increments of 10 to 12 percent over the next few years and to maintain the salary level with cost-of-living increases thereafter. Table 9-1 shows the stipend levels in 2003, which reflect a 10 percent increase over 2002 and a 12 percent increase from 2001 to 2002. While these salary levels apply only to the NRSA, they form a guideline for individuals supported by other mechanisms, including research grants. However, PIs of large research programs have often found it difficult to follow these guidelines because their research grants (which are typically multiyear with budgets that are set years earlier) do not have sufficient funds for both this purpose and the goal of carrying out the research mission of the project. Aside from the increased compensation in the form of salaries for NRSA recipients, they are disadvantaged by the fact that they are not considered employees at many institutions and therefore are not eligible for standard benefits. This is an issue of growing concern as tenure in these positions has lengthened, and NIH is urged to correct the situation, as previously suggested in other reports.[8]

Compensation is not the only issue of concern to postdoctoral trainees. Even with the formation of local postdoctoral organizations, postdoctoral offices in institutions, and the NPA, the environment in the laboratory poses challenges. Postdoctoral trainees supported on research grants are often seen less as trainees and more as employees of the PI. The nation's grant structure, therefore, tends to pose obstacles to generalized postdoctoral training, as opposed to training specifically related to the goals of a given grant project. In large laboratories with many postdoctoral trainees, there is seldom an opportunity for generalized training, and real mentoring by the PI is too often missing. Too many trainees end up with long tenures in these types of laboratory positions with little opportunity to establish their own research agendas.

These concerns about the nature of postdoctoral training should not be taken as an argument against the need for large

TABLE 9-1 Postdoctoral Stipends for the NRSA Program

| Years of Experience | 1999 | 2000 | 2001 | 2002 | 2003 |
|---|---|---|---|---|---|
| 0 | $26,256 | $26,916 | $28,260 | $31,092 | $34,200 |
| 1 | $27,720 | $28,416 | $29,832 | $32,820 | $36,108 |
| 2 | $32,700 | $33,516 | $35,196 | $38,712 | $40,920 |
| 3 | $34,368 | $35,232 | $36,996 | $40,692 | $42,648 |
| 4 | $36,036 | $36,936 | $38,772 | $42,648 | $44,364 |
| 5 | $37,680 | $38,628 | $40,560 | $44,616 | $46,404 |
| 6 | $39,348 | $40,332 | $42,348 | $46,584 | $48,444 |
| 7 or more | $41,268 | $42,300 | $44,412 | $48,852 | $50,808 |

SOURCE: NIH program announcements.

numbers of postdoctoral positions to facilitate the research needs of the country. In addition, we should not view postdoctoral positions as "waiting stations" for Ph.D.s unable to obtain faculty positions or other forms of employment.[9] Not only are years of postdoctoral training often required to obtain the knowledge and skills need for modern-day science, such positions are increasingly valued for the opportunity they afford new researchers to establish a record of publications and scientific output. Thus, at present, postdoctoral positions are populated by a mixture of doctoral recipients waiting for a suitable faculty or other position to come available and doctoral recipients choosing to extend their prejob period for the purposes of training and producing a record of scientific accomplishment.

The fact that the expected boom in the biotech industry in the 1990s did not fully materialize is a key factor underlying the increase in the number of biomedical postdoctorates in the 1980s and 1990s (see Figure 2-4 in Chapter 2). However, Ph.D. production began leveling off in the late 1990s, when there was a decline in the number of doctorates planning postdoctoral study, and growth in postdoctoral positions slowed from 1997 to 1999. In 2001 there was a decline in all employment sectors, which may have been due, in part, to increasing employment opportunities at higher pay outside academia and to a better understanding of postdoctoral working conditions.

Figure 9-2 shows trends over time in the length of postdoctoral training by giving the percentage of doctorates in the biomedical sciences from a two-year post-Ph.D. cohort still in postdoctoral positions.[10] For example, 54 percent of

---

[6]National Postdoctoral Association Web site. Available at *http://www.nationalpostdoc.org/about/*. Accessed on 10/22/2004.

[7]National Research Council. 2000a.

[8]FASEB News June 3, 2004.

[9]Regets, M. C. 1998.

[10]This analysis uses the Survey of Doctorate Recipients and groups doctorates into two-year Ph.D. cohorts, since the survey is conducted every two years. The proportion of doctorates in a postdoctoral position for the one- to two-year cohort is about 50 percent and is less than the 70 percent seen in Appendix Table E-1 for two reasons: (1) a doctorate with a definite commitment for a postdoctoral position might not take the position, and (2) a doctorate in a cohort that takes a position for only one year and is more than one year from the time of their doctorate at the time of the survey will not be captured in such a position.

the doctorates who received their degrees in the 1995–1996 academic years were in postdoctoral positions in 1997, and in 1999 about 35 percent of that cohort was still in postdoctoral positions. Figure 9-3 shows a steady increase in the 1980s and 1990s in the percentage of doctorates still in postdoctoral positions several years after receipt of their degrees and a decline in recent years. The decline in 2001 for the 3- to 4-year cohort is partially due to the decline in the 1-

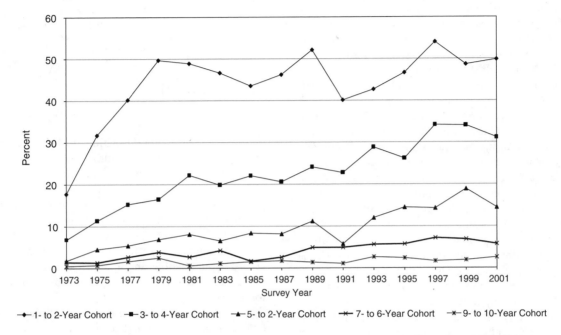

FIGURE 9-2 Proportion of biomedical doctorates in academic postdoctoral positions by Ph.D. cohort year, 1973–2001.
SOURCE: National Science Foundation Survey of Doctorate Recipients.

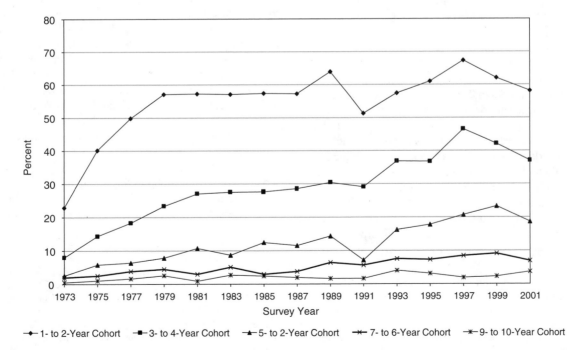

FIGURE 9-3 Proportion of biomedical doctorates with postdoctoral positions in all employment sectors by cohort year, 1973–2001.
SOURCE: National Science Foundation Survey of Doctorate Recipients.

TABLE 9-2 Sector or Type of Employment for Doctorates in Postdoctoral Positions 2 Years Earlier

| Status in Year | Tenure or Tenure Track Faculty (%) | Non-Tenure Track Faculty (%) | Non-Faculty Academic Appointment (%) | All Postdoctoral Appointments (%) | All Non-Academic Employment (%) |
|---|---|---|---|---|---|
| 1995 | 11.9 | 6.1 | 16.4 | 49.5 | 16.2 |
| 1997 | 14.0 | 6.3 | 10.1 | 53.6 | 16.0 |
| 1999 | 10.9 | 3.5 | 10.9 | 54.7 | 19.9 |
| 2001 | 10.6 | 7.0 | 12.4 | 47.6 | 22.4 |

SOURCE: National Science Foundation Survey of Doctorate Recipients.

to 2-year cohort in 1999, and there was a definite decline in 2001 for the 5- to 6-year cohort. It is interesting to note that the data do not show the commonly believed situation that there are large numbers of doctorates in postdoctoral positions 7 and 8 years after receiving a degree. If all postdoctoral positions are taken into consideration, the decline in recent years is even more apparent, as shown in Figure 9-3. The economy in 2001 and tighter budgets in the nonacademic sector may have had an effect here as well.

An examination of data for 1995 to 2001 for U.S. doctorates in the biomedical sciences, from the perspective of their career progression, also shows a decline in 2001 in the proportion of postdoctorates continuing their postdoctoral training and an increase in the portion moving into nonacademic employment (see Table 9-2). In 1997, individuals who had been in postdoctoral positions in 1995 went on to nonacademic employment at a rate of 16.0 percent and continued their postdoctoral training at a rate of 53.6 percent. However, the 2001 data for the 1999 postdoctoral appointees show a decline of 6 percent for those continuing postdoctoral training to a rate of 47.6 percent and an increase in nonacademic employment to 22.4 percent. By contrast, the data show a decline in faculty appointments and an increase in nonfaculty academic appointments. The general growth in nonfaculty positions is also seen in the earlier cohort analysis where the five- to six-year post-Ph.D. cohort in these positions increased from 12.4 in 1999 to 17.7 in 2001. The increase in the number of doctorates in nonfaculty positions and the decline in the number of tenure-track faculty positions (see Appendix E) raises the question as to whether bright young talent in the biomedical sciences can find positions where they can develop their own ideas and become independent researchers. While nonacademic employment is a viable career path, individuals trained in the academic environment may see the freedom and security that a tenure-track professorship can bring as a more attractive option, and will hope and wait for a position to come available.

Higher salaries may be an influencing factor in shortening postdoctoral appointments (see Table 9-3). The median salaries for academic postdoctorates are similar to the stipends given by NRSA (Table 9-1). The increased salary levels for NRSA recipients may have carried over to post-

doctoral appointments on research grants and reduced the number of individuals who could be supported.

The situation in the behavioral and clinical sciences is less clear, since fewer doctorates are in postdoctoral positions and the proportion of doctorates in later cohorts has fluctuated over time. A downward trend in the proportion of doctorates in the later cohorts from 1999 to 2001 may be similar to the stronger pattern found in the biomedical sciences.

## TRANSITION AND CAREER DEVELOPMENT

An important step in career progression is the transition from postdoctorate status to independent researcher. The dilemma in the biomedical sciences, described in the preceding section, is a problem that developed along with the advances made in biomedical research. The increase in funding created a need for personnel to carry out the research and led to increases in graduate enrollments and Ph.D. production. At the same time, there was essentially zero faculty growth in educational institutions combined with many senior faculty members continuing in their roles beyond the traditional retirement age. Both factors contributed to an increase in the postdoctoral pool. Although a larger pool is not by itself a cause for concern, it is a problem that too many postdoctoral appointees receive little help or guidance in making the dif-

TABLE 9-3 Median Salaries for Academic Postdoctorates in the Biomedical Sciences by Cohort Years from Doctorate

| Survey Year | 1- to 2-Year Cohort | 3- to 4-Year Cohort | 5- to 6-Year Cohort | 7- to 8-Year Cohort |
|---|---|---|---|---|
| 1993 | $22,500 | $25,600 | $27,000 | $30,000 |
| 1995 | $25,000 | $28,000 | $30,000 | $30,800 |
| 1997 | $25,600 | $29,000 | $30,000 | $31,650 |
| 1999 | $27,000 | $30,000 | $31,000 | $35,000 |
| 2001 | $30,000 | $35,000 | $37,000 | $40,000 |

SOURCE: National Science Foundation Survey of Doctorate Recipients.

ficult transition out of this pool.[11] This leads to the concern that institutions (and in some cases federal granting agencies) do not typically allow postdoctoral trainees to apply for grant support as individual researchers. Consequently, key productive research years are spent working on someone else's project. Under these conditions, the experience that would allow postdoctoral trainees to develop their own research agenda is not provided, nor do they receive the type of generalized training needed to realize an independent research career. These factors highlight the tension between (1) the need for postdoctoral researchers to carry out the research missions of PIs and laboratories and (2) the inadequate work conditions faced by, and the inadequate training received by, postdoctoral researchers. The importance of the first factor should not supersede attention to the problems posed by the second. Future generations should not be discouraged or impeded from becoming productive, independent researchers, and the best-possible training should not be withheld from them.

Another important part of the career progression involves the issue of productivity, for time to degree and the lengthening of postdoctoral appointments affect the productive years of research scientists. NIH has generated data on its Web site (*http://grants1.nih.gov/grants/award/trends/prin inv.htm*) to show the changing age distribution for the principal investigators it supports with R01, R29, and R37 grants. The striking features of these data are the decline in the proportion of awards to individuals under the age of 36 and the increase in awards to the over 55 age group. This shift is in part due to the aging of the biomedical workforce. For example, the percentage of awards to the over 55 age group doubled in the period from 1980 to 2001, but that population also doubled (see Table 9-4). In addition, the distribution of awards has changed over the years. In 1980 the proportion of awards to the youngest age cohort (under 36) was consistent with the academic biomedical population at about 26 percent. However, by 2001 about 16 percent of this population was under 36 but received only 5 percent of the research awards; the 36- to 40-year age group received a proportion of the awards that matched their population; the next older cohort (41 to 55), received awards in greater proportion than their population. One reason for this shift is the increase in postdoctoral positions. If the postdoctorates are not included in the under 36 age group, the proportion of the population drops to 7 percent and is more consistent with the 5 percent award level.

By comparison, less complete data are available for the behavioral and clinical sciences. In 1981, 12 percent of the behavioral and 13 percent of the clinical science Ph.D. researchers were over the age of 55, percentages that grew to 29 and 23 percent, respectively, in 2001. In 1981 about 25 percent of the doctorates in these fields were in the under 36

**TABLE 9-4** Comparison of the Population Distribution of Researchers in the Biomedical Sciences and NIH Principal Investigators (Percentage Across Cohorts)

Age Cohorts of Ph.D.s in the Biomedical Sciences in Academic Institutions (Including Postdoctorates)

|      | Under 36 (%) | 36–40 (%) | 41–45 (%) | 46–50 (%) | 51–55 (%) | Over 55 (%) |
|------|------|------|------|------|------|------|
| 1981 | 27 | 25 | 16 | 11 | 11 | 11 |
| 1985 | 21 | 22 | 20 | 12 | 10 | 15 |
| 1991 | 18 | 22 | 19 | 18 | 10 | 13 |
| 1995 | 17 | 19 | 18 | 16 | 14 | 16 |
| 2001 | 16 | 17 | 16 | 15 | 13 | 22 |

Age Cohorts of Principal Investigators for R01, R29, and R37 Research Grants

|      | Under 36 (%) | 36–40 (%) | 41–45 (%) | 46–50 (%) | 51–55 (%) | Over 55 (%) |
|------|------|------|------|------|------|------|
| 1980 | 26 | 29 | 17 | 10 | 8 | 9 |
| 1985 | 20 | 28 | 24 | 13 | 7 | 9 |
| 1990 | 11 | 25 | 23 | 21 | 9 | 10 |
| 1995 | 7 | 18 | 25 | 22 | 16 | 12 |
| 2001 | 5 | 14 | 21 | 22 | 18 | 20 |

SOURCE: National Science Foundation Survey of Doctorate Recipients.

age group, a percentage that fell to 11 percent in the behavioral sciences and 9 percent in the clinical sciences in 2001. Thus, a marked shift in age demographics has occurred in the behavioral and clinical sciences as well.[12]

The declining research support in the early age groups is related to three factors. One is the increased age at which individuals receive their doctorates. Since the early 1980s, age at degree increased by about 1.5 years. This is due to three incremental increases: a small increase of about a quarter of a year for the age at which they enter graduate school, an increase of about 1 year of actual graduate study, and an increase of about one-quarter of a year out of study during a graduate program (see Appendix E). The second factor is the increasing time researchers spend in postdoctoral positions (e.g., as illustrated in Figure 9-2 by the proportion of a Ph.D. cohort in a postdoctoral position for three or more years). There may be signs of a decrease in the length of postdoctoral positions in recent years, but they are still much longer than in the early 1980s. The third reason for this trend is the changing requirements NIH study sections have established for initial research grants. NIH has recognized the problem associated with the lack of preliminary data and has instituted a check box on the proposal sheet to alert reviewers to proposals that come from individuals who have never had NIH support. Generally, preliminary data are now required

---

[11]National Research Council. 1998c.

[12]Unpublished tables from the Survey of Doctorate Recipients.

for proposals.[13] Consequently, new independent investigators may be several years into independent positions before receiving an NIH grant.

While there is a need for postdoctoral training, especially for individuals seeking academic research careers, the prospects for such positions are not good. Given that there were approximately 20,000 postdoctoral positions in 2001, with new Ph.D.s entering postdoctoral positions each year, and faculty positions have remained constant at about 38,000, it is unlikely that a majority of postdoctoral trainees will find faculty positions. The use of postdoctorate training as an employment option while awaiting an academic position varies greatly by field, but ideally the postdoctorate training system would allow the best and the brightest to move into faculty positions.[14] Nevertheless, the postdoctorate is a necessary and important stage in the research career path and should be maintained in a relatively stable form over the long term. Therefore, cuts are not advisable.

That said, something must be done to ameliorate the negative aspects of these positions, including what sometimes is poor training outside the grant topic, research experience that may disappoint potential future scientists, lack of full employment benefits, and obstacles to establishment of an independent research career. There have been a variety of efforts to move people from postdoctoral training to research status. *Enhancing the Postdoctoral Experience for Scientists and Engineers*, a report published by the National Academies Committee on Science, Engineering, and Public Policy, recommends several action points to improve the conditions of postdoctoral trainees, including steps to improve this transition to career.[15] Among the guiding principles presented is the need to ensure that appointments are beneficial to all concerned. There are other notable models that are part of the efforts to move people from postdoctoral training to research status. The Markey Charitable Trust, no longer in operation, developed a program to assist young scholars in making this transition, and the Burroughs Welcome Fund currently has a program modeled after the Markey program. The American Heart Association has a similar program directed at holders of an M.D. or M.D./Ph.D. who are interested in cardiovascular or stroke research. Indeed, NIH's postdoctoral training programs are noteworthy in providing such opportunities for minority postdoctorates as well. Each of these programs provides a few years of supervised training at the postdoctoral level and additional years of support in a faculty position. While they address the issue of career transition and development, they also have a goal of identifying the best researchers at an early age and of providing sufficient funds so an individual can comfortably pursue

research, but only a few doctorates are supported each year since the support levels are reasonably high.

The NIH has developed an award series, called the K awards, to assist researchers in making career transitions. The awards in this series fall into three categories:

### Career development for M.D.s in clinical research

Mentored Clinical Scientist Development Award (K08)
Mentored Clinical Scientist Development Program Award (K12)
Mentored Patient-Oriented Research Career Development Award (K23)
Mid-career Investigator Award in Patient-Oriented Research (K24)

### Skills development

Academic Career Award (K07)
Career Enhancement Award for Stem Cell Research (K18)
Mentored Quantitative Research Career Development Award (K25)
Mid-career Investigator Award in Mouse Pathobiology Research (K26)
Clinical Research Curriculum Award (K30)

### Career transition

Mentored Research Scientist Development Award (K01)
Independent Scientist Award (K02)
Senior Scientist Award (K05)
Career Transition Award (K22)

The *career development* awards are directed at individuals with an M.D. and were discussed in Chapter 4. Some of the *skills development* awards are also directed at clinical research but are generally designed to support training in a specific area or curriculum development. The *career transition* awards are available to Ph.D.s and provide support while learning a new field or transitioning from training to research status. However, in this last group only the K22 is designed to facilitate the transition from a postdoctoral to a faculty position. The K01, at most of the NIH institutes and centers, is designed to support reentry or retraining experiences for fully trained scientists to significantly expand their expertise in their current field. The K02 and K05 are for established investigators who might benefit from a sustained period of support and release time. Table 9-5 shows the number of awards each year from 1994 to 2002, and it is clear that most of the support in the K series is directed at clinical research or career development for established investigators.

The K22 award is relatively new, with the first awards in 1999 and the number roughly doubling each year to 92 in 2002. Many but not all institutes and centers offer this award, and they vary in type and support level. Application for the

---

[13] National Academies Workshop: Bridges to Independence. June 16, 2004.

[14] Regets. 1998. op. cit.

[15] National Research Council. 2000. op. cit.

TABLE 9-5 Number of Awards for Current K Grant Programs, 1994–2002

| Award | 1994 | 1995 | 1996 | 1997 | 1998 | 1999 | 2000 | 2001 | 2002 |
|-------|------|------|------|------|------|------|------|------|------|
| **Clinical Research Training** | | | | | | | | | |
| K08 | 736 | 791 | 929 | 1045 | 1174 | 1155 | 1208 | 1140 | 1161 |
| K12 | 42 | 41 | 39 | 34 | 41 | 49 | 75 | 80 | 107 |
| K23 | 0 | 0 | 0 | 0 | 1 | 142 | 327 | 496 | 664 |
| K24 | 0 | 0 | 0 | 0 | 0 | 81 | 158 | 215 | 261 |
| Total | 778 | 832 | 968 | 1079 | 1216 | 1427 | 1768 | 1931 | 2193 |
| **Skills and Curriculum Development** | | | | | | | | | |
| K07 | 150 | 158 | 144 | 142 | 149 | 137 | 138 | 122 | 131 |
| K25 | 0 | 0 | 0 | 0 | 0 | 0 | 8 | 31 | 53 |
| K26 | 0 | 0 | 0 | 0 | 0 | 0 | 3 | 8 | 10 |
| K30 | 0 | 0 | 0 | 0 | 0 | 35 | 57 | 57 | 59 |
| Total | 150 | 158 | 144 | 142 | 149 | 172 | 206 | 218 | 253 |
| **Ph.D. Career Development** | | | | | | | | | |
| K01 | 51 | 58 | 90 | 155 | 233 | 319 | 419 | 530 | 603 |
| K02 | 147 | 152 | 193 | 225 | 257 | 277 | 298 | 294 | 278 |
| K05 | 132 | 132 | 131 | 132 | 127 | 110 | 100 | 90 | 80 |
| K22 | 0 | 0 | 0 | 0 | 0 | 5 | 27 | 54 | 92 |
| Total | 330 | 342 | 414 | 512 | 617 | 711 | 844 | 968 | 1053 |

SOURCE: NIH IMPACII Database.

K22 usually occurs when an individual in a postdoctoral position seeks support for an additional period of training in either that position or a new appointment. It typically provides 2 or 3 years of additional support, followed by support in a faculty position for a total of 5 years. Sometimes this period is required to be intramural at the NIH, and there may be restrictions on the number of years of postdoctoral training prior to receiving it. Basic research could be conducted on the K22. It is usually related to the research area of the awarding institute or center, and support for basic research is limited. While the basic mission of NIGMS is to support students at the predoctoral level and the institute has some postdoctoral traineeships, it does not offer K22 awards. The application process is complicated by the different requirements, as reported in "Science: Next Wave," which discusses the problems incurred by several people who tried to get advice.[16] The K22 award is a step forward in the effort to assist in the transition from trainee to investigator, but it may have more potential that could be explored by NIH. The 93 awards given in 2002 had little impact on the overall postdoctoral picture.[17] Fewer restrictions on the field of research and a mechanism that allows for a significant expansion of the K22 program would be helpful in addressing the problem of getting young investigators through postdoctoral positions and into independent research careers.

---

[16]*Science:* Next Wave. 2002.
[17]*Federal Corner.* 2002.

There is at least one category of researchers that does not seem well served by this potpourri of K grants—namely, researchers who have already received extensive scientific training, sometimes through a postdoctoral period, and then choose for personally important reasons to leave the scientific workforce. The typical example is a women scientist who decides to have children and raise a family but does not find it possible to do so while simultaneously fulfilling all of the demands of a normal scientific/academic career that includes teaching, research, and service. Many highly trained, excellent scientists fall into this category but are forced to forego active research for a large enough number of years that they find it difficult, if not impossible, to resume the path to a research career. Retraining programs, such as the NIH supplement to existing research grants, do not always address their needs and would help too few scientists to deal with the problem. The nation invests a large amount of training in these scientists, who are ready to make significant contributions, and cannot afford to see them leave the scientific workforce. NIH should consider a new form of K awards that would allow such individuals to reduce their overall workload for a time but continue their scientific research until they are ready to resume a full-time career.

## FOREIGN RESEARCHERS

The U.S. scientific research enterprise has benefited from the immigration of foreign-born scientists and engineers. They come for doctoral education, postdoctoral training, or employment in educational institutions, government laboratories, and industrial research facilities. Their numbers are significant in most fields and notably high in certain fields. For example, in recent years more than half of the doctorates in engineering have been temporary residents. These numbers increased particularly rapidly in the 1990s, when many researchers entered the country on H1-B visas (part of other highly skilled academic entry visas) during the high-tech Internet boom. Some thought there might be a decline in the number of foreign students and foreign workforce entrants as technological advances were made in other countries, on the theory that U.S.-trained doctorates might return to their home country universities and workforce. Until recently, there has been little support for this prediction. However, new immigration policies following 9/11 have made entry from countries with the largest number of foreign immigrants more difficult. The new immigration policies pose a serious potential threat to the research mission of this country, a point that will be addressed again shortly.

Participation of foreign researchers across the three broad fields in this study is quite different. Since 1996, about 24 percent of the doctorates in the biomedical sciences went to temporary visa holders, and the averages are about 7 percent and 20 percent in the behavioral and clinical sciences, respectively. Table 9-6 shows the percentage of non-U.S. citizens with doctorates across the three broad fields. In addi-

TABLE 9-6 Percentage of Doctorates by Citizenship Status, 1993–2003

| | 1993 (%) | 1994 (%) | 1995 (%) | 1996 (%) | 1997 (%) | 1998 (%) | 1999 (%) | 2000 (%) | 2001 (%) | 2002 (%) | 2003 (%) |
|---|---|---|---|---|---|---|---|---|---|---|---|
| **Biomedical Sciences** | | | | | | | | | | | |
| Citizens | 69.1 | 66.4 | 65.2 | 62.5 | 65.8 | 66.7 | 66.9 | 68.0 | 70.2 | 69.9 | 68.7 |
| Permanent residents | 6.3 | 13.3 | 16.5 | 15.2 | 10.7 | 10.2 | 9.3 | 6.8 | 6.5 | 6.2 | 5.2 |
| Temporary residents | 24.7 | 20.3 | 18.3 | 22.3 | 23.5 | 23.2 | 23.8 | 25.1 | 23.3 | 23.9 | 26.1 |
| **Behavioral and Social Sciences** | | | | | | | | | | | |
| Citizens | 88.6 | 88.6 | 88.2 | 88.4 | 89.1 | 89.2 | 90.8 | 89.6 | 90.1 | 90.1 | 89.1 |
| Permanent residents | 3.5 | 3.8 | 4.4 | 4.1 | 3.7 | 3.4 | 2.8 | 3.2 | 2.9 | 3.0 | 2.5 |
| Temporary residents | 7.9 | 7.6 | 7.5 | 7.4 | 7.2 | 7.5 | 6.3 | 7.3 | 7.0 | 7.0 | 8.4 |
| **Clinical Sciences** | | | | | | | | | | | |
| Citizens | 75.2 | 74.6 | 71.7 | 71.8 | 73.2 | 74.1 | 73.6 | 75.4 | 73.5 | 74.3 | 75.6 |
| Permanent residents | 5.9 | 7.6 | 8.5 | 7.2 | 6.2 | 6.3 | 6.4 | 5.2 | 5.5 | 4.4 | 4.1 |
| Temporary residents | 18.9 | 17.8 | 19.7 | 21.0 | 20.6 | 19.6 | 19.9 | 19.4 | 21.0 | 21.2 | 20.3 |

SOURCE: Survey of Earned Doctorates.

tion, about 1 percent of the M.D. graduates each year are temporary residents, but it is difficult to estimate how many might pursue research careers.[18]

The training of temporary residents is important on two separate grounds. First, trainees who return to their home countries play an important role in advancing health care knowledge in those countries. Since disease does not respect political boundaries, it is vital to our own interests that the best health research, knowledge, and treatment occur worldwide. Second, we have not found it possible to carry out our domestic health care research at the required highest levels of quality without the contributions of the best foreign researchers. This fact is undoubtedly related to the high percentage of foreigners who arrive in the United States with excellent backgrounds in technical and mathematical areas.

There is no database that tracks these individuals, but studies by Finn[19] have identified individuals from the Doctorate Records File who at specific times after their doctorate have paid Social Security taxes. Findings for the life sciences, which include both the biomedical and clinical sciences, show that temporary resident doctorates in the late 1990s were staying in the United States in a greater proportion than graduates in the earlier part of the decade (see Table 9-7). The increase is not (yet) seen in the behavioral sciences, where the rates are about the same for doctorates in the 10-year period.

There may be some problems in interpreting these data due to the Chinese Student Protection Act, which gave permanent residency to students from China in the mid-1990s who would have normally graduated with temporary resident status. Since students from China have the highest stay

rate for temporary residents (about 95 percent), the stay rates for temporary residents might even be higher.

These U.S.-trained foreign scientists stay in the United States 5 to 10 years after receipt of their doctorates and are very likely to remain and join the workforce as permanent residents and citizens. One would expect stay rates for doctorates 1 or 2 years after their degrees to be even higher, as is the case in the biomedical/clinical sciences where 77 percent of the 1999 doctorates were in the United States in 2000 and 74 percent stayed in 2001. In the behavioral sciences, about 47 percent of the 1999 doctorates stayed in 2000 and 2001. Some of these short-term stays were probably for additional training in a postdoctoral position, but based on the 5- and 10-year data, many graduates remain in this country after a postdoctoral appointment.

TABLE 9-7 Stay Rates for Doctorates with Temporary Resident Visas at Time of Receipt of Doctorate (%)

| | Year of Doctorate | 5 Years Later (%) | 10 Years Later (%) |
|---|---|---|---|
| Biomedical/clinical sciences | 1987 | 36 | 39 |
| Biomedical/clinical sciences | 1992 | 39 | 67 |
| Biomedical/clinical sciences | 1996 | 62 | NA |
| Behavioral sciences | 1987 | 30 | 29 |
| Behavioral sciences | 1992 | 31 | |
| Behavioral sciences | 1996 | 33 | NA |

NA = not applicable.

SOURCE: Tabulation by Michael Finn from the Doctorate Records File.

---

[18]American Association of Medical Colleges. 2004.
[19]Finn, M. 2003.

Based on the number of temporary resident doctorates and the above stay rates, about 700 of the 1996 and 900 of the 1999 biomedical doctorates remained in the United States in 2002. When compared to the data in Chapter 2 (see Table 2-5) on the citizenship of academic postdoctoral appointees, this means that most of the 10,000 temporary residents have foreign doctorates. How many of these temporary resident postdoctorates eventually stay in this country is difficult to estimate, but data from the National Center for Educational Statistics show that 4 percent of the biomedical faculty had temporary residency in 1999. However, the data do not identify individuals who have converted their status from temporary residency to naturalized citizen. Considering these numbers, it is clear that foreign citizens have made a real contribution to biomedical research. The contribution of foreign scientists to the behavioral and social sciences workforce is comparatively smaller, with only 6 percent of the doctorates going to temporary residents and only about 30 percent of those doctorates staying. However, putting aside changes in immigration policy, the general trend of increased foreign participation in the research workforce seems to apply to all the health-related sciences.

The large number of foreign researchers who stay in this country is in no way meant to imply a problem. It is in this country's interest to gain the best foreign scientists as citizens. What problem there is lies in the opposite domain, when foreign countries lose an important human intellectual resource. Given the worldwide nature of most health problems, at least some thought needs to be given to the potential problem that foreign countries could experience an insufficient number of high-quality health researchers. If the U.S. immigration policies put in place after 9/11 are not altered, the obstacles placed in the path of foreign researchers at every level may drive them to seek training and employment elsewhere, posing a serious threat to the research effort in this country.

There are already indications of a slowdown in the supply of foreign scientists. In the fall of 2003 the Council of Graduate Schools (CGS) conducted a survey of graduate schools and found a 47 percent decline in international enrollments for the fall of 2003 compared to the fall of 2002.[20] One reason for this decline may be the time required to complete security checks associated with visa applications. A 2003 U.S. Government Accountability Office (GAO) report found that between April and May of 2003 it took an average of 67 days to complete such checks.[21] Another CGS survey in February 2004 found that graduate school applications declined by 32 percent and that 90 percent of the surveyed institutions saw a decline. The latest survey in June 2004 on applications and acceptances for the fall 2004 term found that in the agricultural and life sciences applications had declined by 24

percent and admissions by 19 percent over 2003, and in the social and behavioral sciences applications were down 20 percent and admissions were down by 13 percent. The fear of double-digit declines in actual enrollment were allayed by a final CSG survey in the fall of 2004 which overall saw a 6 percent decline in first year enrollments by foreign students and a 10 percent decline in the life sciences.[22] Even though this is the third straight year for a decline in foreign enrollments, it might be a temporary occurrence caused by the visa problems highlighted in the GAO report or the beginning of a long-term trend brought on by global competition and international perceptions of America. In either case, the loss of foreign graduate students to U.S. programs could affect research capacity in this country.

The career implications for U.S.-trained citizens and permanent residents due to the influx of foreign scientists are difficult to determine. Foreign students makeup 22 percent of the graduate students and 26 percent of the doctorates in the biomedical sciences, and over 50 percent of the postdoctorates in academic institutions. Changes in these percentages could affect career opportunities and the availability of qualified students for doctoral programs. The Committee at the National Academies is Studying the Policy Implications of International Graduate Students and Postdoctoral Scholars, and its report will be issued in the spring of 2005.

## UNDERREPRESENTED MINORITY SCIENTISTS

Minority participation in the biomedical, clinical, and behavioral and social sciences continues at a rate lower than their respective population proportions. The overall percentage of minority doctorates is very low. Recently, minorities have comprised about 9 percent of the biomedical and clinical sciences doctorates and about 17 percent in the social and behavioral sciences (see Table 9-8).

In addition to participation levels, the attrition rate of minority scientists from graduate school is a concern. In each of the three fields, the percentage of full- and part-time minority students is greater than the graduation rate. The disparity between graduate student and doctorate rates is likely caused by some combination of two factors: (1) higher than normal dropout rate among minority students or attrition (2) a decision to conclude the training process at a lower level (such as the master's degree). These factors may be due in part to debt incurred up to this point in the education process, as fewer minorities than whites graduate debt free at the baccalaureate level.[23] In either case the result is low participation by minorities in the research workforce.

The problem of retaining minority students in the pipeline from high school to the doctorate has been addressed by many organizations, including the NIH. NIH has a number

[20]Council of Graduate Schools. 2004.
[21]Government Accountability Office. 2003.

[22]Council of Graduate Schools. 2004.
[23]Rapoport, A. 1999.

TABLE 9-8 Comparison of Doctorates Awarded to the Graduate Student Population, 1997–2002

| | 1997 (%) | 1998 (%) | 1999 (%) | 2000 (%) | 2001 (%) | 2002 (%) |
|---|---|---|---|---|---|---|
| **Percentage of Minority Doctorates**[a] | | | | | | |
| Biomedical sciences | 6.5 | 6.9 | 7.9 | 7.9 | 9.2 | 9.4 |
| Clinical sciences | 8.6 | 8.9 | 10.4 | 10.1 | 10.0 | 9.4 |
| Behavioral sciences | 11.4 | 12.7 | 13.6 | 13.8 | 14.7 | 15.5 |
| **Percentage of minority students in doctoral-ranking institutions**[b] | | | | | | |
| Biomedical sciences | 10.1 | 10.3 | 9.9 | 10.3 | 10.5 | 10.8 |
| Clinical sciences | 11.5 | 12.3 | 13.0 | 12.8 | 14.4 | 14.4 |
| Behavioral sciences | 13.9 | 14.2 | 14.9 | 16.5 | 16.9 | 17.4 |

[a]National Science Foundation Survey of Earned Doctorates.

[b]Survey of Graduate Students and Postdoctorates in Science and Engineering.

of programs that are monitored by the National Center on Minority Health and Health Disparities. There are 61 different programs at NIH, every institute having at least one. They range from the Minority Access to Research Careers (MARC) program to supplement awards on research grants. The MARC program has been in existence from 1975 and is administered by the NIGMS. It offers awards from the four-year college level to senior faculty fellowships, and each is designed to assist students with their education or to provide existing faculty members with support for retaining or development of a research project. The MARC program was evaluated in 1997 with no conclusive results as to its effectiveness, but it has supported a large number of individuals and is the core of NIH's activities in this area. Most other programs at NIH are small and are directed by individual institutes and centers. These are usually designed to promote the research interests of the institute or center by providing support at the predoctoral or postdoctoral levels as an individual or institutional award. Each institute- or center-based program supports only a few individuals. Although they do assist students with their education, it is unclear whether they support significant numbers of students beyond those that would have been supported by other mechanisms. These programs are currently being evaluated by another NRC study with the hope of identifying effective models that truly increase minority participation.

Although many minority programs are institute and center based, there is a supplemental research grant program that cuts across the NIH institutes and centers and provides additional funds on a research grant to support a student or a faculty member. The intent of this program is to interest students in a particular research area or to develop the research skills of a faculty member. This program could be highly effective in creating opportunities for minority participation.

Looking at the various programs in place at NIH, one is struck by their focus on relatively late stages of the training/academic career. It will be difficult to increase minority participation later in the path if there are too few students at the precollege level with the requisite academic background and interest to pursue a scientific research career. The MARC awards and some of the other institutional programs that support students at the undergraduate level and aim programs at college-level students are one step toward helping minority students pursue advanced degrees and research careers. However, to make a real difference, intervention needs to take place at the precollege level with programs that properly prepare students and capture their interest in the biomedical, behavioral, and clinical sciences.

## CONCLUSION

The road map for career development in scientific research is appropriately multifaceted. Opportunities exist at all levels, as does the need for improvement. The development of a research scientist begins at a very early age. Outreach programs and encouragement are needed well before undergraduate and graduate programs enter the picture. This is particularly true for minorities but includes the entire population. An effective pipeline of students is needed to enter the professional education that begins with graduate training. This situation notwithstanding, it is also true that strong efforts are needed for training and recruitment at the graduate level.

Postdoctoral training is becoming a requirement for all fields, and this trend is likely to continue as the complexity of the research enterprise increases. The existence of this large training pool is in fact desirable in terms of both training opportunities and research accomplishments. However, the status and working conditions of postdoctoral candidates need to be improved. Moreover, training and opportunities for advancement to independent research positions must be enhanced. The flow of foreign scientists into the system at this level should be encouraged as an opportunity to improve both training and research in this country. In the case of physicians, programs are needed that permit research training without major disruption of clinical duties.

The recommendations presented here should be regarded as only a small part of the integrated effort over all agencies, at all levels, that is needed for the enhanced development of research personnel in this country.

## RECOMMENDATIONS

**Recommendation 9-1: The committee recommends that career development grants (currently K awards) be maintained but be restructured such that fewer mechanisms are established and consistently implemented across NIH.**

The concept of K awards is meritorious, but the large variety of K awards and inconsistent usage across NIH institutes and centers makes it difficult for applicants to use the opportunities that exist optimally. Furthermore, the program would be enhanced if K awards were given by a greater number of institutes and centers than is currently the case.

**Recommendation 9-2: The committee recommends that the restructured K awards include the following: (1) a transition award to span senior postdoctoral status and an independent research position; (2) beginning faculty awards to free certain classes of investigators from non-research duties; (3) senior scientist awards for the purpose of faculty moving into new research areas; (4) awards to allow faculty and other researchers to maintain research careers during periods when personal demands (e.g., child rearing) prevent full employment status; and (5) clinical science awards to provide research training for clinical faculty/personnel.**

The committee recognizes that the above categories, except for the fourth one, are included among existing K awards. However, uniform presentations and criteria across NIH would make these awards more accessible. This list is not meant to be inclusive, but in any event, it is important to delineate clearly what mechanisms are available, who is eligible, and how applications can be made.

**Recommendation 9-3: The committee recommends that NIH develop a mechanism for support such that NRSA postdoctoral fellows receive the employee benefits of the institutions at which they are located.**

Although NRSA postdoctoral fellows are selected through a highly competitive process, they are often at a financial disadvantage with regard to postdoctoral employees paid directly through research grants. In particular, health insurance benefits are not always readily provided. This need not be a major budget issue if a portion of the current supplemental allocation is used for this purpose. This usage of the supplemental allowance could even be required if health in-

surance is not provided by other means. In terms of the normal fringe benefits package provided by institutions, a lower rate should be possible for postdoctoral fellows since they are very seldom able to utilize the retirement portion of the package due to vesting requirements, typically 5 years.

**Recommendation 9-4: The committee recommends that supplements to existing training grants be made available for the purpose of developing outreach programs for undergraduates and high school students from underrepresented minorities and for the secondary school teachers serving them.**

Training resources for minorities at the doctoral and postdoctoral levels is clearly insufficient. The pool of suitable candidates is far too small by the time the doctoral level is reached. It is critical that NIH find new ways to encourage members of underrepresented groups to pursue research careers well before the doctoral level. Furthermore, updating and training for secondary school teachers are critical for this effort. By utilizing existing training programs, already evaluated for their excellence, a quality environment is assured and resources can be rapidly dispersed. Among the programs envisioned are summer research experiences, weekend training sessions, and direct interaction of training grant personnel with students.

**Recommendation 9-5: The committee recommends that NIH work with other federal agencies to find ways to encourage students at precollege levels to pursue training in technical, computational, mathematical, and scientific areas that are necessary precursors for careers in science.**

In recent years the need for researchers trained in such areas has been filled by an influx of foreign scientists. This influx may change due to immigration laws or changes in the support structure in foreign countries. It is a slow and long process to change the education structure in a way that will produce larger numbers of students capable and willing to pursue careers in science.

# 10

# Final Comments

The committee has been given the task of assessing present and future demands for research personnel over the entire spectrum of health-related sciences, including the areas of basic biomedical, behavioral, clinical, oral health, nursing, and health services. This chapter puts the task in perspective by considering the issues in a larger context. In addition, what has been done and what is needed for future considerations are assessed.

In a world with an ever-growing and continually aging population that travels and intermixes to an ever-increasing degree, a very safe prediction is that the nation's and the world's vital need for scientific research in health-related areas will continue to grow rapidly. New health problems and rapidly propagating diseases will continue to threaten the entire world, including the United States. It is difficult to conceive of a scenario in which the need for health research will not continue to accelerate.

Given this picture of the future, the distinction between *need* and *demand* for research personnel needs to be clarified. The *need* for improved health care, which ultimately requires research, will continue to grow. However, this committee and its predecessors have been forced to consider *demand*, rather than *need*. *Demand* refers to the research positions that society decides are of sufficient value to fund. It is determined by many variables, including the state of the economy and the extent of perceived threats to the nation's health. The present demand can be estimated by various models, and extrapolations can be made into the future. These estimates, however, are only valid if all factors remain stable, an unlikely prospect. This committee believes it much more likely that demand will grow, rather than decline, relative to the projections from static models.

Manpower models have been developed for the fields of basic biomedical, clinical, and behavioral and social sciences research. Although the quality and quantity of data available for this purpose are limited, the available information suggests that this committee have a system that is roughly in balance: low unemployment currently exists, and extrapola-

tion into the future suggests this will continue. Importantly, the bulge of personnel in postdoctoral positions appears to be dissipating. The committee harbors reservations about the ability to extrapolate into the future, either on the basis of the model or personal judgment, but it is likely that trained researchers will continue to find positions in their fields, at least for the near future. This current situation has been created on the basis of training commitments made over the past 5 to 10 years. Because the committee believes that a healthy environment exists in terms of training possibilities and job opportunities, this committee has recommended that the number of trainees be no less than its level in 2003. However, this committee has made a number of recommendations with regard to modifications in training, stressing the needs of the future and the importance of flexibility.

In the fields of oral health and nursing the data are insufficient to carry out a workforce model, but it is clear that research efforts and research personnel are not at the level that is optimal for maintaining a vital research effort. Breaking out of this situation will require an input of funding and great creativity on the part of the professions and professional schools.

In the committee's consideration of the present and past training of biomedical research personnel, it has become apparent that adequate data are not available for a thorough analysis. In many cases this could be remedied by the National Institutes of Health (NIH) creating and maintaining reliable databases gleaned from the annual reports associated with their research and training programs. Given the importance of biomedical research and the maintenance of a highly skilled workforce, the committee believes that NIH would be well served in establishing procedures to provide workforce data that would facilitate future assessment of the National Research Service Award (NRSA) program. Improved mechanisms for supplying data and coordinating data collection are needed if future estimates of workforce needs are to be more accurate.

Given the present training capabilities in this country and

around the world, particularly the existing university systems and research in health-related industries, market forces are an important factor in determining the choices of research careers. Thus, the supply of trained research personnel tends to adjust to the demand. A significant phase difference of several years or more may be required to adjust the differences between supply and demand, but history suggests that this adjustment inevitably occurs. The present training capability is determined by a mixture of federal, state, and private research grants, various group and individual training grants, training received by individuals pursuing professional degrees, and research carried out by for-profit private institutions. This mix of training venues is highly varied and flexible and can adjust to local fluctuations in demand, as long as they are not too extreme. Given this situation, it is probably less useful to base decisions about adjusting training personnel on the basis of stable states of the world than it is to have a system that can respond rapidly to unusual changes. Partly for this reason, the committee recommends that a standing independent committee be established to continually monitor research personnel and to recommend adjustments when needed. This would be more effective than the current method of convening a new committee every four years.

When discussing the supply of research personnel, it is critical to move past discussion of sheer numbers. The quality and skills of research personnel are of paramount importance. Research is continually used to justify far-reaching health decisions that affect large segments of the population. The accuracy, reliability, and validity of such research must be as high as can be reached. In addition, new advances in health treatment are dependent on the creativity and insight of the world's best researchers. This committee has therefore made recommendations to ensure that the training of researchers and of those who will provide training for future researchers is of the highest attainable quality.

The committee is particularly concerned about career development opportunities for research personnel. Although its research efforts are the best in the world, this country may be losing individuals with special talents, especially among underrepresented groups and young people with responsibilities other than research that prevent them from achieving their full potential. Consequently, the committee encourages NIH to continue its efforts to provide unique career development programs, albeit in a more integrative fashion across NIH than is currently being done.

Any large research organization, such as NIH, must necessarily divide itself into units based on categories of related science. The benefits of this type of organization are obvious, but clearly some drawbacks also are present. Such an organization promotes research and research training that tend toward the center of each unit's discipline. Such tendencies work against inter- and multidisciplinary research and research training, despite the well-recognized fact that major breakthroughs in medical research often occur at the interfaces between and across traditional areas. Because of such tendencies, the committee has tailored several recommendations to promote vital inter- and multidisciplinary training.

Both in the past and in the present report, considerable effort has been devoted to analysis of and recommendations concerning training in the form of NRSAs. However, this training, while vital for the nation, is only a small part of research training in this country. A major segment of research training is supported by research grants, as is deemed appropriate by this committee. Even within the subset of training in the university community, NRSA awards are restricted to U.S. citizen and green card holders. This leaves out the training of foreign personnel, which typically occurs on research grants, and the vital role played by foreign personnel in the overall research effort. Ultimately, a significant number of foreign personnel remain in this country and become an important part of the training and research community. This committee has tried to place its recommendations in a larger context, containing both domestic and foreign researchers and the important roles played by each group. In this regard, the committee is concerned about recent visa restrictions that may restrict the entry of foreign students and research personnel into this country. The input of foreign personnel is essential for the vitality of the research and training community. In fact, if the restrictions on foreign researchers continue, the demand for domestic researchers may significantly outstrip the supply.

Finally, the committee notes that this nation does not exist in isolation. Disease and health problems do not respect political borders. It is in the nation's vital interest that health solutions and health services extend to the world at large and that research and research training take place in the larger context of the world's scientific community. Although this committee did not believe its mandate extended this far and time and resources did not permit full consideration of research training in the world at large, some of our recommendations are made with such issues in mind.

It is hoped that this report, with its analyses and recommendations, will serve as a useful guide to NIH in the consideration of research training for both the present and the immediate future and that it will provide a foundation for our successors.

## RECOMMENDATIONS

**Recommendation 10-1: The committee recommends that a standing independent committee be created to monitor biomedical, clinical, and behavioral and social sciences research personnel needs, to evaluate the training of such personnel, to assess the number and nature of research personnel that will be required in the future, to assist in the collection and analysis of appropriate data, and to make recommendations concerning these matters to NIH.**

An assessment of the availability and need for biomedical, clinical, and behavioral research personnel is essential for the health enterprise of the nation and the world. An appropriate pool of researchers in appropriate numbers must be continuously available. The training of new research personnel to meet anticipated short- and long-term future demands, in terms of both area of expertise and number, is important enough to merit independent review and recommendations. It is not sufficient to constitute a new committee every five years. Each committee must analyze vast amounts of data, relearn old lessons, and duplicate past work and is pressed for time in completing its task.

A standing committee, established by and advisory to the NIH, could develop long-term procedures for collecting relevant data, could generate methods for analyzing the data in productive ways, could analyze the research personnel from all sources (i.e., universities, business, and government, both domestic and foreign), could assess the appropriateness of training procedures, and could make reasonable projections about needs and ways to meet those needs in future years.

A standing committee could coordinate with NIH and other agencies to establish regular procedures for data collection and to put in place continually updated databases. Useful databases would include, for example, accurate information about the total number of students and postdoctorals supported by federal funding and knowledge of whether they are foreign or domestic. Surveys, including condition of employment surveys, might be initiated from time to time.

A standing committee would greatly improve the quality, validity, and scope of the recommendations and projections produced.

**Recommendation 10-2: The committee recommends that the NIH implement a data collection system for tracking the career outcomes of its recipients of research training support. A minimum set of outcomes would include sector of employment, involvement in research, and subsequent NIH awards.**

At the very least, the data should include individuals funded under all training awards and research grants. The lack of data on the career outcomes of NRSA recipients has been noted in previous chapters of this report. A similar scarcity of data on the career outcomes and trajectories of biomedical, behavioral, and clinical scientists in general has been identified by other personnel study groups. Although the NIH currently collects some information on the outcomes of trainees and fellows, it is not in a form amenable to aggregation and further analysis. Moreover, no career outcome information is routinely collected for trainees on research grants. This lack of information works against making progress toward addressing which training mechanisms and strategies will best ensure a talented and productive research workforce.

# References

Agency for Healthcare Research and Quality. 1998. Innovation Incentive Award. AHRQ Publication No. 00-P044. Rockville, MD. Available at *http://www.ahrq.gov/fund/incentiv.htm.* Accessed October 22, 2004.

Agency for Healthcare Research and Quality. 2001. AHRQ Research Training and Career Development Databook: 1986 to 1998. AHRQ: Rockville, MD

Agres, T. 2002. NIMH shifts research priorities: Scientists fear curtailed funding for basic social and behavioral research. The Scientist Daily News. September 30, 2004. Available at *http://www.biomedcentral. com/news/20040930/03.* Accessed October 22, 2004.

Ahrens, E. H. Jr. 1992. The Crisis in Clinical Research, Overcoming Institutional Obstacles. New York: Oxford University Press.

Aiken, L. H. et al. 2002. Hospital nurse staffing and patient mortality, nurse burnout, and job dissatisfaction, Journal of the American Medical Association 288:16(October):1987–1993.

American Association of Colleges of Nursing. 2003a. 2002–2003 Enrollment and graduations in baccalaureate and graduate programs in nursing. Washington, D.C. Available at *http://www.aacn.nche.edu/IDS/ EnrlTOC.htm.*

American Association of Colleges of Nursing. 2003b. Faculty Shortages in Baccalaureate and Graduate Nursing Programs: Scope of the Problem and Strategies for Expanding the Supply. Available at *http://www.aacn. nche.edu/Publications/WhitePapers/TFFFWP.pdf.* Accessed 10/10/ 2003.

American Association of Colleges of Nursing. 2004. Nursing Faculty Shortage Fact Sheet, May. Available at *www.aacn.nche.edu/Media/Back grounders/facultyshortage.htm.* Accessed 5/20/2004.

American Association of Medical Colleges. 2004. AAMC Web site facts—applicants, matriculants, and graduates. Available at *www.aamc.org/ data/facts/archive/famg92002.htm* Accessed 10/22/2004.

American Dental Association. 1999. The 1998 Survey of Dental Practice: Dentists in Solo and Nonsolo Practice. Chicago, IL: American Dental Association.

American Dental Association. 2001. Future of Dentistry.Report. Chicago, IL: American Dental Association.

American Dental Association. 2002. 2001–2002 Survey of Predoctoral Dental Education: Tuition, Admission, and Attrition. 2:36. Chicago, IL: American Dental Association.

American Dental Association.2002. 2001–2002 Trends In Advanced Dental Education. Chicago, IL: American Dental Association.

American Dental Education Association. 2001. Faculty Salary Survey, Summary Report 1999–2000. Washington, D.C.

American Nurses Association 1985. Directions for Nursing Research: Toward The Twenty-First Century. D-79 (May):1–6.

Arias, I. M. 2004. Bridge building between medicine and basic science:

contributions of the Markey Trust. National Research Council. Washington D.C.: National Academies Press, pp. 45–60.

Babco, E. L. 2003. Trends in African American and Native American participation in stem higher education. Commission on Professionals in Science and Technology. (May).

Bowen, W.G. and N.L. Rubenstine. 1992. In Pursuit of the PhD. Princeton, NJ: Princeton University Press.

Center for Public Policy and Advocacy American Dental Education Association (ADEA). 2003. Dental Education At-A-Glance 2003. Available at *http://www.adea.org/CPPA_Materials/default.htm.* Accessed October 22, 2004.

Coggeshall, P., and P. W. Brown. 1984. The Career Achievements of NIH Predoctoral Trainees and Fellows. Washington, D.C.: National Academy Press.

Council of Graduate Schools. 2004. Council of Graduate Schools Finds Decline in New International Graduate Student Enrollment for the Third Consecutive Year, November 4, 2004.News Release.

Council of Graduate Schools. 2004. Findings from U.S. Graduate Schools on International Graduate Students' Admissions Trends. 2004. Available at *http://www.cgsnet.org/pdf/Sept04FinalIntlAdmissionsSurvey Report.pdf.*

Council on Scientific Affairs (I-99). 1998. Summary of Report of the Graylyn Development Consensus Conference, November 1998, from Report 13 of the, Update on Clinical Research. Available online at: *http://www.ama-assn.org/ama/pub/article/2036-2392.html.*

Donaldson, S. K. and Crowley, D. M. 1978. The discipline of nursing. Nursing Outlook 26(February):113–120.

Draft Report of the Working Group of the NIH Advisory Committee to the Director on Research Opportunities in the Basic Behavioral and Social Sciences, *http://obssr.od.nih.gov/Activities/Basic%20Beh%20Report_ complete.pdf,* Accessed December 2, 2004.

Ebert-Flattau, P. 1981. Some preliminary data on the health services research labor force in the United States. Systems Science in Health Care, C. Tilquin ed. New York: Pergamon Press

FASEB News June 3, 2004. FASEB President Wells Testifies on NIH Funding Issues Federation of American Societies for Experimental Biology. Bethesda, MD. 37(3):1 Available at *http://www.faseb.org/opa/newsletter/6x04/june_nl_web.pdf.* Accessed October 22, 2004.

Federal Corner 2002. *Deciphering NIH K Awards—Inside Tips from an NIH Expert.* Available at *http://nextwave.sciencemag.org/cgi/content/ full/2002/12/30/5* Accessed 10/22/2004.

Federation of American Societies for Experimental Biology. Bethesda, MD. 37(3):1 Available at *http://www.faseb.org/opa/newsletter/6x04/june_ nl_web.pdf* Accessed October 22, 2004.

Finn, M. 2003. Stay Rates of Foreign Doctorate Recipients from U.S. Universities 2001. Oak Ridge Institute for Science and Education. Oak Ridge TN: Government Printing Office.

Freeman, R. B., et. al. 2001. Careers and rewards in bio sciences: the disconnect between scientific progress and career progression. The American Society for Cell Biology, August 2001. Available at: *http://www.ascb.org/newsroom/careers_rewards.pdf 1*. Accessed October 22, 2004.

Gentile, N. D., et al. 1987. Research Activity of Full-Time Faculty in Departments of Medicine: Final Report. Washington, D.C.: Association of Professors of Medicine and Association of American Medical Colleges.

Goldman, E. and E. Marshall. 2002. Research funding NIH grantees: where have all the young ones gone? Science 298:5591(October):40–41.

Government Accountability Office. 2004. *Border Security: Improvements Needed to Reduce Time Taken to Adjudicate Visas for Science Students and Scholars.* GAO-04-371 February 2004. Washington, D.C: Government Printing Office.

Grady P. A. Report to the nursing panel of the committee to monitoring the changing needs for biomedical and behavioral research personnel. August 5, 2003. Atlanta, GA.

Gray, M. L. and J. Bonventre. 2002. Training Ph.D. researchers to translate science to clinical medicine: closing the gap from the other side. Nature Medicine. May; 8(5):433–436.

Haden, N. K., R. G. Weaver, and R. W. Valachovic. 2002. Meeting the demand for future dental school faculty: trends, challenges, and responses. Journal of Dental Education 66(September):1102–1113.

Hinshaw, A. S. 2001. A continuing challenge: the shortage of educationally prepared nursing faculty. Online Journal of Issues in Nursing. Available at http://nursingworld.org/ojin/topic14/tpc14_3.htm. 6(January):3.

Hussey, P. S., et al. 2004, How does the quality of care compare in five countries? Health Affairs 23(3)89–111.

Institute of Medicine. 1994. Careers in Clinical Research: Obstacles and Opportunities. Washington, D.C.: National Academy Press.

Institute of Medicine. 1995. Health Services Research: Workforce and Educational Issues. Washington, D.C.: National Academy Press.

Institute of Medicine. 1997. The Lessons and the Legacy of the Pew Health Policy Program. Washington D.C.: National Academy Press.

Institute of Medicine. 1999. To Err Is Human: Building a Safer Health System. Washington D.C.: National Academy Press.

Institute of Medicine. 2001. Crossing the Quality Chasm: A New Health System for the 21st Century. Washington, D.C.: National Academy Press.

Institute of Medicine. 2004. Insuring America's Health: Principles and Recommendations. Washington, D.C.: The National Academies Press.

Ley, T. J. and L. E. Rosenberg 2002. Removing career obstacles for young physician-scientists—loan-repayment programs. The New England Journal of Medicine 346:368–372.

Lohr, K. N. and D. M. Steinwachs 2002. Health services research: an evolving definition of the field. Health Services Research 37(1):7–9.

Massy, W. F. and C. A. Goldman. 1995. The production and utilization of science and engineering doctorates in the United States. Stanford Institute for Higher Education Research Discussion Paper, Stanford, CA.

Massy, W. F. and C. A. Goldman, 2001. The PhD Factory. Boston, MA: Anker Publishing Company.

Massy, W. F., and C. A. Goldman, 1995. The Production and Utilization of Science and Engineering Doctorates in the United States. Stanford Institute for Higher Education Research Discussion Paper. Stanford, CA.

May, G. S. and D. E. Chubin. 2003. A retrospective on undergraduate engineering success for underrepresented minority students. Journal of Engineering Education 83(January):1–13.

McEwen, M., and G. Bechtel. 2000. Characteristics of nursing doctoral programs in the United States. Journal of Professional Nursing. 16(5):282-292.

McGlynn, E. A., et al. 2003. The quality of health care delivered to adults in the United States. New England Journal of Medicine 348:26(June): 2635–2645.

Nathan, D. G. 2002. Careers in translational clinical research—Historical perspectives, future challenges. Journal of the American Medical Association 287(18):2424–2427.

Nathan, D. G. and J. D. Wilson. 2003. Clinical Research and the NIH—A Report Card. The New England Journal of Medicine 349(19).

National Academies Workshop: Bridges to Independence: Fostering the Independence of New Investigators in the Life Sciences June 16, 2004. Washington, D.C. Available at *http://dels.nas.edu/bls/bridges.html*.

National Center for Health Statistics Health, United States. 2003. Online Health United States. Hyattsville, Maryland: Public Health Service. Table 27 p. 133. Available at *http://www.cdc.gov/nchs/data/hus/tables/2003/03hus027.pdf*. Accessed June 30, 2004.

National Institute for Mental Health. 2001. The numbers count: mental disorders in America: A summary of statistics describing the prevalence of mental disorders in America. Available at *http://www.nimh.nih.gov/publicat/numbers.cfm*. Accessed June 30, 2004.

National Institute for Nursing Research 2003. Research produces a successful school health promotion program to prevent cardiovascular disease-and the effects may last a lifetime, Making a Difference. Online. Available at *http//www.ninr.nih.gov/ninr/news-info/pubs/makinga difference.pdf*. Accessed May 18, 2004.

National Institute of General Medical Sciences. 1998. The Careers and Professional Activities of Graduates of the NIGMS Medical Scientist Training Program. Publication No. 93-4363. Bethesda, MD: NIH.

National Institutes of Health Office of Extramural Research. 2003. Data communicated August 4, 2003. Trends in training and fellowships—fiscal years 1976–2002.

National Institutes of Health. 1986. Effects of the National Research Service Award Program on Biomedical Research and Teaching Careers. Bethesda, MD:NIH.

National Institutes of Health. 1997. Director's Panel on Clinical Research. Report to the Advisory Committee to the NIH Director. Available on *http://www.nih.gov/news/crp/97report*. Accessed October 22, 2004.

National Institutes of Health. 1997. Implementing the Recommendations in the 1994 Report from the National Academy of Sciences: Meeting the Nation's Needs for Biomedical and Behavioral Scientists. Report to U.S. House of Representatives, Subcommittee on Labor, Health and Human Services, and Education, Committee on Appropriations. Bethesda, MD: NIH.

National Institutes of Health. 1998. The Early Career Progress of NRSA Predoctoral Trainees and Fellows. Bethesda, MD:NIH.

National Opinion Research Center. 2001. Survey of earned doctorates. Unpublished special reports generated for the American Association of Colleges of Nursing. Chicago, IL: AACN.

National Postdoctoral Association. Web site. Available at *http://www.nationalpostdoc.org/about/*. Accessed 10/22/2004.

National Research Council and Institute of Medicine 1995. Preventing HIV Transmission: The Role of Sterile Needles and Bleach. Washington, D.C.: National Academy Press.

National Research Council. 1975. Personnel Needs and Training for Biomedical and Behavioral Research. Washington, D.C.: National Academy Press.

National Research Council. 1975. Report of the committee on a feasibility study on national needs and training for biomedical and behavioral research personnel. Washington, D.C.: National Academy of Sciences.

National Research Council. 1976. Research Training and Career Patterns of Bioscientists: The Training Programs at the National Institutes of Health. Washington, D.C.: National Academy Press.

National Research Council. 1978. Personnel Needs and Training for Biomedical and Behavioral Research. Washington D.C.: National Academy Press.

National Research Council. 1994. The Funding of Young Investigators in the Biological and Biomedical Sciences. Washington, D.C.: National Academy Press, National Research Council.

National Research Council. 1995. Reshaping the Graduate Education of Scientists and Engineers. Washington, D.C.: National Academy Press.

National Research Council. 1996a. Understanding Risk: Informing Decisions in a Democratic Society. Washington, D.C.: National Academy Press.

National Research Council. 1996b. Understanding Violence Against Women. Washington, D.C.: National Academy Press.

National Research Council. 1998a. Preventing Reading Difficulties in Young Children. Washington, D.C.: National Academy Press.

National Research Council. 1998b. Protecting Youth at Work: Health, Safety, and Development of Working Children and Adolescents in the United States. Washington, D.C.: National Academy Press.

National Research Council. 1998c. Trends in the Early Careers of Life Scientists. Washington, D.C.: National Academy Press.

National Research Council. 1999. Work-Related Musculoskeletal Disorders. A Review of the Evidence; Work-Related Musculoskeletal Disorders Report. Workshop Summary, and Workshop Papers. Washington, D.C.: National Academy Press.

National Research Council. 2000a. Addressing the Nation's Changing Needs for Biomedical and Behavioral Scientists. Washington, D.C.: National Academy Press.

National Research Council. 2000b. Enhancing the Postdoctoral Experience for Scientists and Engineers. Washington D.C.: National Academy Press.

National Research Council. 2001a. Educating Children with Autism. Washington, D.C.: National Academy Press.

National Research Council. 2001b. Informing America's Policy on Illegal Drugs: What We Don't Know Keeps Hurting Us. Washington, D.C.: National Academy Press.

National Research Council. 2004a. Facilitating Interdisciplinary Research. Washington D.C.: The National Academies Press.

National Research Council. 2004b. Reducing Underage Drinking: A Collective Responsibility. Washington, D.C.: The National Academies Press.

National Research Council. 2005. Bridges to Independence: Fostering the Independence of New Investigators in Biomedical Research. Washington, D.C.: The National Academies Press.

National Science Foundation. 1997. Characteristics of Doctoral Scientists and Engineers in the United States: 1995. Division of Science Resources Studies, NSF 97-319. Arlington, VA.

National Science Foundation. 2002. Survey of Graduate Students and Postdoctorates in Science and Engineering: Division of Science Resources Statistics WebCASPAR Database. Available at *http://caspar. nsf.gov/TableBuilder;jsessionid=B9D03B124DD406744DB4355 BE3DB1C94.* Accessed October 22, 2004.

National Science Foundation. 2004. Research and Development in Industry, 1993 and Science and Engineering Indicators.

National Science Foundation. 2004. Survey of Industrial Research and Development: 1994. NSF 96-304 and National Science Foundation, InfoBrief: Industrial R&D Employment in the United States and U.S. Multinational Corporations, NSF 05-302, December.

Pion, G. M. 2000. Office of Extramural Research, National Institutes of Health. The Early Career Progress of NRSA Predoctoral Trainees and Fellows. Bethesda, MD: NIH.

Rapoport, A. 1999. Does the educational debt burden of science and engineering doctorates differ by race/ethnicity and sex? Division of Science Resources Studies Issue Brief. NSF 99-341 1999. Arlington, VA: National Science Foundation.

Regets, M. C. 1998. Has the use of postdocs changed? Division of Science Resources Studies Issue Brief. NSF 99-310 12/2/98. Arlington, VA: National Science Foundation.

Reinhardt, U. E., P. S. Hussey, and G. F. Anderson 2002. Cross-national comparisons of health systems using OECD data 1999. Health Affairs 21(3).

Rosenfield, P. L. 1992. The potential of transdisciplinary research for sustaining and extending linkages between the health and social science, Social Science & Medicine 35, 1343–1357.

Science: Next Wave. 2002. The Grant Doctor. Available at *http:// nextwave.sciencemag.org/cgi/content/full/2002/10/10/2.* and *http:// nextwave.sciencemag.org/cgi/content/full/2002/10/23/8.* Accessed 10/ 22/2004.

Shulman, L. E. 1996. Clinical Research 1996: Stirrings from the Academic Health Centers. Academic Medicine, 71(4):362–63, 398.

Sung, N. S., et al. 2003. Central challenges facing the national clinical research enterprise. Journal of the American Medical Association. 289(October):1278–1287.

Tabulations from the Higher Education Research Institute and the U.S. Department of Education.

Tsapogas, J. 2001. Retention of the Best Underrepresented Minority Graduates in Science and Engineering. Making Strides: Quarterly Research Newsletter. American Association for the Advancement of Science. 3(January):1–12.

U.S. Congress, 1976. Health Research and Health Services Amendments of 1976, H.R.7988: P.L. 94–278. 94th Cong., 2nd sess., 22 April 1976.

U.S. Congress, 1978. Health Services Research, Health Statistics, and Health Care Technology Act of 1978. P.L. 95-623, Section 3. 95th Cong., 2nd session, 9 November 1978.

U.S. Congress, 1985. Health Research Extension Act of 1985, P.L. 99–158. 99th Cong., 1st sess., 20 November 1985.

U.S. Congress, 1988. Health omnibus programs extension of 1988. P.L. 100–607. Title I, Section 151. Title VI, Section 635. 102 Statutes 3058, 3148. 100th Cong., 2nd sess., 4 November 1988.

U.S. Congress, 1993. National Institutes of Health Revitalization Act Of 1993. P.L. 103-43. Title XVI, Section 1601, 1602, 1632, 1641. Title XX, Section 2008(b)14. 107 Statutes 181, 186, 211. 103rd Congress, 10 June 1993.

U.S. Congress, Senate, 1973. Committee on Labor and Public Welfare. National Research Service Award Act of 1974. 93rd Cong., 1st sess., S. Rept. 93-381.

U.S. General Accounting Office, 1987. Division of Human Resources. Medical research: national research service awards for research in primary medical care. A report to the chairman, Subcommittee on Health and the Environment, and the Committee on Energy and Commerce. House of Representatives. Washington, D.C.: Government Printing Office.

U.S. Department of Education. 2000. Table 140. National Center for Education Statistics, Sources: High School and Beyond. First follow-up surveys: 1990 High School Transcript Study, and National Education Longitudinal Study of 1988, Second follow-up surveys: 1994 High School Transcript Study, and 1998 High School Transcript Study.

Weaver, R. G., K. Haden, and R. W. Valachovic. 2002. Annual ADEA survey of dental school seniors: 2001 graduating class. Journal of Dental Education 66(October):1209–1222.

Weaver, R. G., K. Haden, and R. W. Valachovic. 2002. Annual ADEA survey of dental school seniors: 2002 graduating class. Journal of Dental Education 66(December):1388–1404.

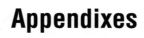

# Appendixes

# Appendix A

# Biographical Sketches of Committee and Panel Members

**Gordon G. Hammes, Ph.D. (Committee Chair), (NAS)** is the University Distinguished Service Professor of Biochemistry at Duke University. He joined the faculty at Duke in 1991 and served as Vice Chancellor for Medical Center Academic Affairs from 1991 to 1998. He was a faculty member at MIT and Cornell University prior to his appointment at Duke University. Dr. Hammes' awards and honors include an award in Biological Chemistry from the American Chemical Society (1967), Member of the National Academy of Sciences (1973), Member of the American Academy of Arts and Sciences (1974), National Institutes of Health Fogarty Scholar (1975–1976), and the 2002 William C. Rose award of the American Society for Biochemistry and Molecular Biology. He has published more than 225 scientific publications, including two books on chemical kinetics, a book on enzyme catalysis and regulation, a book on thermodynamics and kinetics for the biological sciences, and a book on spectroscopy for the biological sciences. Dr. Hammes received his doctorate in 1959 from the University of Wisconsin, Madison, and was a NSF Postdoctoral Fellow at the Max Plank Institute, Göttingen, Germany, from 1959 to 1960. During his professional career, Dr. Hammes has been involved in various education and training programs, was president of the American Society for Biochemistry and Molecular Biology, and served on NIH training grant and research panels.

**Michael M. E. Johns, M.D. (Committee Vice-Chair), (IOM)** is Executive Vice President for Health Affairs at Emory University, Director of the Robert W. Woodruff Health Sciences Center and Professor in the Department of Surgery, Emory University School of Medicine. He began his career in the Medical Corp of the U.S. Army as assistant chief of the Otolaryngology Service at Walter Reed Army Medical Center, 1975 to 1977. He joined the Department of Otolaryngology and Maxillofacial Surgery at the University of Virginia Medical Center in 1977 and moved to Johns Hopkins University as professor and chair of Otolaryngol-

ogy-Head and Neck Surgery in 1984. He served 6 years as Dean of the Johns Hopkins School of Medicine and Vice President for Medical Affairs at Johns Hopkins University. Dr. Johns is recognized for his work as a cancer surgeon of head and neck tumors and his studies of treatment outcomes. He is the editor of the *Archives of Otolaryngology* and serves on the editorial board of the *Journal of American Medical Association*. He is fellow of the American Association for the Advancement of Science. He is a member of the Institute of Medicine, and currently sits on the Council of the Institute of Medicine. He is a member of the National Research Council Governing Board, Chairman of the Association of Academic Health Centers, and is immediate past president of the American Board of Otolaryngology. Dr. Johns obtained his M.D. with honors from the University of Michigan Medical School. During his career, he has been actively involved in the development of educational programs, and was instrumental in the revamping of the Johns Hopkins medical school curriculum to meet changing health care needs. He has expert knowledge in the areas of health care research and in the special issues of clinical research.

**Richard Shiffrin, Ph.D., (Committee Vice-Chair), (NAS)** is a Distinguished Professor, and the Luther Dana Waterman Professor of Psychology at Indiana University. He joined the faculty at Indiana University after earning his doctorate in Experimental and Mathematical Psychology from Stanford University in 1969. During his tenure at Indiana University he has held visiting professorships at Rockefeller University, University of Queenstown, Brisbane, Australia; and University of Amsterdam, The Netherlands. Dr. Shiffrin has exploited an adroit combination of experimental discovery and mathematical models to initiate major new developments. His theories of short-term memory, of automatic and controlled processes in attention, and of the processes of retrieval from long-term memory have profoundly influenced the course of cognitive psychology. He is a member of the National Academy of Sciences and the American Academy of Arts and Sciences, and has served as officer of many professional societies. He is a Guggenheim Fellow, a Warren Medalist of the Society for Experimental Psychology, and has received the Rumelhart Prize for distinguished accomplishments in Cognitive Science. As a co-PI on an NIH NIMH training grant, he has the understanding and knowledge of NIH—NRSA training programs.

**Larry Bumpass, Ph.D. (NAS)** is Professor Emeritus of Sociology, and Co-Director of the National Survey of Families and Households. His research focuses on the social demography of the family, including cohabitation, marriage, the stability of unions, contraception and fertility, and the implications of these processes for children's living arrangements and subsequent life-course development. He is a member of the National Academy of Sciences. Dr. Bumpass holds a Ph.D. (1968) and an M.A. (1965) in Sociology from the University of Michigan. His knowledge of demographic methods and national databases contributed to the estimation of the current number of researchers in the three major areas, and in making projections about the future need for personnel.

**Christine K. Cassel, M.D., MACP (IOM)** is Dr. Cassel is President and CEO of the American Board of Internal Medicine and ABIM Foundation in Philadelphia. She is the former Dean of the School of Medicine and Vice President for Medical Affairs at Oregon Health and Science University in Portland, Oregon. She is a leading expert in geriatric medicine, medical ethics and quality of care. Among her many professional leadership positions, Dr. Cassel is immediate past-Chair of the ABIM Foundation Board of Trustees, served as Chair of the Board of the Greenwall Foundation, which supports work in bioethics; immediate past-President of the American Federation for Aging Research; and was a member of the Advisory Committee to the Director at the National Institutes of Health. She is a member of the Institute of Medicine Governing Council and has served on previous IOM committees responsible for influential reports on quality of care and medical errors, chaired a recent report on end-of-life care, and co-chaired a report on public health.

**William T. Greenough, Ph.D. (NAS)** is Swanlund Chair and Center for Advanced Study Director and Professor of Psychology at the University of Illinois in Urbana-Champaign. His research focuses on neural mechanisms of learning and memory; neurobiology of fragile X syndrome; mechanisms of brain-behavioral development; neurobiology of the aging process; recovery from developmental brain damage, and plasticity of metabolic support components of the brain. Dr. Greenough's awards and honors include AAAS fellow (1985), NIMH MERIT award (1989), member of the National Academy of Sciences (1992), Fragile X Foundation William Rosen Award for Outstanding Research (1998), University of Illinois Oakley-Kunde Award for Un-

dergraduate Teaching (1998), American Psychological Society William James Fellow Research Award (1998) and the American Psychological Association Distinguished Scientific Contribution Award (1999). He obtained his Ph.D. from the University of California at Los Angeles in 1969. He brought to the committee his knowledge of the neuropsychology and learning processes, which is an important area of NIH research. He also has a broad knowledge of training and research issues through his research support from the National Institute of Aging, National Institute of Mental Health, and National Institute on Alcohol Abuse and Alcoholism and his directorship of a pre- and postdoctoral training grant from NICHHD.

**James Jackson, Ph.D., (IOM)** is the Daniel Katz Distinguished University Professor of Psychology and Director of the Institute for Social Research at the University of Michigan at Ann Arbor. Dr. Jackson's Research efforts include carrying out a number of national and surveys of black populations focusing on issues of racial and ethnic influences on life course development, attitude change, reciprocity, social support, and coping and health. He obtained his Ph.D. in Social Psychology from Wayne State University. Dr. Jackson is a recognized authority on African American life, and currently has major grants from the National Institute of Mental Health and the National Institute on Aging to assess the physical, emotional, mental, and economic health of a nationally representative sample of more than 7,000 African American and Black Caribbean adults. He has expert knowledge of issues related to the underrepresentation of minority groups in biomedical, behavioral, and clinical research.

**Lynn Landmesser, Ph.D., (NAS)** is currently the Arline H. and Curtis F. Garvin Professors and chair of the Department of Neurosciences in the School of Medicine at Case Western Reserve University. She joined the Case Western Reserve faculty in 1993 as a professor in the Department of Neurosciences. She has also been a served as a faculty member at the University of Connecticut and Yale University. Her professional activities include, service as president of the Society for Developmental Biology and secretary of the Society for Neuroscience, president-elect of the Neuroscience Section of the American Association for the Advancement of Science, member of the National Advisory Council of the National Institute of Neurological Disorders and Stroke (NIH), and a fellow of the American Academy of Arts and Sciences. Her research, conducted over the past 30 years, has established basic principles of how nerve cells make accurate connections with other cells, such as muscles, skin or other neurons. She earned her Ph.D. in neurophysiology at the University of California in 1969 and received additional postdoctoral training in physiology at the University of Utah College of Medicine. She contributed valuable knowledge on research and training issues as the holder of two National Institutes of Health research awards and as the principal investigator on an NIH Predoctoral Neurosciences Training Grant and co-principal investigator on an NIH Developmental Biology Training Grant.

**William J. Lennarz, Ph.D., (NAS)** is the Distinguished Professor and Chairman of the Department of Biochemistry and Cell Biology at Stony Brook University, State University of New York. Dr. Lennarz' research focuses on the Biosynthesis of glycoproteins and the role of cell surface glycoproteins in fertilization and early development. Using the techniques of biochemistry, cell and developmental biology, and more recently, molecular biology, he has made contributions of great importance in biological science. These contributions have been in three principal areas: membrane structure and function; the structure, biosynthesis, and function of glycoproteins; and the role of cell surface proteins in fertilization and embryonic development. He is a member of the National Academy of Sciences and earned a Ph.D. from the University of Illinois. Dr. Lennarz is a department chair and researcher in a discipline in which a significant number of doctorates are training through the NRSA program.

**Joseph B. Martin, M.D., Ph.D., (IOM)** is Dean of the Harvard Faculty of Medicine. Prior to returning to the Harvard medical community in July of 1997, he served as Chancellor of the University of California, San Francisco for four years. Dr. Martin initially went to UCSF in 1989 as Dean of the School of Medicine. He began his academic career at McGill University where he became Chair of the Department of Neurology and Neurosurgery. Following his tenure at McGill University he joined the faculty of the Harvard Medical School in 1978 as Bullard Professor of Neurology and Chief of Neurology service at Massachusetts General Hospital. His research has focused on hypothalamic regulation of pituitary hormone secretions and on application of neurochemical and molecular genetics to better understand the causes of neurological and neurodegenerative disease. He is a member of the Institute of Medicine. He has served on the editorial boards of the *New England Journal of Medicine*, *Annals of Neurology*, and *Science*. He received his premedical and medical education at the University of Alberta, Edmonton, receiving the M.D. degree in 1962. He completed a residency in neurology in 1966 and fellowship in neuropathology in 1967 at Case Western Reserve University in Cleveland, Ohio, and earned his Ph.D. in anatomy from the University of Rochester in 1971. He has experience at UCSF and Harvard in the establishment of innovative programs of research and education and in investigating career options open to researchers in the biomedical, behavioral and clinical sciences.

**Barbara J. Meyer, Ph.D., (NAS)** is a Howard Hughes Medical Institute Investigator and Professor of Genetics and Development at the University of California at Berkeley. She received her Ph.D. training with Mark Ptashne at Harvard

University and her postdoctoral training with Sydney Brenner at the MRC Laboratory of Molecular Biology in Cambridge, UK, Prior to her current position, she was a tenured faculty member at MIT. Her research is directed toward understanding basic issues in development: how choices are made between alternative cell fates, how cells become restricted in developmental potential prior to differentiation, and how regulatory gene hierarchies control developmental decisions. She also investigates the control of X-chromosome-wide gene expression through the process of dosage compensation and its mechanistic link to higher-order chromatin structure and chromosome segregation during meiosis and mitosis. She is a member of the National Academy of Sciences and the American Academy of Arts and Sciences. She has experience in training issues as well as the perspective of a Howard Hughes Investigator in assessing the NRSA and other training programs at NIH.

**Georgine Pion, Ph.D.** is Research Associate Professor of Psychology and Human Development and Senior Fellow with the Vanderbilt Institute for Public Policy Studies at Vanderbilt University. She received her Ph.D. in social-environmental psychology from Claremont Graduate School in 1980 and did postdoctoral research training in the Division of Methodology and Evaluation Research at Northwestern University. She has served on committees involved in the evaluation of research and health professional training programs and gender differences in the career development of scientists for the National Research Council, the National Science Foundation, and the National Institute of Mental Health. In addition to conducting an evaluation of the NRSA predoctoral training program, she has been involved in several studies related to graduate education and the employment of new doctorates. An Associate of the National Academy of Sciences, she also received a Merit award from the National Institutes of Health for her work on a large-scale survey of NIH applicants and was awarded an Outstanding Leadership Award from Peabody College at Vanderbilt University. Currently, she is involved in directing an evaluation of the neuroscience peer review process at the NIH, evaluating the outcomes of new instructional strategies in biomedical engineering education, and assessing the outcomes of postdoctoral research training programs sponsored by the Burroughs Wellcome Fund and other foundations.

**Edward H. Shortliffe, M.D., Ph.D., (IOM)** is Deputy Vice President for Information Technology at Columbia University Medical Center and Professor and Chair of the Department of Biomedical Informatics at Columbia's College of Physicians and Surgeons. During the early 1970s, Dr. Shortliffe was principal developer of the medical expert system MYCIN. He also spearheaded the formation of Stanford University's graduate degree program in medical informatics. He served as Principal Investigator for Stanford's SUMEX-AIM and CAMIS Computing Resources, which shared research facilities that supported medical informatics research and training from the early 1970s until 1997. Dr. Shortliffe is a member of the Institute of Medicine, American Society for Clinical Investigation, American College of Medical Informatics, American College of Physicians (Master), Association of American Physicians, American Association for Artificial Intelligence (Fellow), American Institute for Medical and Biological Engineering, and the American Clinical and Climatological Association. He has a broad range of interests in biomedical informatics, especially decision-support systems, integrated workstations for clinicians, and web-based information dissemination. Education and training in the field are of particular concern. He received his M.D. from Stanford University School of Medicine in 1976, and in 1975 he earned his Ph.D. in Medical Information Sciences from Stanford University. His expertise was used in guiding the analysis of data for this study and in addressing education and training issues in the clinical sciences.

## DENTAL PANEL

**Robert J. Genco, D.D.S., Ph.D. (Panel Chair), (IOM),** is a currently Distinguished Professor in the Department of Oral Biology, School of Dental Medicine, and in the Department of Microbiology, School of Medicine and Biomedical Sciences University at Buffalo, State University of New York. He has served as Chair of the Department of Oral Biology and Provost at the University at Buffalo, State University of New York. He is currently Vice President for Research (Interim) and Director of the Office of Science, Technology Transfer, and Economic Outreach (STOR). He is the Editor-in-Chief of the Journal of Periodontology and Annals of Periodontology. He received his D.D.S., cum laude, from the State University of New York at Buffalo School of Dentistry, 1963. He also received a Ph.D. from the University of Pennsylvania, in Microbiology and Immunology in 1967, and he completed residency training in Periodontology at the University of Pennsylvania in 1967. Dr. Genco's recognition includes: Basic Research in Oral Science Award (IADR), Deans Medal, George Thorn Award, Research in Periodontal Disease Award (IADR), and Gold Medal for Excellence in Research (American Dental Association). Dr. Genco has over 315 publications and has edited 11 books or Proceedings of Symposia, and has been awarded 9 patents. His current research areas include tissue engineering; developing regenerative procedures using growth factors and other materials for regeneration of osseous tissues; and a series of studies on the effects of infectious diseases and inflammatory mediators on atherosclerotic diseases, and diabetes and its complications. Dr. Genco has been a member of the Institute of Medicine since 1988.

**Charles N. Bertolami, D.D.S., D.Med.Sc.** is Dean of the School of Dentistry at the University of California, San Fran-

cisco where he has served in this capacity since 1995. He has served as president of the American Association for Dental Research (2003–03) and is a nationally recognized expert in the field of connective tissue repair and treatment disorders of the temporomandibular joint. Dr. Bertolami is a member of several editorial boards, including the *Journal of Oral and Maxillofacial Surgery,* and he has more than 25 years of experience with and commitment to the oral health community. He is a diplomat of the American Board of Oral and Maxillofacial Surgeons, a fellow of the American College of Dentists and a fellow of the International College of Dentists. He received his D.D.S. degree, summa cum laude, from Ohio State University in1974 and his Doctor of Medical Sciences degree from Harvard in 1979. He served as chief resident at the Massachusetts General Hospital where he did his residency training in oral and maxillofacial surgery. In national and oral health community service, Dr. Bertolami co-chaired the NIDCR Blue Ribbon Panel on Research Training and Career Development (2000) and the NIDCR Workshop on Biometrics, Tissue Engineering and Biomaterials (1998). He served as a member of the dental panel for the Committee on Monitoring the Changing Needs for Biomedical Research Personnel of the National Research Council/The National Academies.

**Chester Douglass, D.M.D., Ph.D.** is Professor and Chair of the Department of Oral Health Policy and Epidemiology in the Harvard School of Dental Medicine and Professor of Epidemiology in the Harvard School of Public Health where he is Director of the Harvard University Oral Epidemiology Doctoral Training Program. Currently, Dr. Douglass is the principal investigator of an NIH study relating water fluoridation and topical fluoride use to the occurrence of osteosarcoma. This national collaborative study is coordinating data collection efforts in ten orthopedic surgery departments throughout the United States. Other major epidemiological studies in which this program is participating include the International Collaborative Study of Children's Dental Caries. Dr. Douglass also presently serves as the Chief of Service for Dentistry and Oral Surgery in the Cambridge (Massachusetts) Health Alliance which includes 3 hospitals, 2 health departments, and 21 ambulatory care centers in Cambridge, Somerville, and Everett, Massachusetts. A major component of Professor Douglass' research over the past decade has been the development of methods for combining epidemiological data, demographic trends and patient utilization behavior to document current movements and future expectations regarding the need and demand for dental services. Contrary to initial expectations during the early 1980s of reduced need, his analyses have instead demonstrated that the use of dental services increased during the 1980s and 1990s and that this trend should continue well into the 21st century. His application of behavioral, epidemiological and public health data to this problem was the first to demonstrate the impact of the aging population on future dental caries and periodontal disease patterns.

**Marjorie K. Jeffcoat, D.M.D.,** is Dean and Professor of Periodontics at the University of Pennsylvania School of Dental Medicine. Dr. Jeffcoat is the school's first woman dean and the eleventh in its 125-year history. Prior to her appointment with Penn Dental in July 2003, Dr. Jeffcoat served as Assistant Dean of Research and Professor and Chair of the Department of Periodontics at the University of Alabama at Birmingham School of Dentistry. A 1976 graduate of the Harvard School of Dental Medicine, Dr. Jeffcoat also taught periodontology there for 10 years. Among her national committee posts, Dr. Jeffcoat is currently a member of the National Institutes of Health-NIDCR Advisory Committee for Research on Women's Health, the National Institutes for Dental Research National Advisory Committee, and the American Academy of Periodontology Clinical Trials Committee, the Academy of Osseointegration Board of Directors, and the International Association for Dental Research Board of Directors. In addition, Dr. Jeffcoat is president of the Academy of Osseointegration and a past president of both the American Association for Dental Research and the International Association for Dental Research. Dr. Jeffcoat also serves on the editorial boards of the *Journal of Periodontology*, the *Current Opinion in Dentistry*, and the *Journal of Periodontal Research*, and from 2001–2004, was editor of the *Journal of the American Dental Association*.

## NURSING PANEL

**Ada Hinshaw Ph.D., (Panel Chair), (IOM),** is a nationally recognized contributor to nursing research, and is Dean and Professor at the University of Michigan School of Nursing. Before coming to the University of Michigan, Dr. Hinshaw was the first permanent director of the National Institute of Nursing Research (NINR) at the National Institutes of Health in Bethesda, Maryland. Dr. Hinshaw led the Institute in its support of valuable research and training in many areas of nursing science, such as disease prevention, health promotion, acute and chronic illness, and the environments that enhance nursing care patient outcomes. Her current research involves an anticipated turnover study for nursing staff and the validity of ratio scales for subjective nursing concepts. From 1975 to 1987, Dr. Hinshaw served as Director of Research and Professor at the University of Arizona College of Nursing in Tucson, and as Director of Nursing Research at the University Medical Center's Department of Nursing. She has also held faculty positions at the University of California, San Francisco, and the University of Kansas. Dr. Hinshaw received her Ph.D. and M.A. in Sociology from the University of Arizona, an MSN from Yale University, and a B.S. from the University of Kansas. Her major fields of study included maternal-newborn health, clinical nursing and nursing administration, and instrument development and testing.

She was Vice Chair of the Keeping Patients Safe: Transforming the Work Environment of Nurses IOM Committee on the Patient Safety Board on Health Care Services. Dr. Hinshaw currently serves on the 2003 Institute of Medicine Council and has been a member of the Institute of Medicine since 1989.

**Sue Karen Donaldson, Ph.D., (IOM)** is a Professor of Physiology at The John Hopkins University School of Medicine and is Dean and Professor of Nursing at the School of Nursing. She received her Ph.D. from the University of Washington and her MSN from Wayne State University. Her areas of scholarly expertise and interest are biophysics, physiology and muskuloskeletal diseases. Dr. Donaldson has been a member of the Institute of Medicine since 1993.

**Margaret McLean Heitkemper, R.N., Ph.D., FAAN** is Chairperson, Department of Biobehavioral Nursing and Health Systems, School of Nursing, Corbally Professor in Public Service, and Adjunct Professor, Division of Gastroenterology, School of Medicine, University of Washington. She is also Director of the NIH/NINR-funded Center for Women's Health and Gender Research at the University of Washington and Director of an NCCAM supported Educational Program. Dr. Heitkemper received her BSN in 1973 from Seattle University, her MN in gerontological nursing from the University of Washington in 1975, and her Ph.D. in Physiology and Biophysics from the University of Illinois in 1981. Her research related to women's health, stress, and gastrointestinal function has been continuously funded by NIH since 1983. She is the author of two nursing textbooks and approximately 100 data-based papers. In 2003, Dr. Heitkemper received the AGA/Janssen award for research in gastroenterology.

**Marla Salmon, Ph.D., (IOM)** is Dean and Professor of the Nell Hodgson Woodruff School of Nursing, and Director of the Lillian Carter Center for International Nursing, at Emory University. She formerly served as Director of the Division of Nursing for the U.S. Department of Health and Human Services and as Chair of the Global Advisory Group on Nursing and Midwifery for the World Health Organization. Dr. Salmon's research interests have included health policy, administration, and national and international health workforce development, with particular emphasis on the importance of nursing and public health. She is a member of the Institute of Medicine, member of the Board of Trustees of the Robert Wood Johnson Foundation, and the Board of Directors of the National Center for Healthcare Leadership and is both nationally and internationally recognized for her contributions to health policies influencing health care delivery systems. Dr. Salmon is a Fellow in the American Academy of Nursing and has received numerous awards, including the Presidential Meritorious Executive Award and the U.S. Public Health Special Service Award.

# Appendix B

# Ruth L. Kirschstein National Research Service Award Training Grants and Fellowships

The National Institutes of Health (NIH), the Agency for Health Care Policy and Research, and the Health Resources and Services Administration provide predoctoral and post-doctoral research training support through a number of National Research Service Award (NRSA) programs. At each level the programs are distinguished by whether they are made directly to individuals, who use the support at an institution of their choice, or to institutions, which in turn make awards to individuals in their programs. The following is a list of programs encompassed by the NRSA.

## INDIVIDUAL AWARDS

### National Research Service Award Individual Predoctoral Fellowships (F30)

The National Institute of Mental Health, the National Institute on Drug Abuse, the National Institute on Alcohol Abuse and Alcoholism, and the National Institute of Environmental Health Sciences provide NRSA predoctoral training to individuals working toward the combined M.D./Ph.D. degree. This fellowship program is designed to help ensure that highly trained physician-scientists will be available in adequate numbers and in the appropriate research areas and fields to meet the nation's mental health, drug abuse and addiction, alcohol abuse and alcoholism, and environmental health sciences research needs. In addition, this mechanism has the potential to train clinical investigators who wish to focus their research endeavors on patient-oriented studies.

### National Research Service Awards Individual Predoctoral Fellowships (F31)

This fellowship program is directed at the following different groups:

- **The National Research Service Award Predoctoral Fellowship for Minority Students.** This award provides up to five years of support for research training leading to the Ph.D. or equivalent research degree, the combined M.D./Ph.D. degree, or other combined professional degree and research doctoral degree in biomedical, behavioral, or health services research. These fellowships are designed to enhance the racial and ethnic diversity of the biomedical, behavioral, and health services research labor force in the United States. Accordingly, academic institutions are encouraged to identify and recruit students from underrepresented racial and ethnic groups who can apply for this fellowship. Support is NOT available for individuals enrolled in medical or other professional schools UNLESS they are also enrolled in a combined professional doctorate/Ph.D. degree program in biomedical, behavioral, or health services research.

- **The NRSA Predoctoral Fellowship for Students with Disabilities.** This award provides up to five years of support for research training leading to the Ph.D. (or equivalent research degree) or the combined M.D./Ph.D. degree (or other combined professional research doctoral degrees) in the biomedical or behavioral sciences. The intent of this predoctoral fellowship program is to encourage students with disabilities to seek graduate degrees and thus further the goal of increasing the number of scientists with disabilities who are prepared to pursue careers in biomedical and behavioral research.

- **The NRSA Individual Predoctoral Fellows.** This fellowship award is provided by the National Institute on Alcohol Abuse and Alcoholism, the National Institute on Deafness and Other Communication Disorders, the National Institute on Drug Abuse, the National Institute of Mental Health, and the National Institute of Neurological Disorders and Stroke. These institutes award NRSA individual predoctoral fellowships (F31) to promising applicants with the potential to become productive, independent investigators in the scientific mission areas of these institutes. This program will provide predoctoral training support for doctoral candidates who have successfully completed their comprehensive examinations or the equivalent by the time of the award and will be performing dissertation research and training.

## National Research Service Award Individual Postdoctoral Fellowship (F32)

This fellowship is designed to provide individuals who have received a Ph.D., M.D., D.O., D.C., D.D.S., D.V.M., O.D., D.P.M., Sc.D., Eng.D., Dr. P.H., D.N.S., N.D., Pharm.D., D.S.W., Psy.D., or equivalent degree with postdoctoral training that broadens their scientific background and promises applicants the potential to become productive, independent investigators in fields related to the mission of the NIH constituent institutes and centers. Research is to be conducted at a sponsoring institution under the direction of an individual who will serve as a mentor and who will supervise the training and research experience. Individuals may receive up to three years of aggregate NRSA support at the postdoctoral level, including any combination of support from institutional training grants and individual fellowship awards.

## National Research Service Award Senior Postdoctoral Fellowship (F33)

The NIH awards NRSA senior fellowships to experienced scientists who wish to make major changes in the direction of their research careers or broaden their scientific background by acquiring new research capabilities. These awards will enable individuals with at least seven years of research experience beyond the doctorate, and who have progressed to the stage of independent investigator, to take time from regular professional responsibilities for the purpose of receiving training to increase their scientific capabilities. In most cases this award is used to support sabbatical experiences for established independent scientists. This program is not designed for postdoctoral-level investigators seeking to prove their research potential prior to independence. Senior fellowship support may be requested for a period of up to two years. However, no individual may receive more than three years of aggregate NRSA support at the postdoctoral level, including any combination of support from institutional and individual awards.

## Minority Access to Research Careers Faculty Fellowships (F34)

These fellowships are for advanced research training of selected faculty members at eligible institutions, in which student enrollments are drawn substantially from minority groups.

## Intramural National Research Service Award Postdoctoral Fellowships (F35)

The purpose of these fellowships is to allow physicians, dentists, and veterinarians with limited research experience an opportunity to prepare for careers in biomedical or behav-

ioral laboratory research through training on the NIH campus.

## INSTITUTIONAL AWARDS

### National Research Service Award Institutional Training Grants (T32)

The institutional research training grants provide support to training programs at institutions of higher education and are designed to allow the director of the program to select the trainees and develop a curriculum of study and research experiences necessary to provide high-quality research training. The grant offsets the cost of stipends and tuition support for the appointed trainees. The following types of training can be supported by this grant:

- **Predoctoral Training.** Predoctoral research training leads to the Ph.D. degree or a comparable research doctoral degree. Students enrolled in health professional training programs who wish to postpone their professional studies in order to engage in full-time research training may also be appointed to an institutional research training grant. Predoctoral research training emphasizes fundamental training in areas of biomedical and behavioral sciences. Awards may not be used to support studies leading to the M.D., D.O., D.D.S., or a similar professional degree unless the trainee is enrolled in a combined-degree (e.g., M.D./Ph.D.) program. In addition, they may not be used to support residencies or other nonresearch clinical training.
- **Postdoctoral Training.** Postdoctoral research training is for individuals who have received a Ph.D., D.V.M, D.D.S., M.D., or comparable doctoral degree from an accredited domestic or foreign institution. Research training at the postdoctoral level must emphasize specialized training to meet national research priorities in the biomedical, behavioral, or clinical sciences. Research training grants are a mechanism for the postdoctoral training of physicians and other health professionals who may have extensive clinical training but limited research experience. For such individuals the training may be a part of a research degree program. In all cases, postdoctoral trainees should agree to engage in at least two years of research, research training, or comparable activities beginning at the time of appointment. It has been shown that the duration of training is strongly correlated with retention in posttraining research activity.
- **Short-Term Research Training for Health Professional Students.** Applications for institutional research training grants may include a request for short-term predoctoral positions reserved specifically to provide full-time, health-related research training experiences during the summer or other off-quarter periods. Such positions are limited to medical students, dental students, students in other health professional programs, and graduate students in the physical

or quantitative sciences. Short-term appointments are intended to provide such students with opportunities to participate in biomedical and/or behavioral research in an effort to attract them to health-related research careers. Short-term positions should be requested in the application and approved at the time of award. Normally, short-term positions are not to be used for individuals who have already earned a doctoral degree. Short-term research training positions should last at least 8 but no more than 12 weeks. Individual health professional students or students in the quantitative sciences selected for appointment should be encouraged to obtain multiple periods of short-term, health-related research training during the years leading to their degree. Such appointments may be consecutive or may be reserved for summers or other off-quarter periods. It should be noted that not all NIH institutes and centers permit short-term positions. Applicants interested in such positions should contact the awarding institute or center prior to completing their application.

## Minority Access to Research Careers (MARC) Undergraduate Institutional Grants (T34)

The MARC Branch of the Division of Minority Opportunity in Research of the National Institute of General Medical Sciences provides awards for biomedical research to selected institutions to support the undergraduate education of minority students who can compete successfully for entry into graduate programs leading to a Ph.D. degree in the biomedical or behavioral sciences. Biomedical research includes such areas as cell biology, biochemistry, physiology, pharmacology, genetics, and behavioral research as well as the more quantitative areas such as mathematics, physics, chemistry, and computer sciences, necessary to analyze biological phenomena. The MARC Undergraduate Student Training in Academic Research (U-STAR) program supports institutional training grants for underrepresented minority junior and senior honors students in any of the above-cited science areas to improve their preparation for graduate training in the biomedical/behavioral sciences. In addition,

MARC U-STAR grants provide an allowable cost support to improve the research training environment for MARC trainees and pre-MARC students (freshmen and sophomores) and science faculty development at MARC-supported institutions. Currently, progress in many subdisciplines in the biological sciences (e.g., structural biology, bioinformatics, modeling of complex systems, population genetics, evolution) is dependent on the use of information and methodologies from diverse disciplines of science such as mathematics, biophysics, computer science, and engineering. Thus, the MARC U-STAR program specifically encourages the development of pedagogical tools for incorporating quantitative concepts, computational skills, and principles of modeling complex biological phenomena in pre-MARC and MARC student science curricula. To this end, the MARC U-STAR program will also provide funds for the development of needed course materials for the curricular changes proposed, as well as for faculty training required for introducing the use of such materials in the different science courses.

## Short-Term Training Awards (T35)

NRSA Short-Term Institutional Research Training Grants (T35) are made to eligible institutions to develop or enhance research training opportunities for individuals interested in careers in biomedical and behavioral research. Many of the NIH institutes and centers use this grant mechanism exclusively to support intensive, short-term research training experiences for students in health professional schools during the summer. In addition, the Short-Term Institutional Research Training Grant can be used to support other types of predoctoral and postdoctoral training in focused, often emerging, scientific areas relevant to the mission of the NIH funding institute or center. The proposed training must be in either basic or clinical aspects of the health-related sciences. The training should be of sufficient depth to enable the trainees, upon completion of the program, to have a thorough exposure to the principles underlying the conduct of research.

# Appendix C

# Classification of Ph.D. Fields

## C-1. CLASSIFICATION OF BASIC BIOMEDICAL SCIENCES PH.D. FIELDS

Anatomy
Bacteriology
Biochemistry
Bioinformatics
Biological Immunology
Biological Sciences, General
Biological Sciences, Other
Biomedical Engineering
Biomedical Sciences
Biophysics
Biotechnology Research
Cell Biology
Developmental Biology/Embryology
Endocrinology
Genetics, Human and Animal
Medicinal/Pharmaceutical Chemistry
Microbiology
Molecular Biology
Neuroscience
Nutritional Sciences
Parasitology
Pathology, Human and Animal
Pharmacology, Human and Animal
Physiology
Toxicology
Veterinary Medicine
Zoology

## C-2. CLASSIFICATION OF PH.D. FIELDS IN THE BEHAVIORAL AND SOCIAL SCIENCES

Anthropology
Audiology and Speech Pathology
Demography/Population Studies
Sociology

## Psychology

Clinical
Cognitive and Psycholinguistics
Comparative
Developmental and Child
Educational
Experimental
Industrial and Organizational
Personality
Psychology, General
Psychology, Other
Psychometrics
Physiological/Psychobiology
Quantitative
Social

## C-3. CLASSIFICATION OF PH.D. FIELDS IN THE CLINICAL SCIENCES

Biometrics and Biostatistics
Environmental Health
Epidemiology
Exercise Physiology/Science
Health Sciences, General
Health Sciences, Other
Health Systems/Services Administration
Nursing
Pharmacy
Public Health
Rehabilitation/Therapeutic Services
Physicians in Academic Departments of Schools of
    Medicine

# Appendix D

# Demographic Projections of the Research Workforce, 2001–2011

Are universities educating enough research scientists in the biomedical, clinical, and behavioral fields, or are they educating too many or, perhaps, too few? These questions underlie this attempt to project the research workforce. To determine how this workforce will grow, projections are created by taking the current workforce data in these fields and extrapolating over 10 years. Then this projected workforce is compared with estimates of the demand for future researchers.

This analysis only deals with the workforce in the aggregate form looking at the major fields of biomedical, clinical, and behavioral research and does not seek to provide complete answers. In particular, it does not tell whether the workforce will be adequate in specific disciplines. It says nothing about the quality of the workforce, although that is a critical variable. It can be used to evaluate projected quantity in relation to the expected numbers of positions, which could be altered were it essential to national goals.

A demographic model for the current workforce in each field is created by adding graduates year by year (these numbers are estimated with regression models based on data from past decades) and then subtracting retirees and decedents. From these calculations a picture of how the workforce may evolve is developed. Provision is also made in the model for immigrants who arrive with Ph.D.s in these fields, who move from employment to unemployment and back, and for graduate students, who take nonscience jobs and possibly move into science jobs late. The original model is described fully in Appendix D of the last report on the scientific workforce in these fields, *Addressing the Nation's Changing Needs for Biomedical and Behavioral Scientists* (National Research Council, 2000).[1] For this report, the model has been updated with new data and the addition of new groups.

This appendix will address the following issues:

1. fields covered and the data used: more than those in the previous application of the model;
2. current workforce: its components and characteristics, with some attention to recent trends and how they might be extrapolated;
3. workforce projections: over a decade; and
4. parallel projections of research positions: by sector that may become available.

## COVERAGE AND DATA

For this report the definition of the behavioral field has been expanded to include clinical psychologists—a substantial expansion which means that current results for this field cannot be compared with previous results because the projections for 1995–2005 in the previous report did not include this category. The major field of clinical research was also added and includes Ph.D.s in clinical areas (except psychology) and M.D.s engaged in clinical research. Data for the clinical Ph.D.s are available from the same sources as for biomedical and behavioral Ph.D.s. For the M.D.s, only limited data are available; thus, it is only possible to speculate about orders of magnitude.

The disciplines included in biomedical and behavioral sciences include fields from anatomy to zoology; the behavioral sciences cover psychology, sociology, anthropology, demography, and speech-language pathology and audiology. The clinical sciences include all medical disciplines that are not considered biomedical. These categories have not changed from those covered in the previous report except for the addition of clinical psychology in the behavioral sciences.

Data on the U.S.-trained Ph.D. workforce in these fields were obtained from the Survey of Doctorate Recipients (SDR), a longitudinal biennial survey. Data on graduates were obtained from the Survey of Earned Doctorates—an

---

[1]National Research Council. 2000. Addressing the Nation's Changing Needs for Biomedical and Behavioral Scientists. Committee on National Needs for Biomedical and Behavioral Scientists, Education and Career Studies Unit, Office of Scientific and Engineering Personnel. Washington, D.C.: National Academy Press

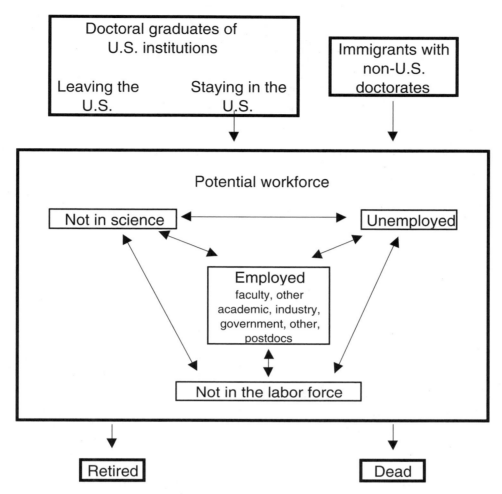

FIGURE D-1 The potential research workforce.

annual, virtually complete census of doctoral graduates in the United States.[2] Data on foreign-trained Ph.Ds in the United States were obtained from the National Survey of College Graduates—rounds of this survey were conducted in 1993, 1995, 1997, and 1999, following up the migrants originally identified in the 1990 census. For clinical M.D.s, data were gleaned from the national roster of medical school faculty from the American Association of Medical Colleges (AAMC). These AAMC data allow some inferences about numbers of researchers, but projections are generally not possible. Therefore issues relating to this group are discussed further below.

---

[2]See Appendix D in *Addressing the Nation's Changing Needs for Biomedical and Behavioral Scientists* (National Research Council 2000a) for more details on these surveys.

## CURRENT WORKFORCE AND RECENT TRENDS

The active workforce of Ph.D. and M.D. researchers includes all those employed in research. The potential workforce is broader and includes those unemployed, those neither employed nor looking for work (provided they are not retired), and those with jobs outside science (see Figure D-1). Some proportion of each of these groups returns to the active research workforce every year.

To avoid confusion, the term "employed" is used instead of "active workforce" and refers to those employed in science jobs. Those employed in nonscience jobs are not counted in the employed group but are referred to as being outside science. The unemployed and those not in the labor force are referred to together as "not working" and combined with those outside science as "not active" in research.

The potential workforce is incremented—in this model on an annual basis—by entering graduates and migrants with

## BOX D-1
## How Accurate Were Previous Projections?

Are the previous projections, for 1995–2005, consistent with current workforce data? The answer to this question is limited by the following:

- 2001 is the last date for which reported data are available at this writing.
- Biomedical researchers only are included because the definition of behavioral researchers has changed and clinical researchers were not previously projected.
- U.S.-trained researchers only are included because (as is discussed below) there is no solid current data on the foreign-trained postdoctorates for comparison purposes.
- Those employed outside science who were not previously counted in the potential workforce are excluded.

To make the comparison, the earlier projections are rerun excluding the foreign-trained researchers but not changing any other assumptions.

The projections, shown in Table D-A, up to 2001 for male and female biomedical researchers were 2-3 percent too low. By comparison with actual growth, this is not a large error. For males the error is smaller than growth in the workforce between 2000 and 2001; and, for females only a sixth of 2000-2001 growth. The error is also small relative to the uncertain number of foreign-trained researchers in the workforce. Nevertheless as small as this error is, it is not easy to explain.

Looking at the number of graduates, the most important component of the projections, it can be seen that the medium projection

TABLE D-A Comparison of Projected with Reported 2001 Workforce in Biomedical Research

| Biomedical researchers | Males | Females |
| --- | --- | --- |
| Reported, excluding nonscience employment | 71,209 | 33,988 |
| Projected from 1995 | 76,604 | 37,455 |
| Projected excluding migrants | 68,956 | 33,350 |
| Ratio of projected (without migrants) to reported | 0.968 | 0.981 |

SOURCE: Addressing the Nation's Changing Needs for Biomedical and Behavioral Scientists. Washington, D.C.: National Academy Press (National Research Council 2000a); and the National Science Foundation Survey of Doctorate Recipients

from 1995 did not capture the fluctuations in reported numbers but is reasonably close. The estimates of male graduates are slightly too high rather than too low.

Another possible explanation for projection error has to do with stay rates, the proportions of graduates assumed to stay and work in the U.S., based on their stated intentions. The 1995 projections assumed constant stay rates, whereas rates actually rose, so that by the year 2001 males were 93 percent instead of the projected 90 percent. This still would not account for more than a quarter of the error. Other possibilities may include retirement or death rates being slightly too high, relatively too much assumed movement toward jobs outside science, or even errors in the data (such as errors in age distribution) that could affect projections. Because the projections seem generally accurate, many of these errors, if they exist, probably cancel each other out.

doctoral degrees. It is decremented by retirements and deaths. Movements within the workforce are also modeled, such as those between employment and unemployment. The most common movements are those in both directions between science employment and nonscience employment.

The biomedical and behavioral fields include only Ph.D.s. The clinical field includes Ph.D.s and M.D.s. The distinction between Ph.D.s and M.D.s is relevant partly for methodological reasons as the kinds of data available for each are quite different. Therefore, these groups are discussed sepa-

rately. Similarly, a distinction between U.S.-trained and foreign-trained researchers is important because the types of data differ.

The components of the current potential workforce, as illustrated in Figure D-1, are given in the following order: U.S.-trained Ph.D. researchers; M.D. researchers; foreign-trained Ph.D. researchers; entrants into the workforce, meaning migrants and graduates; and movements within the workforce and exits from it. Current levels as well as recent trends that suggest possible approaches to projection are

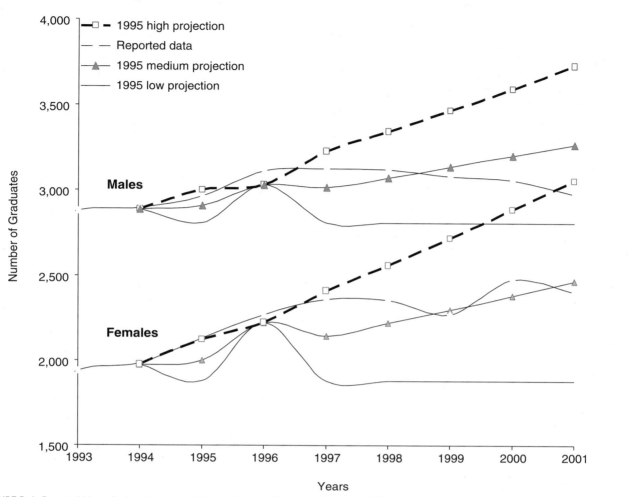

FIGURE D-A Reported biomedical graduates and high, medium, and low projections from 1995, by sex.
SOURCE: *Addressing the Nation's Changing Needs for Biomedical and Behavioral Scientists*. Washington, D.C.: National Academy Press (National Research Council 2000a); and the National Science Foundation Survey of Doctorate Recipients.

taken into consideration in the discussion. The characteristics of each group will be addressed below.

## U.S.-Trained Ph.D. Workforce

### Numbers

Table D-1 shows the U.S.-trained potential workforce of Ph.D.s in 2001 as determined from the Survey of Doctoral Recipients. The size of the workforce is essentially equal in both the biomedical and behavioral fields, at 113,000 to 114,000 each, but much smaller in the clinical field, at 19,100. Between 87 and 90 percent of the potential workforce in each major field is employed in science, and 7 to 9 percent have jobs outside science. Nonscience jobs are more common among behavioral scientists than the other two groups. Those who are not working, whether they are unemployed or simply not looking for work, comprise 3 to 5 percent in each field. The numbers of Ph.D.s not working are

TABLE D-1 Potential Workforce of U.S.-Trained Ph.D. Graduates in Three Major Fields, by Employment Status and Sex, 2001

| Field and employment status | Number | | | % of Workforce | | |
|---|---|---|---|---|---|---|
| | Males | Females | Total | Males | Females | Total |
| **Biomedical** | | | | | | |
| Potential workforce | 75,866 | 37,422 | 113,288 | 67.0 | 33.0 | 100.0 |
| Employed | 69,156 | 31,106 | 100,262 | 61.0 | 27.5 | 88.5 |
| Postdoctorates | 6,342 | 5,338 | 11,680 | 5.6 | 4.7 | 10.3 |
| Unemployed | 713 | 306 | 1,019 | 0.6 | 0.3 | 0.9 |
| Not in labor force[a] | 1,340 | 2,576 | 3,916 | 1.2 | 2.3 | 3.5 |
| Out of science | 4,657 | 3,434 | 8,091 | 4.1 | 3.0 | 7.1 |
| **Clinical** | | | | | | |
| Potential workforce | 8,149 | 10,956 | 19,105 | 42.7 | 57.3 | 100.0 |
| Employed | 7,526 | 9,654 | 17,180 | 39.4 | 50.5 | 89.9 |
| Postdoctorates | 136 | 279 | 415 | 0.7 | 1.5 | 2.2 |
| Unemployed | 3 | 124 | 127 | 0.0 | 0.6 | 0.7 |
| Not in labor force[a] | 74 | 330 | 404 | 0.4 | 1.7 | 2.1 |
| Out of science | 546 | 848 | 1,394 | 2.9 | 4.4 | 7.3 |
| **Behavioral and Social** | | | | | | |
| Potential workforce | 59,175 | 54,822 | 113,997 | 51.9 | 48.1 | 100.0 |
| Employed | 52,606 | 46,540 | 99,146 | 46.1 | 40.8 | 87.0 |
| Postdoctorates | 759 | 1,377 | 2,136 | 0.7 | 1.2 | 1.9 |
| Unemployed | 280 | 509 | 789 | 0.2 | 0.4 | 0.7 |
| Not in labor force[a] | 647 | 2,771 | 3,418 | 0.6 | 2.4 | 3.0 |
| Out of science | 5,642 | 5,002 | 10,644 | 4.9 | 4.4 | 9.3 |

[a]Not employed, not looking for work, but not retired.

SOURCE: National Science Foundation Survey of Doctorate Recipients.

higher among women: 2 to 3 percent of the total workforce compared to less than 2 percent of men.

## Trends

Over the past three decades, the U.S.-trained workforce in each field has grown steadily. From 1973–2001, the average annual workforce growth rates have been 4.1 percent for biomedical researchers, 6.8 percent for clinical researchers, and 4.8 percent for behavioral researchers (see Figure D-2). Growth in employment outside science has contributed to this (see Figure D-3). When only those employed in science are considered, growth rates would be 0.2 to 0.5 percentage points lower. More recently, from 1991 to 2001, growth rates were lower for the workforce as a whole: 3.7 percent for biomedical, 6.3 percent for clinical, and 2.7 percent for behavioral researchers.

As a proportion of the potential workforce, the percentage of those not working has increased. Their proportion varied roughly between 1.5 and 2.5 percent up to 1990, but the range has since increased to 3.0 to 4.5 percent. These percentages appear small, but the numbers involved have risen rapidly. For example, in the biomedical field, those not working numbered 1,500 in 1989. This increased to 4,900 in 2001. Two major factors contributed to this increase. First, the proportion not working was consistently higher in each field among females, who comprised only 10 to 20 percent of the workforce in the 1970s and increased to 30 to 60 percent in 2001. Second, around 1990, the proportion of males not working began to increase. Nevertheless, total unemployment has not increased by much, neither among males nor females. Notably, most of the increase in those not working has involved people staying out of the labor force. This not-working group represents a small proportion of the workforce, but the absolute numbers have grown rapidly among females, and males in the not-working category began to outnumber the unemployed in the early 1990s (see Figure D-4). People may stay out of the labor force to care for chil-

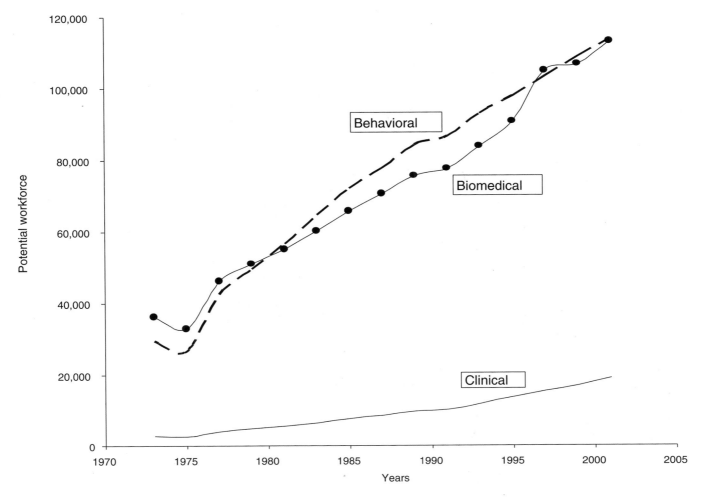

FIGURE D-2  Trends in the U.S.-trained potential workforce by major field, 1973–2001.
SOURCE: National Science Foundation Survey of Doctorate Recipients.

dren, to take a break between jobs, or for other personal reasons, but the extent to which this is voluntary is not evident from the data.

## M.D. Workforce

### Numbers

These data include M.D.s if they also have a Ph.D. from a U.S. institution. There are few data on clinical researchers with only M.D. degrees. Medical school faculty in the year 2000 totaled 90,678, but only a small minority of these should be considered clinical researchers (see Table D-2).

• of the total, only 64 percent have M.D.s, rather than Ph.D.s, M.D./Ph.D.s, or no doctoral degree (M.D./Ph.D.s are

grouped with Ph.D.s because they are included in datasets on Ph.D.s).

• of the M.D.s, 96 percent are in clinical departments and the rest are in biomedical departments (anatomy, biochemistry, microbiology, basic pathology, pharmacology, physiology, and other basic sciences).

• of the clinical M.D.s, only 2,879, or 5.2 percent, have ever had an R01 grant.

Therefore, it is feasible to add the 2,879 M.D. researchers to the 19,105 clinical researchers in the workforce. This number allows for M.D.s who are not currently doing research but have done so in the past, yet it is still a substantial underestimate for three reasons. First, R01 grants are not the only possible type of grant; research funds from pharmaceutical companies, foundations, and other sources compose a sig-

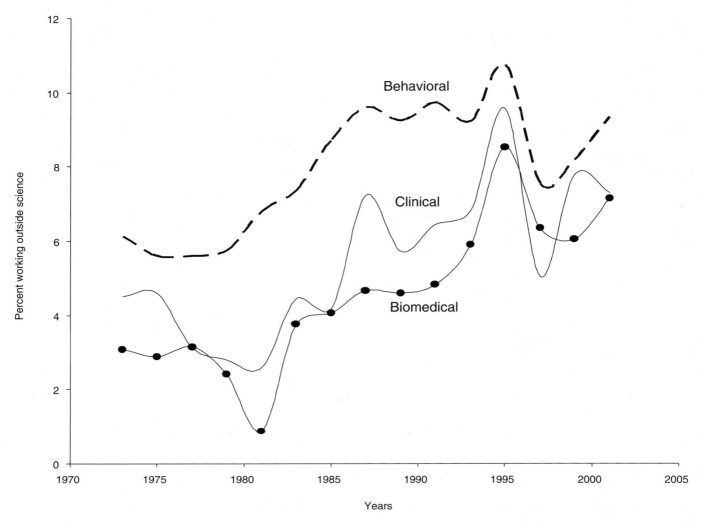

FIGURE D-3 Percent in conscience jobs by major field, 1973–2001.
SOURCE: National Science Foundation Survey of Doctorate Recipients.

nificant part of the research enterprise. Second, M.D. researchers may not be on medical faculties. Third, some additional (though very small) number currently may not be working or may be employed outside science. While one could argue that all M.D.s not in research should be categorized as "outside science" in the workforce, the discussion here is limited by the available data. Fourth, the criterion that requires evidence of a research grant may be too strict as Ph.D.s may not have had a research grant but are still counted in the potential workforce.

Of the Ph.D.s and M.D./Ph.D.s in clinical departments, 3,860 have had R01 grants. These individuals were included among those counted in the previous U.S.-trained Ph.D. discussion. However, the 13,577 who have not had an R01 grant were also counted. Ph.D.s and M.D./Ph.D.s in clinical departments make up 90 percent of the clinical Ph.D. workforce, although the proportion is somewhat uncertain due to lack of data on the foreign-trained Ph.D. component. These Ph.D.s and M.D./Ph.D.s in clinical departments total 4.5 times the number that have had R01 grants. When this same ratio is applied to the number counted as M.D. clinical researchers, it results in a total of 13,000. While there is some ambiguity in defining the M.D. clinical research workforce, it could be assumed that their numbers are between 3,000 and 13,000. This means that the number of clinical researchers regardless of degree type would have to be increased from the earlier estimate by as little as 16 or as much as 68 percent to incorporate the M.D. researchers who would, however, still

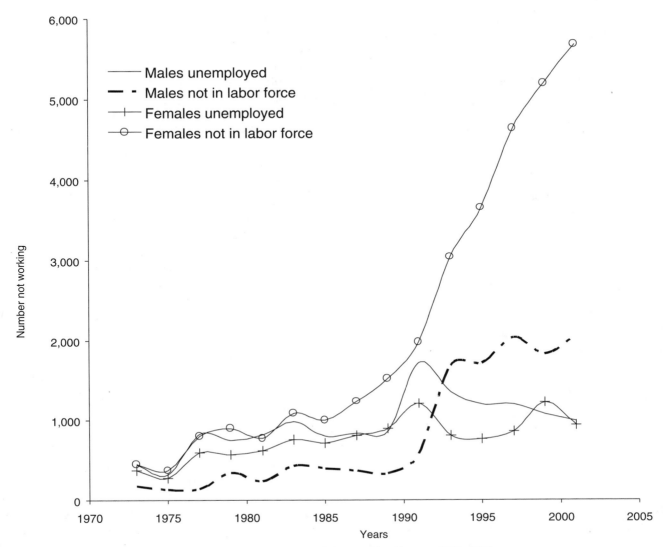

FIGURE D-4 Numbers unemployed and not in labor force for all fields combined by sex, 1973–2001.
SOURCE: National Science Foundation Survey of Doctorate Recipients.

be in the minority. Given the considerable uncertainty in these numbers, no attempt is made to project clinical M.D. researchers other than to make the following observations.

### Trends and Characteristics

The faculty roster data show that M.D.s in clinical departments who have ever had an R01 grant increased from 2,482 in 1993 to 3,090 in 2003, which is an annual rate of increase of 2.4 percent. This is much slower than the rate of increase for clinical Ph.D. researchers of 6.3 percent annually (from 1991 to 2001) and slightly slower than faculty growth in clinical departments. However, M.D. clinical researchers

with other types of grants or those not on medical faculties might have increased more rapidly.

There is a striking contrast between the male-female ratios for both M.D. and Ph.D. clinical researchers. Ph.D. clinical researchers are 57 percent female (see Table D-1). However, M.D. clinical researchers on medical faculties who have had R01s are 84 percent male. In each clinical discipline, male faculty with M.D.s and R01 experience outnumber equivalent female faculty by at least 2 to 1 and often much more. This is true from anesthesiology to surgery, including such fields as family medicine, pediatrics, and obstetrics and gynecology. Since Ph.D. clinical faculty with R01s are also largely male (71 percent), the mechanisms by

TABLE D-2  Medical School Faculty, by Major Field and Degree, and Number and Percent Having Had an R01 Grant, 2000

|  | Total | Biomedical | Clinical | Behavioral |
|---|---|---|---|---|
| **Faculty** |  |  |  |  |
| Total | 90,678 | 14,583 | 76,073 | 22 |
| M.D.s | 58,104 | 2,285 | 55,819 | 0 |
| Ph.D.s | 23,759 | 11,030 | 12,715 | 14 |
| M.D./Ph.D.s | 5,706 | 983 | 4,722 | 1 |
| Other | 3,109 | 285 | 2,817 | 7 |
| **Faculty who have ever had an R01 grant** |  |  |  |  |
| Total | 11,824 | 5,033 | 6,787 | 4 |
| M.D.s | 3,183 | 304 | 2,879 | 0 |
| Ph.D.s | 6,960 | 4,191 | 2,767 | 2 |
| M.D./Ph.D.s | 1,585 | 490 | 1,093 | 2 |
| Other | 96 | 48 | 48 | 0 |
| **Percent who have ever had an R01** |  |  |  |  |
| Total | 13.0 | 34.5 | 8.9 | 18.2 |
| M.D.s | 5.5 | 13.3 | 5.2 | a |
| Ph.D.s | 29.3 | 38.0 | 21.8 | a |
| M.D./Ph.D.s | 27.8 | 49.8 | 23.1 | a |
| Other | 3.1 | 16.8 | 1.7 | a |

aFewer than 20 base cases.

NOTE: Major field is defined by department, which may not agree exactly with field definitions in Table D-1.

SOURCE: American Association of Medical Colleges Faculty Roster.

which medical faculty obtain R01s may have something to do with the small proportion of females.

Foreign-trained M.D.s on faculty rosters represented 15 percent of those with R01s in 1993, rising slightly to 17 percent by 2002. It is important to distinguish between the data on Ph.D.s discussed in the previous section, which only included U.S.-trained Ph.D.s, and this section, which integrates an estimate of foreign-trained Ph.D.s. The following discussion will address this issue of the number to add for foreign-trained Ph.D.s.

## Foreign-Trained Ph.D. Workforce

### Numbers and Trends

Foreign-trained Ph.D.s are an important component of the workforce. However, the data are limited and provide uncertain results. The data for foreign-trained Ph.D.s come from the National Survey of College Graduates. This survey covers only those identified in the 1990 U.S. census. Therefore the numbers for those who migrated since 1990 and for attrition up to 2001 needed to be determined. This was done in several steps. First, those identified in the 1993 survey by

date of entry into the United States are broken down and then are "reverse survived" by age group for each field and sex to obtain estimates of their original numbers at entry going back as far as 1980. Second, this flow of migrants, from 1980 to 1990, is projected forward to 2001 using regression models. Third, by taking the distribution of the foreign trained in 1993 as roughly equivalent to the 1990 Census cohort, they are projected forward from 1990 to 2001 by adding, year by year, the estimated flow of migrants. This same projection model is used just as in the main exercise, although in this case it deals only with migrants and not U.S. graduates. This model allows for the accumulating numbers of migrants and for attrition. These rates are similar to those described below for the workforce as a whole.

Figure D-5 shows data and results in the biomedical field. The stock of foreign-trained biomedical Ph.D.s in the 1993 survey (at the left end of the middle line) was 8,800. This stock declined in subsequent surveys since migrants after 1990 were not added to the sample. The slight increase in 1999 occurred because survey nonresponse was reduced. Working backward from these levels, the migrant flow over the 1980s is estimated, shown by the line on the lower left. This flow, referred to as "entrants" to distinguish them from the stock of migrants, rose from 400 to over 700 annually during the 1980s. These entrants are added to the stock to give the projected stock of foreign-trained Ph.D.s, which doubled from 1993 to 2001, when it reached 17,400.

This projected stock analysis relies on the trends of the 1980s entrants. There are no data that allow direct assessment of whether changes in the flow took place in the 1990s. However, there are data on postdoctorates that permit a similar exercise to be conducted. Assuming that foreign-trained postdoctorates entered the United States just before accepting their posts, their dates of entry must have been more recent, on average, than those of migrants captured in the 1990 Census. Again, the data used are from the Graduate Student Survey, which includes numbers of postdoctorates by calendar year and field. Those with M.D.s rather than Ph.D.s are eliminated. Those with U.S. rather than foreign doctoral training are determined by applying ratios of temporary residents to U.S. citizens and permanent residents. In addition, stay rates are estimated for graduates. Both of these will be discussed further below. An estimate is made of when each postdoctorate started, using data on the duration an individual spent as a postdoctorate, and the assumption is made that this date is identical to the date of migration.

Figure D-6 resembles Figure D-5 (and is drawn to the same scale to facilitate comparison). The middle line shows the stock of foreign-trained postdoctorates, and the bottom line shows entrants estimated, as described above, from this stock. The stock numbers in Figure D-6 are consistent with those in Figure D-5, at least to the extent of indicating a smaller number of foreign-trained postdoctorates than foreign-trained researchers generally. The entrant numbers, however, are inconsistent, which suggests that more foreign-

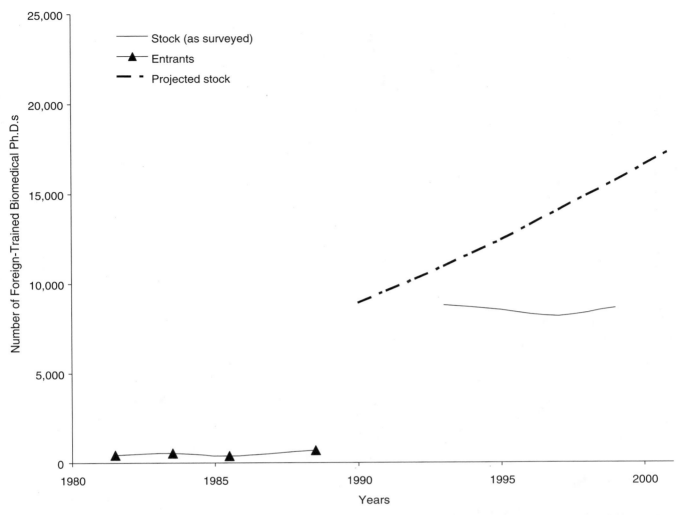

FIGURE D-5 Proportion of temporary residents among graduates and proportion of each group intending to stay in the United States: Means for 1997–2001.
SOURCE: National Science Foundation Survey of Earned Doctorates.

trained Ph.D.s entered the U.S. to take postdoctorates than the total number of entering foreign-trained Ph.D.s.

The reasons for this inconsistency are not clear. Either the data or the assumptions must be incorrect in Figure D-5 or Figure D-6, but it is not possible to determine which. One scenario would be to take the estimated entrants in Figure D-6, add a minimal 10 percent to allow for entrants who do not take postdoctorates, and apply the trend to 1993 stock numbers for all foreign-trained Ph.D.s. This results in a projected stock shown in the top line in Figure D-6. Note that these numbers are higher than those in Figure D-5 by 40 percent in the year 2001. Consequently, both estimates referring to the projected stock in Figure D-5 will be termed "medium" estimates, while those in Figure D-6 will be termed "high" estimates.

Similar results can be produced for foreign-trained clinical Ph.D.s. As for biomedical Ph.D.s, estimates based on surveyed migrants are lower than estimates based on reported postdoctorates. The former are obtained by working backwards from a stock of 2,200 foreign-trained researchers in 1993. This results in just under 200 annual entrants in the 1980s but follows an upward trend. Projections based on this trend would result in foreign-trained researchers tripling during the 1990s and reaching 6,200 by 2001. However, using reported postdoctorates results in an estimate that is 30 percent higher by 2001. Again, the former is considered a medium estimate and the latter a high estimate.

In contrast, foreign-trained behavioral researchers have a different picture. In 1993 this group was almost 50 percent more than clinical researchers, but proportionally more of

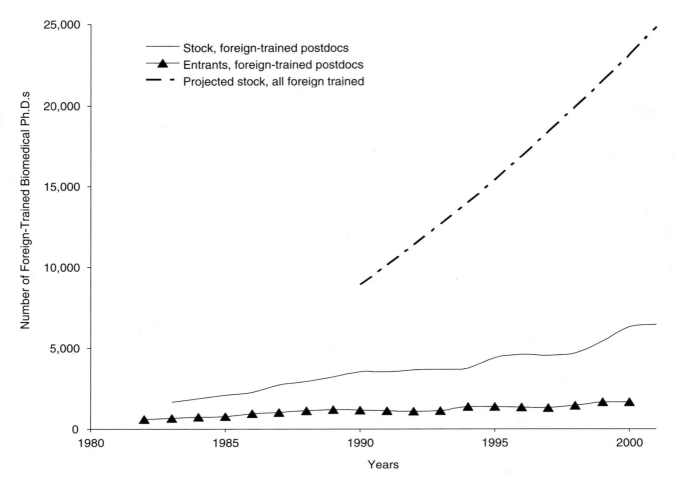

FIGURE D-6 Foreign-trained biomedical Ph.D.s: postdoctorates, postdoctoral entrants, and projected total stock.
SOURCE: National Science Foundation Survey of Graduate Students and Postdoctorates in Science and Engineering; and National Science Foundation National Survey of College Graduates.

them arrived before 1980, and during the 1980s entrants were few topping off at 100 annually. Projections based on this flow would indicate an increase in the stock to 4,300 by 2001. Foreign-trained postdoctorates are very few. As a result, the stock averages about 100 over two decades. For this group the projected stock from the migrant survey gives the high estimate, and the medium estimate is created by assuming a constant inflow of 100 per year.

## Characteristics

The estimates for 2001 of foreign-trained Ph.D.s in each field-broken down by sex and employment status based on the 1993 survey-are shown in Table D-3. In the biomedical field there are between 17,400 and 24,800 foreign-trained

Ph.D.s who make up 13 to 18 percent of the entire workforce. Although the number of foreign-trained Ph.D.s in the clinical field is smaller, they comprise between 25 and 30 percent of the workforce, which is a larger proportion; only 17 percent of the M.D. clinical researchers are on medical faculties. Finally, in the behavioral field they are much less consequential, at 3.0 to 3.6 percent of the entire workforce.

The distribution of foreign-trained Ph.D.s by employment status resembles that for U.S.-trained Ph.D.s with one exception: female biomedical researchers appear substantially more likely to be out of the labor force. The balance between males and females differs somewhat by field. In clinical research, foreign-trained Ph.D.s are more likely to be male than the U.S.-trained Ph.D.s, but the reverse appears to be the case in the other two fields (among M.D. clinical re-

TABLE D-3  Potential Workforce of Foreign-Trained Ph.D.s In Three Major Fields, By Employment Status, 2001: Medium and High Estimates

| Field and Employment Status | Number | | % Distribution by Status | | % Males Among Foreign Trained | | % Foreign Trained of Total Workforce | |
|---|---|---|---|---|---|---|---|---|
| | Medium | High | Medium | High | Medium | High | Medium | High |
| **Biomedical** | | | | | | | | |
| Potential workforce | 17,443 | 24,795 | 100.0 | 100.0 | 55.6 | 52.5 | 13.3 | 18.0 |
| Employed | 14,629 | 20,514 | 83.9 | 82.7 | 61.9 | 59.3 | 12.7 | 17.0 |
| Unemployed | 105 | 140 | 0.6 | 0.6 | 53.3 | 49.3 | 9.3 | 12.1 |
| Not in labor force[a] | 1,478 | 2,423 | 8.5 | 9.8 | 5.2 | 4.2 | 27.4 | 38.2 |
| Out of science | 1,231 | 1,718 | 7.1 | 6.9 | 42.1 | 39.2 | 13.2 | 17.5 |
| **Clinical** | | | | | | | | |
| Potential workforce | 6,197 | 8,133 | 100.0 | 100.0 | 79.1 | 78.8 | 24.5 | 29.9 |
| Employed | 5,846 | 7,683 | 94.3 | 94.5 | 79.8 | 79.4 | 25.4 | 30.9 |
| Unemployed | 17 | 21 | 0.3 | 0.3 | 52.9 | 52.4 | 11.8 | 14.2 |
| Not in labor force[a] | 30 | 38 | 0.5 | 0.5 | 30.0 | 28.9 | 6.9 | 8.6 |
| Out of science | 304 | 391 | 4.9 | 4.8 | 72.4 | 73.1 | 17.9 | 21.9 |
| **Behavioral** | | | | | | | | |
| Potential workforce | 3,483 | 4,284 | 100.0 | 100.0 | 38.8 | 34.8 | 3.0 | 3.6 |
| Employed | 3,041 | 3,756 | 87.3 | 87.7 | 39.1 | 34.9 | 3.0 | 3.7 |
| Unemployed | 14 | 17 | 0.4 | 0.4 | 21.4 | 17.6 | 1.7 | 2.1 |
| Not in labor force[a] | 105 | 137 | 3.0 | 3.2 | 7.6 | 6.6 | 3.0 | 3.9 |
| Out of science | 323 | 374 | 9.3 | 8.7 | 47.4 | 44.7 | 2.9 | 3.4 |

[a]Not employed, not looking for work, but not retired.

SOURCE: National Science Foundation Survey of Doctorate Recipients.

searchers on medical faculties, the male-female ratio, which heavily favors males, is similar for both the U.S.- and the foreign-trained postdoctorates).

## INFLOWS OF MIGRANTS AND GRADUATES

Every year foreign-trained researchers and graduates of U.S. institutions are added to the workforce. The inflows, and the corresponding outflows of retirees and decedents, constitute the forces that shape and reshape the workforce. Therefore it is important to consider each of these flows carefully, using past trends and alternative assumptions that might be made in projecting the future workforce. As done for projections in the previous report, past trends are used to define high, medium, and low options for numbers of future entrants.

### Migrants

The inflow has largely been described for foreign-trained Ph.D.s, and only a few points need to be added. To project their future flow, projections of migrant flow up to 2001 can be extended for an additional decade as described above. For

each field this gives a medium and a high option. A low option is defined for biomedical and clinical researchers by keeping the number of entrants constant at the 2001 value and for behavioral researchers by reducing it to 90 percent of that value.

### Numbers of Graduates

For females the number of Ph.D. graduates entering the workforce has been rising since 1970 in each major field (see Figure D-7). For male graduates the trend is less consistent: male clinical and biomedical graduates have generally risen since the mid-1980s, but male behavioral graduates have clearly fallen. The latter group aside, year-to-year increases are common, but there are exceptions: from 2000 to 2001, male behavioral graduates fell as well as graduates in four of the other five groups. To project graduates from these trends, the total graduates in each group (the proportion who stay in the United States and enter the workforce) and their age distribution need to be considered.

Regressions were run for total numbers of graduates over time in each field by sex, using data that start in 1985, 1990, or 1995 to reflect longer-term and shorter-term trends. For

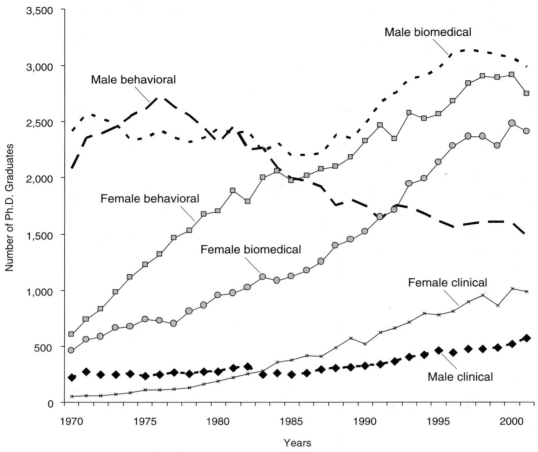

FIGURE D-7 Trends in Ph.D. graduates by major field and sex, 1970–2001.
SOURCE: National Science Foundation Survey of Earned Doctorates, 2001.

the 1985 regressions, a quadratic term was used. Pre-1985 data were not used because breaks in the trend appear for some groups. In addition, as noted below, age patterns of graduates also shifted slightly around that time.

Table D-4 shows the regression results. The longer-term regressions appear to fit better, probably because year-to-year fluctuations have proportionally less of an impact than in shorter-term regressions. The regression equations are used to define possible future paths, as illustrated in Figure D-8 for female behavioral graduates, and an additional path is defined by keeping the numbers of graduates constant at the average of the past five years (1997–2001). For female behavioral researchers and the other groups generally, the linear regression from 1985 provides the greatest increase in graduates, whereas holding graduates constant provides the least optimistic option. Conversely, numbers of male behavioral graduates are declining and, as noted by the 1985 linear regression, are the least optimistic. The 1985 linear regres-

sion defines a high option for graduates in general and a constant flow as the low option, except for male behavioral graduates, for which these are reversed. A medium option is then defined as the average of these two.

## Stay Rates Among Graduates

Not all Ph.D. graduates enter the U.S. workforce. In particular, non-U.S. citizens with temporary visas are less likely to stay in the country after graduation. These temporary residents represent a variable proportion of graduates across major fields, ranging over time from 3 to 40 percent. Unlike U.S. citizens and permanent residents, 95 to 99 percent of whom express an intention to stay in the United States, temporary residents express a similar intention only 25 to 80 percent of the time. In any year and field when the proportion of temporary-resident graduates is high, they are slightly more likely to intend to stay, but their inclusion among

TABLE D-4 Regressions For Total Ph.D. Graduates By Major Field and Sex

| | From 1985 | | From 1985 | | From 1990 | | From 1995 | |
|---|---|---|---|---|---|---|---|---|
| | B | t-test | B | t-test | B | t-test | B | t-test |
| **Male biomedical** | | | | | | | | |
| Year | 66.356 | 10.53 | 16400.811 | 4.04 | 47.245 | 4.66 | −3.742 | −0.28 |
| Constant | −129516 | −10.31 | −16406702 | −4.05 | −91351 | −4.52 | 10542 | 0.39 |
| $R^2$ | 0.881 | | 0.945 | | 0.685 | | 0.015 | |
| **Female biomedical** | | | | | | | | |
| Year | 92.043 | 20.38 | 8291.131 | 2.26 | 86.031 | 9.63 | 40.635 | 2.87 |
| $Year^2$ | −2.057 | −2.23 | | | | | | |
| Constant | −181592 | −20.17 | −8351933 | −2.28 | −169586 | −9.52 | −78864 | −2.79 |
| $R^2$ | 0.965 | | 0.974 | | 0.903 | | 0.623 | |
| **Male clinical** | | | | | | | | |
| Year | 19.002 | 25.63 | −329.462 | −0.47 | 19.968 | 13.70 | 17.746 | 4.38 |
| $Year^2$ | 0.087 | 0.50 | | | | | | |
| Constant | −37479 | −25.36 | 309764 | 0.45 | −39407 | −13.55 | −34969 | −4.32 |
| $R^2$ | 0.978 | | 0.978 | | 0.949 | | 0.794 | |
| **Female clinical** | | | | | | | | |
| Year | 40.917 | 21.34 | 1808.031 | 1.03 | 40.441 | 11.00 | 35.361 | 3.84 |
| $Year^2$ | −0.443 | −1.01 | | | | | | |
| Constant | −80850 | −21.16 | −1841769 | −1.06 | −79901 | −10.89 | −69752 | −3.80 |
| $R^2$ | 0.968 | | 0.970 | | 0.924 | | 0.747 | |
| **Male behavioral** | | | | | | | | |
| Year | −26.591 | −8.69 | −6125.923 | −2.56 | −18.257 | −4.36 | −10.710 | −1.30 |
| $Year^2$ | 1.530 | 2.55 | | | | | | |
| Constant | 54699 | 8.97 | 6132646 | 2.57 | 38060 | 4.55 | 22973 | 1.40 |
| $R^2$ | 0.834 | | 0.887 | | 0.655 | | 0.252 | |
| **Female behavioral** | | | | | | | | |
| Year | 62.020 | 14.17 | 6678.112 | 1.78 | 52.806 | 6.49 | 38.210 | 1.80 |
| $Year^2$ | −1.660 | −1.77 | | | | | | |
| Constant | −121132 | −13.88 | −6714028 | −1.80 | −102732 | −6.33 | −73559 | −1.73 |
| $R^2$ | 0.930 | | 0.943 | | 0.808 | | 0.393 | |

SOURCE: Analysis based on data from the National Science Foundation Survey of Earned Doctorates.

graduates contributes to a lower proportion for those intending to stay among graduates as a whole.

Around 1990, temporary residents increased as a proportion of all graduates, particularly in the biomedical field. Since then their proportion has fluctuated with no clear trend. Their stay rate—the proportion intending to stay in the U.S.—may have increased since 1995 but only after an apparent decline earlier in the 1990s. It is not certain how to extrapolate from these trends and trend reversals, given the apparent volatility of the stay rates. For projection purposes the assumption is made that both the percentage of temporary residents and the stay rate remain constant, by field and sex, at the average level for the past five years. This assumption gives overall stay rates (for U.S. citizens and noncitizens combined) of between 87 and 96 percent (see Table D-

5). For biomedical researchers these levels are slightly higher than those used in the 1995-2005 projections.

Some evidence suggests, however, that actual stay rates for temporary resident science and engineering Ph.D.s rose during the 1990s. This is supported by Finn (2003), who followed up 1991, 1996, and 1999 cohorts using Social Security data.[3] Actual stay rates tend to match stated intentions to stay. For instance, temporary resident behavioral graduates clearly have lower stay rates than temporary resident biomedical graduates. However, whether the relatively short-

[3]Hecker, D. E. 2001. Occupational employment projections to 2010. *Monthly Labor Review* (Nov.): 57–84.

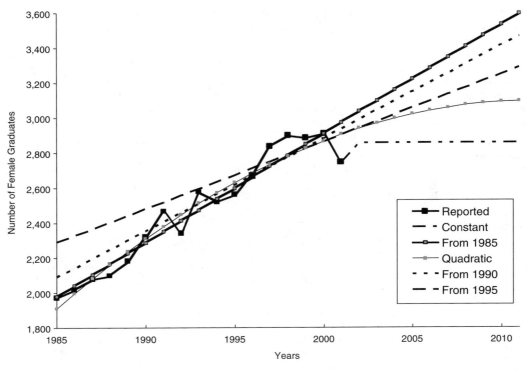

FIGURE D-8 Female behavioral graduates projected using various equations.
SOURCE: National Science Foundation Survey of Earned Doctorates, 2001.

TABLE D-5 Proportion of Temporary Residents Among Graduates and Proportion of Each Group Intending To Stay In The U.S.: Means For 1997–2001

| Indicator | Biomedical | | Clinical | | Behavioral | |
| --- | --- | --- | --- | --- | --- | --- |
| | Male | Female | Male | Female | Male | Female |
| Proportion of temporary residents | 0.257 | 0.209 | 0.294 | 0.151 | 0.099 | 0.054 |
| Proportion intending to stay in the U.S.: | | | | | | |
| U.S. citizens and permanent residents | 0.964 | 0.969 | 0.960 | 0.967 | 0.970 | 0.980 |
| Temporary residents | 0.845 | 0.841 | 0.669 | 0.550 | 0.518 | 0.584 |
| All graduates combined | 0.934 | 0.942 | 0.874 | 0.904 | 0.925 | 0.959 |

SOURCE: National Science Foundation Survey of Earned Doctorates, 2001.

term rise in rates will continue and whether it will be matched with increases or decreases in the proportion of graduates who are temporary residents remain to be determined. There is an alternative method to model the rise in overall stay rates. Linear regressions were run on the 1995-2001 data to extrapolate trends to 2011 for U.S. citizens and noncitizens combined (however, for male clinical researchers, data from 1990 were used to avoid too rapid a rise that would contrast strongly with other groups). The results, compared with the projected constant stay rates shown in Figure D-9, indicate

that stay rates could be as much as five percentage points higher at the end of the projection period.

## Age Distribution of Graduates

Ph.D. graduates in these fields have aged over the years. This major change took place in the mid-1980s, and no clear trend has become evident since then. In the 1970s graduates of these ages accounted for about 45 percent of all graduates in these fields combined. This percentage dropped by five

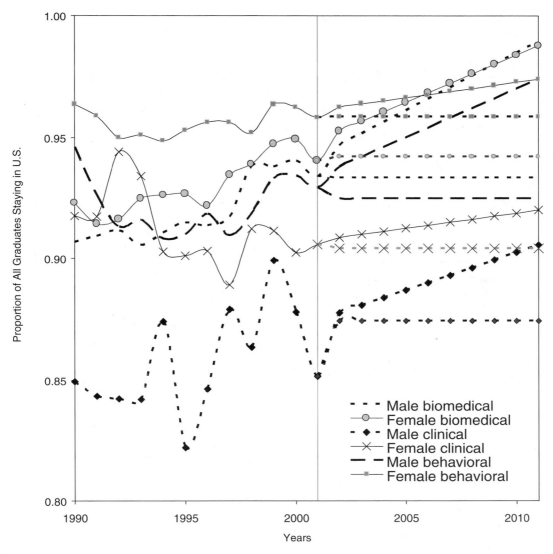

FIGURE D-9 Proportion of all graduates intending to stay and rising and constant projections by major field and sex, 1990–2011.
SOURCE: National Science Foundation Survey of Earned Doctorates, 2001.

points in the early 1980s and again in the late 1980s. Similar reductions took place in the smaller proportions graduating under age 28. Some of these reductions were due to more students graduating at ages 32 to 35, but a larger increase occurred above age 35. Overall, ages 28 through 31 are the peak ages for graduating with a Ph.D.; about 10 percent of graduates are typically of each age. However, this trend did not continue into the 1990s. Some changes in age at graduation did take place in the 1990s but were inconsistent across fields and did not indicate any sustained trends.

Since there is no clear evidence that age at graduation is rising or falling, it is assumed (for projection purposes) that it stays constant at the average levels by field and sex for the past five years. The median ages in these distributions are lowest in the biomedical field and highest in the clinical field.

For males and females, respectively, median ages at graduation are 31.1 and 30.5 in biomedical research, 34.7 and 39.5 in clinical research, and 33.4 and 32.7 in behavioral research.

## OUTFLOWS AND CHANGES IN STATUS

Once in the workforce, individuals may take a job outside science, become unemployed, move out of the labor force, or eventually leave the workforce altogether through retirement or death (they may also emigrate, but these numbers are small and probably unreliable, so they have not been considered). Such changes in status were used to track changes in the potential workforce. The likelihood of most of these movements is estimated from the biennial survey of doctoral recipients for the years 1993 to 2001. When the numbers of cases in various categories are small, data were pooled across surveys and tabulations were produced for employment status initially and again two years later. Table D-6 summarizes these tabulations.

The most common work scenario is for a graduate to be initially employed in science and to still be so employed two years later (note that the data do not indicate whether the job is the same or whether there was a break in employment in between). This holds for 77 to 86 percent of researchers in each major field. By contrast, those with jobs outside science who are still in the same or similar jobs two years later, range from 3 to 6 percent of the entire group. Movement from science to nonscience employment and vice versa involves 4.5 to 8 percent with comparable flows in each direction. Movement toward nonscience employment is more common in the biomedical field. Movement to or from nonscience jobs does not appear to be age related. Median ages of those moving out of or into science from nonscience jobs are close to median ages for those who stay in science employment, and age distributions have similar patterns across these groups.

Those not working (whether unemployed or not in the labor force) tend to be proportionally more numerous among females than males. In the biomedical field they are 7.4 percent among females but only 2.2 percent among males (averaging across initial percentages and percentages two years later). In the clinical field the contrast is between 4.4 and 1.4 percent and in the behavioral field between 5.2 and 1.5 percent. Women are also more likely to still not be working two years later. In each field more than half of females who are initially not working are still not working two years later. Among males the parallel proportions are 10 to 25 percentage points lower. Males are slightly more likely than females to be employed two years later, to take a job outside science, or even to retire.

Retirement is a major transition point that is fairly predictable. At least half of each group retires between the ages of 61 and 70. Females tend to retire slightly earlier than males, especially in the biomedical field.

The SDR data do not provide mortality rates. Consequently, these rates were obtained from TIAA/CREF to represent rates in academia generally. Separate rates are used

TABLE D-6 Initial Employment Status and Status 2-Years Later: Percentages Based On All Cases in Each Field by Sex, Pooled 1993–2001 Data

| Employment Status After 2 Years | Initial Employment Status | | | | | | | |
|---|---|---|---|---|---|---|---|---|
| | Males | | | | Females | | | |
| | Employed | Not Working[a] | Out of Science | All Males | Employed | Not Working[a] | Out of Science | All Females |
| **Biomedical** | | | | | | | | |
| Employed | 86.1 | 1.0 | 2.0 | 89.1 | 77.1 | 2.2 | 2.5 | 81.7 |
| Not working[a] | 1.2 | 0.8 | 0.1 | 2.1 | 2.8 | 4.2 | 0.5 | 7.4 |
| Out of science | 2.5 | 0.2 | 3.5 | 6.1 | 3.4 | 0.7 | 5.2 | 9.4 |
| Retired | 2.2 | 0.3 | 0.2 | 2.6 | 0.9 | 0.3 | 0.3 | 1.5 |
| Total | 91.9 | 2.3 | 5.8 | 100.0 | 84.2 | 7.4 | 8.4 | 100.0 |
| Weighted cases | 185,335 | 4,643 | 11,594 | 201,572 | 68,401 | 6,024 | 6,831 | 81,255 |
| **Clinical** | | | | | | | | |
| Employed | 85.6 | 0.5 | 3.3 | 89.4 | 81.8 | 1.3 | 3.4 | 86.5 |
| Not working[a] | 0.5 | 0.7 | 0.0 | 1.2 | 1.6 | 2.3 | 0.4 | 4.3 |
| Out of science | 2.3 | 0.3 | 3.9 | 6.5 | 3.6 | 0.3 | 3.1 | 7.0 |
| Retired | 2.4 | 0.2 | 0.3 | 2.8 | 1.4 | 0.5 | 0.2 | 2.2 |
| Total | 90.8 | 1.7 | 7.6 | 100.0 | 88.3 | 4.5 | 7.1 | 100.0 |
| Weighted cases | 17,788 | 328 | 1,485 | 19,601 | 19,290 | 990 | 1,556 | 21,836 |
| **Behavioral** | | | | | | | | |
| Employed | 83.3 | 0.6 | 2.7 | 86.7 | 80.4 | 1.5 | 2.8 | 84.7 |
| Not working[a] | 0.7 | 0.5 | 0.2 | 1.4 | 1.9 | 2.8 | 0.4 | 5.2 |
| Out of science | 2.8 | 0.3 | 5.8 | 8.9 | 2.7 | 0.6 | 5.1 | 8.3 |
| Retired | 2.3 | 0.3 | 0.4 | 3.0 | 1.3 | 0.3 | 0.1 | 1.8 |
| Total | 89.1 | 1.7 | 9.2 | 100.0 | 86.4 | 5.2 | 8.4 | 100.0 |
| Weighted cases | 164,788 | 3,204 | 16,992 | 184,984 | 115,366 | 6,975 | 11,186 | 133,527 |

[a]"Not working" includes the unemployed and those not in the labor force.

SOURCE: National Science Foundation Survey of Earned Doctorates, 2001.

for males and females. These mortality rates are slightly lower than those in the 2000 report, reflecting secular improvement in life expectancy.

## WORKFORCE PROJECTIONS

### Scenarios

An analysis of the research workforce provides the base for 10-year projections. The inflows, outflows, and shifts in status provide alternative assumptions for future trends. Various assumptions are combined in order to define three main projection scenarios: (1) high for high numbers of graduates and high numbers of foreign-trained migrants, (2) medium for intermediate numbers in both groups, and (3) low for low numbers in both groups. The medium and low scenarios both start with the lower estimates of the 2001 stock of foreign-trained Ph.D.s, and the high scenario starts with the higher estimates. Additional scenarios will be considered below based on variations in stay rates and migrants.

Table D-7 shows the varying numbers of graduates assumed in each scenario. In the medium scenario, biomedical graduates reach the 6,000 level by 2006. In the high scenario they are at this level by 2002. In the low scenario they never

TABLE D-7  Projected Ph.D. Graduates in Three Major Fields, by Sex: Medium, High, and Low Scenarios

|  | Biomedical | | | Clinical | | | Behavioral | | |
|---|---|---|---|---|---|---|---|---|---|
|  | Total | Male | Female | Total | Male | Female | Total | Male | Female |
| **Medium** | | | | | | | | | |
| 2002 | 5,730 | 3,202 | 2,528 | 1,540 | 535 | 1,005 | 4,459 | 1,514 | 2,945 |
| 2003 | 5,806 | 3,235 | 2,571 | 1,568 | 544 | 1,024 | 4,476 | 1,502 | 2,974 |
| 2004 | 5,888 | 3,269 | 2,619 | 1,599 | 553 | 1,046 | 4,494 | 1,489 | 3,005 |
| 2005 | 5,962 | 3,300 | 2,662 | 1,624 | 559 | 1,065 | 4,511 | 1,477 | 3,034 |
| 2006 | 6,041 | 3,333 | 2,708 | 1,658 | 572 | 1,086 | 4,530 | 1,463 | 3,067 |
| 2007 | 6,122 | 3,366 | 2,756 | 1,690 | 582 | 1,108 | 4,546 | 1,451 | 3,095 |
| 2008 | 6,199 | 3,401 | 2,798 | 1,716 | 593 | 1,123 | 4,568 | 1,439 | 3,129 |
| 2009 | 6,286 | 3,434 | 2,852 | 1,747 | 601 | 1,146 | 4,580 | 1,423 | 3,157 |
| 2010 | 6,363 | 3,466 | 2,897 | 1,779 | 610 | 1,169 | 4,599 | 1,408 | 3,191 |
| 2011 | 6,440 | 3,497 | 2,943 | 1,809 | 618 | 1,191 | 4,619 | 1,398 | 3,221 |
| Total | 60,837 | 33,503 | 27,334 | 16,730 | 5,767 | 10,963 | 45,382 | 14,564 | 30,818 |
| **High** | | | | | | | | | |
| 2002 | 6,003 | 3,327 | 2,676 | 1,632 | 567 | 1,065 | 4,603 | 1,570 | 3,033 |
| 2003 | 6,167 | 3,398 | 2,769 | 1,690 | 582 | 1,108 | 4,663 | 1,570 | 3,093 |
| 2004 | 6,325 | 3,460 | 2,865 | 1,748 | 602 | 1,146 | 4,727 | 1,570 | 3,157 |
| 2005 | 6,481 | 3,526 | 2,955 | 1,809 | 618 | 1,191 | 4,788 | 1,570 | 3,218 |
| 2006 | 6,644 | 3,596 | 3,048 | 1,867 | 639 | 1,228 | 4,847 | 1,570 | 3,277 |
| 2007 | 6,806 | 3,664 | 3,142 | 1,928 | 660 | 1,268 | 4,912 | 1,570 | 3,342 |
| 2008 | 6,956 | 3,729 | 3,227 | 1,992 | 678 | 1,314 | 4,971 | 1,570 | 3,401 |
| 2009 | 7,116 | 3,794 | 3,322 | 2,045 | 698 | 1,347 | 5,040 | 1,570 | 3,470 |
| 2010 | 7,275 | 3,859 | 3,416 | 2,109 | 714 | 1,395 | 5,099 | 1,570 | 3,529 |
| 2011 | 7,434 | 3,927 | 3,507 | 2,166 | 734 | 1,432 | 5,161 | 1,570 | 3,591 |
| Total | 67,207 | 36,280 | 30,927 | 18,986 | 6,492 | 12,494 | 48,811 | 15,700 | 33,111 |
| **Low** | | | | | | | | | |
| 2002 | 5,450 | 3,076 | 2,374 | 1,445 | 505 | 940 | 4,316 | 1,462 | 2,854 |
| 2003 | 5,450 | 3,076 | 2,374 | 1,445 | 505 | 940 | 4,293 | 1,439 | 2,854 |
| 2004 | 5,450 | 3,076 | 2,374 | 1,445 | 505 | 940 | 4,261 | 1,407 | 2,854 |
| 2005 | 5,450 | 3,076 | 2,374 | 1,445 | 505 | 940 | 4,240 | 1,386 | 2,854 |
| 2006 | 5,450 | 3,076 | 2,374 | 1,445 | 505 | 940 | 4,212 | 1,358 | 2,854 |
| 2007 | 5,450 | 3,076 | 2,374 | 1,445 | 505 | 940 | 4,184 | 1,330 | 2,854 |
| 2008 | 5,450 | 3,076 | 2,374 | 1,445 | 505 | 940 | 4,157 | 1,303 | 2,854 |
| 2009 | 5,450 | 3,076 | 2,374 | 1,445 | 505 | 940 | 4,133 | 1,279 | 2,854 |
| 2010 | 5,450 | 3,076 | 2,374 | 1,445 | 505 | 940 | 4,103 | 1,249 | 2,854 |
| 2011 | 5,450 | 3,076 | 2,374 | 1,445 | 505 | 940 | 4,079 | 1,225 | 2,854 |
| Total | 54,500 | 30,760 | 23,740 | 14,450 | 5,050 | 9,400 | 41,978 | 13,438 | 28,540 |

SOURCE: NRC analysis.

TABLE D-8 Projected Inflow of Foreign-Trained Ph.D.s by Major Field: Medium, High, and Low Scenarios

| Field and Year | Biomedical | | | Clinical | | | Behavioral | | |
|---|---|---|---|---|---|---|---|---|---|
| | Medium | High | Low | Medium | High | Low | Medium | High | Low |
| 2002 | 1,003 | 1,785 | 977 | 504 | 724 | 483 | 93 | 200 | 82 |
| 2003 | 1,037 | 1,845 | 978 | 524 | 751 | 478 | 93 | 208 | 83 |
| 2004 | 1,064 | 1,901 | 979 | 548 | 782 | 478 | 94 | 216 | 83 |
| 2005 | 1,095 | 1,949 | 980 | 570 | 818 | 480 | 93 | 222 | 83 |
| 2006 | 1,126 | 2,010 | 983 | 592 | 846 | 480 | 94 | 228 | 83 |
| 2007 | 1,160 | 2,060 | 984 | 615 | 876 | 480 | 95 | 233 | 83 |
| 2008 | 1,190 | 2,123 | 986 | 643 | 909 | 480 | 95 | 240 | 83 |
| 2009 | 1,222 | 2,181 | 986 | 665 | 940 | 479 | 95 | 247 | 83 |
| 2010 | 1,255 | 2,234 | 988 | 685 | 969 | 479 | 95 | 256 | 83 |
| 2011 | 1,283 | 2,287 | 988 | 708 | 1,003 | 479 | 95 | 263 | 83 |
| Total | 11,435 | 20,375 | 9,829 | 6,054 | 8,618 | 4,796 | 942 | 2,313 | 829 |
| Stock, 2001 | 17,437 | 24,787 | 17,437 | 6,178 | 8,115 | 6,178 | 3,469 | 4,269 | 3,469 |

SOURCE: NRC analysis.

reach this level. Variation is also evident for other groups. For example, in the medium scenario behavioral graduates increase by 400 over a decade; in the high scenario they increase by over 900; but in the low scenario they decrease by over 140. Note that some of these graduates are assumed not to enter the U.S. workforce but to move abroad.

Table D-8 shows the assumed number of entrants among foreign-trained Ph.D.s. The biomedical field should have the most entrants—1,000 a year, possibly rising to 2,000. By contrast, in the behavioral field 100 or 200 are projected annually. Total entrants over a decade will be substantial—at least 50 percent and possibly 100 percent of the initial stock of foreign-trained Ph.D.s in 2001, except in behavioral research.

## THE GROWING WORKFORCE

### Numbers

The projected workforce that absorbs these graduates and migrants is shown for each field in the medium scenario in Figure D-10. Projections shown for U.S.-trained Ph.D.s as well as for U.S.- and foreign-trained Ph.D.s combined are consistent with the historical series. Looking at all Ph.D.s by 2001, behavioral researchers increase to 176,400, clinical researchers increase to 41,700, and behavioral researchers increase to 134,500 (see Table D-9). The clinical field shows the fastest growth but is relatively small. Its total increase over 10 years by 16,400 will be only a third of the increase in the biomedical field and slightly smaller than the increase in the slow-growing behavioral field.

These increases are based on a calculated balance between inflows of U.S. graduates and foreign-trained researchers and outflows of retirees and decedents. The combined inflows are projected at 4.5, 6.5, and 3.5 percent of the workforce in the biomedical, clinical, and behavioral fields, respectively, and foreign-trained Ph.D.s represent a significant proportion of the clinical and biomedical research numbers (see Table D-10). Outflows of retirees are in the range of 1.2 to 1.7 percent annually, and deaths represent one-fourth to one-fifth of that number. In total these flows produce average annual growth rates of 3.0, 5.0, and 1.4 percent in biomedical, clinical, and behavioral research, respectively.

In the high scenario, annual increases will be roughly 30 percent larger and in the low scenario about 20 percent smaller. Annual increases will not be uniform across the decade. The behavioral field will experience slowing growth in each scenario, whereas the biomedical and clinical field scenarios will be marked by slowing growth in the low scenario but accelerating growth in the high scenario (see Figure D-11).

### Composition of Growing Workforce

Those employed in science represent the most important component of the workforce, as shown in Table D-9. This table also shows the projected numbers to be roughly 90 percent of the potential workforce. This should be interpreted to mean that this proportion should be available for employment on the basis of the past distribution of the workforce and on the movement between employment status. However, whether these jobs will be available is not being predicted

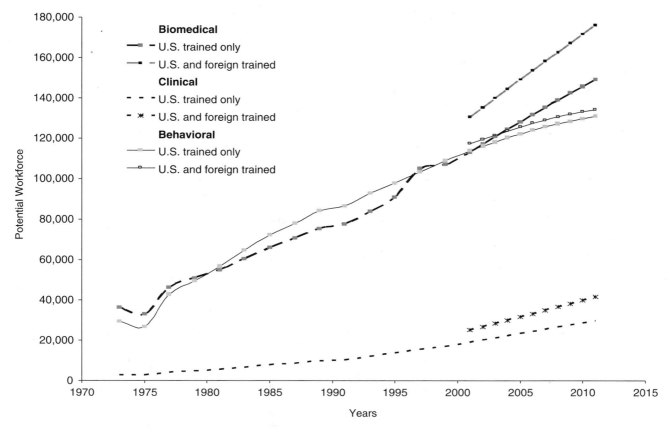

FIGURE D-10 Potential workforce as reported and projected including and excluding foreign trained medium scenario, 1973–2011.
SOURCE: National Science Foundation Survey of Doctorate Recipients and NRC analysis.

and will be discussed in a later section. These projected numbers of employed change in a complex fashion and can increase faster or slower than the workforce. In the biomedical field, annual increases in the employed are projected to be smaller than workforce increases; however, in the behavioral field the reverse will be true in the initial years.

Other components of the workforce, comprising all those not active in research, are shown in Table D-11. Those unemployed (not in the labor force or out of science) are projected to vary only slightly over time as percentages of the potential workforce in the medium scenario (see Figure D-12). Those outside science are the largest group of nonactive researchers. Annually, 1.5 to 1.6 percent of the workforce will move from science to nonscience employment, and an almost equal percentage will move in the other direction (see Table D-10). The variation in the percentage not active in science is due to changes in the age and sex composition of the workforce and not to changes in the probability that researchers become unemployed, exit the labor force, or take nonscience jobs. This probability is fixed in the projection model for each sex and age group and is not allowed to vary.

However, in reality it may vary and whether it will depends on how many research positions are available in these fields; this issue is discussed later.

The composition of the projected workforce by sex is illustrated in Figure D-13, which counts only those in the employed category. Employed males outnumber employed females by more than 40,000 in the biomedical field. This gap will not change much, even though the percentage of employed females will rise from 31 to 35 by 2011. Males slightly outnumber females in clinical research employment, mainly due to foreign-trained Ph.D.s. If foreign-trained doctorates are excluded, females outnumber males by a few thousand with that gap growing. Finally, in the behavioral field, a cross-over is projected by 2004, with females overtaking males to reach 57 percent of the workforce by 2011, which represents 16,000 more females than males.

Median ages for the workforce will generally rise, notably by 4.1 years over a decade for male behavioral researchers, but increases will be substantially less for other main fields. For male clinical researchers, the median age will fall marginally. In each field those age 41 to 60 will decline as a

TABLE D-9  Projected Workforce and Employed Researchers, by Field, Three Main
Scenarios, 2001–2011

| Field and Year | Potential Workforce | | | Employed | | |
|---|---|---|---|---|---|---|
| | Medium | High | Low | Medium | High | Low |
| **Biomedical** | | | | | | |
| 2001 | 130,726 | 138,076 | 130,726 | 114,889 | 120,776 | 114,889 |
| 2002 | 135,505 | 143,922 | 135,215 | 118,379 | 125,111 | 118,172 |
| 2003 | 140,203 | 149,792 | 139,514 | 121,912 | 129,584 | 121,426 |
| 2004 | 144,840 | 155,697 | 143,649 | 125,531 | 134,221 | 124,681 |
| 2005 | 149,446 | 161,663 | 147,654 | 129,236 | 139,019 | 127,941 |
| 2006 | 154,049 | 167,727 | 151,551 | 133,030 | 143,992 | 131,203 |
| 2007 | 158,605 | 173,830 | 155,291 | 136,843 | 149,059 | 134,392 |
| 2008 | 163,113 | 179,975 | 158,881 | 140,649 | 154,191 | 137,484 |
| 2009 | 167,584 | 186,172 | 162,323 | 144,436 | 159,379 | 140,464 |
| 2010 | 172,019 | 192,419 | 165,623 | 148,191 | 164,610 | 143,325 |
| 2011 | 176,400 | 198,703 | 168,770 | 151,889 | 169,864 | 146,046 |
| **Clinical** | | | | | | |
| 2001 | 25,282 | 27,219 | 25,282 | 23,020 | 24,860 | 23,020 |
| 2002 | 26,838 | 29,084 | 26,732 | 24,580 | 26,706 | 24,483 |
| 2003 | 28,439 | 31,025 | 28,175 | 26,125 | 28,566 | 25,881 |
| 2004 | 30,059 | 33,014 | 29,584 | 27,686 | 30,467 | 27,246 |
| 2005 | 31,686 | 35,054 | 30,956 | 29,250 | 32,411 | 28,573 |
| 2006 | 33,332 | 37,138 | 32,292 | 30,818 | 34,382 | 29,856 |
| 2007 | 35,002 | 39,275 | 33,598 | 32,399 | 36,392 | 31,101 |
| 2008 | 36,679 | 41,456 | 34,861 | 33,978 | 38,436 | 32,298 |
| 2009 | 38,352 | 43,659 | 36,068 | 35,542 | 40,485 | 33,429 |
| 2010 | 40,031 | 45,902 | 37,234 | 37,102 | 42,564 | 34,512 |
| 2011 | 41,716 | 48,181 | 38,355 | 38,662 | 44,675 | 35,551 |
| **Behavioral** | | | | | | |
| 2001 | 117,466 | 118,266 | 117,466 | 102,193 | 102,898 | 102,193 |
| 2002 | 119,737 | 120,783 | 119,589 | 104,951 | 105,871 | 104,820 |
| 2003 | 121,833 | 123,174 | 121,499 | 107,302 | 108,476 | 107,005 |
| 2004 | 123,862 | 125,548 | 123,297 | 109,464 | 110,928 | 108,956 |
| 2005 | 125,813 | 127,888 | 124,980 | 111,457 | 113,253 | 110,708 |
| 2006 | 127,670 | 130,178 | 126,526 | 113,319 | 115,491 | 112,288 |
| 2007 | 129,371 | 132,363 | 127,874 | 114,993 | 117,594 | 113,644 |
| 2008 | 130,892 | 134,408 | 128,998 | 116,462 | 119,528 | 114,752 |
| 2009 | 132,244 | 136,343 | 129,919 | 117,747 | 121,333 | 115,648 |
| 2010 | 133,450 | 138,176 | 130,649 | 118,884 | 123,034 | 116,354 |
| 2011 | 134,466 | 139,863 | 131,149 | 119,840 | 124,594 | 116,845 |
| **Ten-year increase** | | | | | | |
| Biomedical | 45,674 | 60,627 | 38,044 | 37,000 | 49,088 | 31,157 |
| Clinical | 16,434 | 20,962 | 13,073 | 15,642 | 19,815 | 12,531 |
| Behavioral | 17,000 | 21,597 | 13,683 | 17,647 | 21,696 | 14,652 |
| **Average annual growth (%)** | | | | | | |
| Biomedical | 3.00 | 3.64 | 2.55 | 2.79 | 3.41 | 2.40 |
| Clinical | 5.01 | 5.71 | 4.17 | 5.18 | 5.86 | 4.35 |
| Behavioral | 1.35 | 1.68 | 1.10 | 1.59 | 1.91 | 1.34 |

SOURCE: NRC analysis.

TABLE D-10 Projected Annual Growth Rates, and Inflow and Outflow Rates (%) for the Potential Workforce, by Major Field, and Medium Scenario, 2001–2011

| Rate | Biomedical | Clinical | Behavioral |
|---|---|---|---|
| Growth | 3.00 | 5.01 | 1.35 |
| Inflow | | | |
| U.S. graduates | 3.72 | 4.54 | 3.39 |
| Foreign trained | 0.79 | 1.98 | 0.08 |
| Outflow | | | |
| Retirements | –1.21 | –1.24 | –1.73 |
| Deaths | –0.30 | –0.26 | –0.39 |
| Shifts within workforce | | | |
| Out of science to employed | 1.40 | 1.67 | 1.55 |
| Employed to out of science | –1.55 | –1.59 | –1.53 |

NOTE: Inflow and outflow rates are calculated annually based on midyear workforce and averaged. Other shifts within the workforce, to *unemployment* and *not in the labor force*, are substantially smaller.

SOURCE: NRC analysis.

proportion of the workforce and essentially be replaced by those older than 60 (see Figure D-14). Additionally as seen in Figure D-13, the increase in older researchers will parallel the increase in the general population—though for age groups that may be off by one year—from Census Bureau projections.

## MIGRANT SCENARIOS

Table D-12 shows how the workforce is divided between U.S.-trained and foreign-trained researchers. Over the decade, the foreign-trained group will increase from 13 to 15 percent for biomedical Ph.D.s and from 24 to 29 percent for clinical Ph.D.s. In behavioral research, which starts at only 3 percent, foreign-trained employed researchers will decline both in absolute numbers and relative to U.S.-trained researchers.

These figures understate the contribution that foreign-trained Ph.D.s make to the workforce. Notably, among

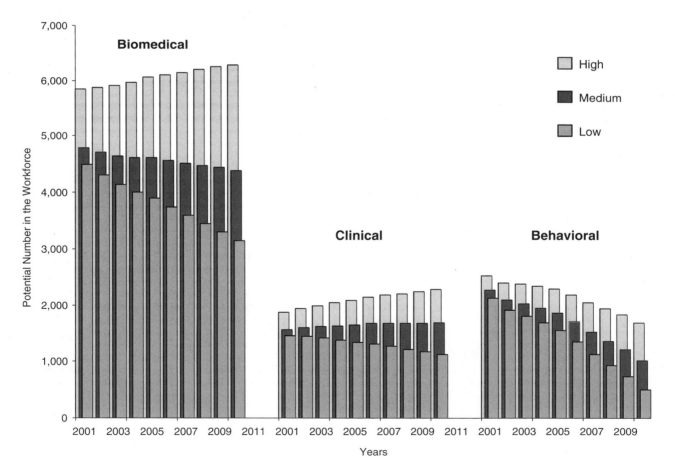

FIGURE D-11 Projected annual increase in the potential workforce in three scenarios by field 2001–2011.
SOURCE: NRC analysis.

TABLE D-11  Projected Workforce Not Active in
Scientific Research, by Major Field, Medium Scenario,
2001–2011

| Field and Year | Out of Science | Unemployed | Not in Labor Force | Total Not Active |
|---|---|---|---|---|
| **Biomedical** | | | | |
| 2001 | 9,323 | 1,125 | 5,389 | 15,837 |
| 2002 | 9,933 | 960 | 6,233 | 17,126 |
| 2003 | 10,425 | 925 | 6,941 | 18,291 |
| 2004 | 10,819 | 916 | 7,572 | 19,307 |
| 2005 | 11,152 | 923 | 8,134 | 20,209 |
| 2006 | 11,462 | 940 | 8,616 | 21,018 |
| 2007 | 11,765 | 963 | 9,033 | 21,761 |
| 2008 | 12,064 | 988 | 9,412 | 22,464 |
| 2009 | 12,356 | 1,013 | 9,779 | 23,148 |
| 2010 | 12,650 | 1,038 | 10,140 | 23,828 |
| 2011 | 12,954 | 1,062 | 10,495 | 24,511 |
| **Clinical** | | | | |
| 2001 | 1,700 | 137 | 426 | 2,263 |
| 2002 | 1,718 | 139 | 402 | 2,259 |
| 2003 | 1,794 | 144 | 375 | 2,313 |
| 2004 | 1,862 | 145 | 366 | 2,373 |
| 2005 | 1,916 | 148 | 371 | 2,435 |
| 2006 | 1,985 | 153 | 376 | 2,514 |
| 2007 | 2,064 | 159 | 381 | 2,604 |
| 2008 | 2,148 | 165 | 386 | 2,699 |
| 2009 | 2,241 | 172 | 397 | 2,810 |
| 2010 | 2,339 | 179 | 410 | 2,928 |
| 2011 | 2,441 | 185 | 426 | 3,052 |
| **Behavioral** | | | | |
| 2001 | 10,957 | 794 | 3,522 | 15,273 |
| 2002 | 10,915 | 577 | 3,293 | 14,785 |
| 2003 | 10,860 | 509 | 3,161 | 14,530 |
| 2004 | 10,816 | 481 | 3,101 | 14,398 |
| 2005 | 10,802 | 466 | 3,087 | 14,355 |
| 2006 | 10,788 | 461 | 3,101 | 14,350 |
| 2007 | 10,768 | 464 | 3,145 | 14,377 |
| 2008 | 10,758 | 469 | 3,202 | 14,429 |
| 2009 | 10,759 | 473 | 3,265 | 14,497 |
| 2010 | 10,761 | 477 | 3,328 | 14,566 |
| 2011 | 10,755 | 478 | 3,393 | 14,626 |

SOURCE: NRC analysis.

U.S.-trained Ph.D.s, as seen in Table D-5, 20 to 25 percent of the biomedical graduates are noncitizens on temporary visas, and an additional undetermined number are noncitizens on permanent resident visas. However, these numbers are uncertain. First, there are statistical uncertainties. There are no data available to distinguish permanent residents from U.S. citizens, and therefore future numbers could be affected by immigration policies. The data used on the foreign trained are very limited compared to the data on U.S.-trained Ph.D.s. Second, there are policy-based uncertainties due to the re-

cent flux in immigration policies. Third, there are behavioral uncertainties because reactions to policy changes by potential immigrants as well as immigrants' decisions to stay in the United States or to emigrate are difficult to predict. Although some statistical information is available, the data are not determinate nor necessarily easy to explain. For these reasons, additional scenarios to reflect possible paths that the inflow of noncitizens might take are addressed below.

There are four possibilities, and each is a variation of the medium scenario. First, stay rates might actually rise, particularly among temporary resident graduates. This possible rise, as discussed earlier, is modeled on the upward trend in stay rates since 1995. Second, stay rates could go in the opposite direction because potential migrants might be discouraged by bureaucratic difficulties, delay, and inconvenience. Therefore, the assumption can be made that temporary resident graduates might increase more slowly, showing a trend that is only 90 percent of the medium scenario. At the same time, the assumption could be made that the flow of foreign-trained migrants would immediately drop to 90 percent of its current estimated level and remain fixed throughout the projection. Third, assuming that immigration restrictions and obstacles are more severe than in the 90 percent scenario, temporary resident graduates could fall to 50 percent of the medium trend, and the flow of foreign-trained migrants could also fall to 50 percent of its current level and stay at that level. Finally, to illustrate an extreme possibility, the flow of both temporary resident graduates and the foreign trained could be reduced to zero.

Table D-13 compares these scenarios with the medium, high, and low scenarios. The behavioral research workforce is little affected by the assumed variations because the number of foreign-trained Ph.D.s are few. The focus instead is on the other two fields. In all fields the scenario of rising stay rates is little different from the medium scenario, giving only a 1 percent larger workforce by 2011. Increases in stay rates in the 1990s, even if they are real, appear to be of little quantitative significance for the workforce in the near term.

The other scenarios produce more variation. As a percentage of all entrants into the workforce (i.e., graduates and migrants), the foreign trained in biomedical research fall from 16 percent in the medium scenario to 13 percent in the 90 percent scenario and in clinical research from 27 to 22 percent. With this reduction of inflow, the 90 percent scenario produces a reduction in the total workforce by 2011 (relative to the medium scenario) of 2 to 4 percent. In other words, there would be a reduction of 3,700 biomedical researchers and 1,900 clinical researchers by 2001. The 50 percent scenario produces substantially more variation, giving workforces that are smaller than in the low scenario. This indicates that a 50 percent reduction in the inflow of foreign-trained and U.S.-trained graduates would affect the workforce more than would cutting back on all graduates from the medium to the low trend. The 0 percent scenario, finally, reduces the workforces in biomedical and clinical research

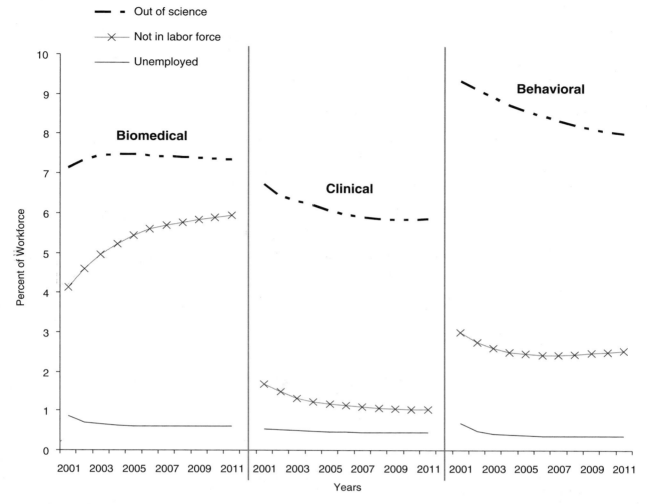

FIGURE D-12 Projected percent of workforce not active in research (out of science, not in the labor force, or unemployed) by field, 2001–2011.
SOURCE: NRC analysis.

by 14 and 20 percent, respectively, relative to the medium scenario. These reductions appear fairly severe, but the workforces would still grow over the decade at annual rates of 1.5 and 2.7 percent.

## EMPLOYMENT PROJECTIONS

An expanding workforce will require a growing number of jobs, which leads to the question of whether enough jobs will be available. This question can be addressed in two ways. First, the trends in employment by sector are reviewed using some of the same data as in the workforce projections, but instead of looking at inflows and outflows by age and sex, only positions by broad sectors are looked at. Second,

government projections for the national labor force and its components are looked at in an attempt to identify where the jobs will be in the future by industry and occupation.

### Sectoral Trends and Projections

The Survey of Doctorate Recipients shows numbers employed by sector. These data come with caveats. The survey does not cover the foreign trained. The number of positions could also be underestimated from these data if some positions were unfilled.

In Figure D-15 six sectors are distinguished as listed below: faculty; other academic positions, excluding postdoctorates; industry, including self-employment; government;

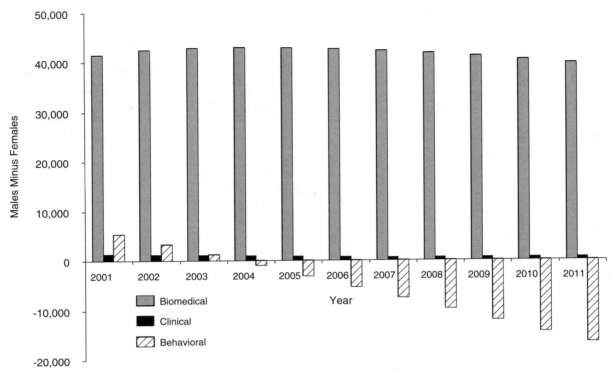

FIGURE D-13 Difference between numbers of employed males and females by field, 2001–2011.
SOURCE: NRC analysis.

other employment, mainly nonprofit groups; and all postdoctorate positions combined, around 75 percent of which are in academia. The largest of these sectors, in each of the three major fields, is faculty. However, industry appears to be catching up fast in the behavioral and biomedical fields. Other sectors have smaller numbers and show slower growth. Sector employment generally moves upward over time, apart from a discontinuity in the late 1980s or early 1990s. In this period, faculty employment in the biomedical and behavioral fields appears to have declined first, followed a few years later by a decline in industrial employment. Nonprofit employment and postdoctorate positions also showed declines. Since the early 1990s, all employment sectors show sustained growth, except for postdoctorates.

Beginning in the late 1990s, postdoctorate employment began to decline, so that by 2001 the numbers had regressed to about the levels of five years earlier (note that foreign-trained postdoctorates are not included here). Even before the decline the numbers of postdoctorates in the clinical and behavioral fields were small, but in the biomedical field employment of U.S.-trained postdoctorates was over 14 percent of total employment and 18 percent of academic employment at its peak.

Employment trends can be extrapolated from the 1990s, avoiding the earlier discontinuities. Specifically, by extrapolating from the five-year trend and using 1997–2001 data, the recent slowdown in growth in behavioral employment may be captured (though for biomedical and clinical employment, using 1991–2001 data would produce the same results). However, one may question whether it is right to ignore discontinuities around 1990 and whether such sectoral employment declines might not reoccur. A second extrapolation is produced from the 20-year trend, using 1981–2001 data, which captures the effects of the discontinuities. Since it is not possible to assign a possible employment decline to any particular future period, this extrapolation in effect reduces growth in each year in the future by a constant factor.

Table D-14 shows the regressions that were run, by major field and sector, with five-year (1997–2001) and 20-year (1981–2001) data. Applying the regression results gives projected 10-year increases in positions by sector shown in Table D-15 (the table also shows estimates based on Bureau of Labor Statistics projections, to be discussed next).

In projections based on the five-year trend, total employment of biomedical researchers appears to grow 2.6 percent annually from 2001 to 2011; employment of clinical researchers grows somewhat faster at 3.7 percent annually; and employment of behavioral researchers grows slowest at 1.7 percent annually. In projections based on the 20-year trend, overall employment growth is reduced for biomedical

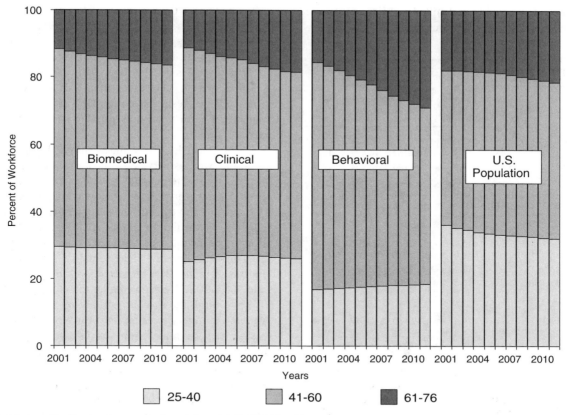

FIGURE D-14 Age distribution (percent) of workforce by field, 2001–2011.
SOURCE: NRC analysis.

and clinical researchers but increased for behavioral researchers. If sectors were combined instead of distinguishing them before running regressions, results would actually be similar.

## BUREAU OF LABOR STATISTICS PROJECTIONS

The projected growth rates can be compared with growth rates from the Bureau of Labor Statistics (BLS; see Table D-16). BLS produces national labor force projections covering a decade or so, the two latest covering 2000–2010 and 2002–2012.[4,5] The dates do not exactly match this study's workforce projections, but there is a bigger problem in matching

occupational categories. BLS does not classify occupations by educational qualifications. Nevertheless, it is possible to roughly equate some of the BLS categories with the ones created for this report. The BLS category of "biological scientists" probably corresponds roughly to what is classified here as "biomedical researchers" (around 2000). The BLS category has about 90 percent as many individuals as the biomedical researchers category. Weaker comparisons can be made between BLS "medical scientists" and this report's category of clinical researchers since the former are more than double the latter. The clinical researcher category includes only Ph.D.s and not M.D.s. The BLS categories of "psychologists," "other social scientists" (which in the later BLS projections is expanded into two categories: "sociologists" and "miscellaneous social scientists and related workers"), and "speech-audio pathologists" are comparable to behavioral researchers. "Psychologists" alone compose 50 percent more than behavioral researchers, presumably because many without Ph.D.s are included, whereas "other social scientists" are few, fewer even than speech-language

[4]Hecker, D. E. 2004. Occupational employment projections to 2012. *Monthly Labor Review* (Feb.):80–105.

[5]Horrigan, M. W. 2004. Employment projections to 2012: Concepts and context. *Monthly Labor Review* (Feb.):3–22.

TABLE D-12 Projected U.S.-Trained and Foreign-Trained Workforce and Employed Researchers by Field, Medium Scenario, 2001–2011

| Field and Year | Potential Workforce | | | Employed | | |
|---|---|---|---|---|---|---|
| | U.S. Trained | Foreign Trained | % Foreign | U.S. Trained | Foreign Trained | % Foreign |
| **Biomedical** | | | | | | |
| 2001 | 113,289 | 17,437 | 13.3 | 100,262 | 14,627 | 12.7 |
| 2002 | 117,175 | 18,330 | 13.5 | 103,148 | 15,231 | 12.9 |
| 2003 | 120,953 | 19,250 | 13.7 | 105,851 | 16,061 | 13.2 |
| 2004 | 124,661 | 20,179 | 13.9 | 108,544 | 16,987 | 13.5 |
| 2005 | 128,335 | 21,111 | 14.1 | 111,305 | 17,931 | 13.9 |
| 2006 | 131,992 | 22,057 | 14.3 | 114,147 | 18,883 | 14.2 |
| 2007 | 135,590 | 23,015 | 14.5 | 117,010 | 19,833 | 14.5 |
| 2008 | 139,135 | 23,978 | 14.7 | 119,875 | 20,774 | 14.8 |
| 2009 | 142,632 | 24,952 | 14.9 | 122,730 | 21,706 | 15.0 |
| 2010 | 146,082 | 25,937 | 15.1 | 125,564 | 22,627 | 15.3 |
| 2011 | 149,482 | 26,918 | 15.3 | 128,361 | 23,528 | 15.5 |
| **Clinical** | | | | | | |
| 2001 | 19,104 | 6,178 | 24.4 | 17,180 | 5,840 | 25.4 |
| 2002 | 20,177 | 6,661 | 24.8 | 18,281 | 6,299 | 25.6 |
| 2003 | 21,273 | 7,166 | 25.2 | 19,344 | 6,781 | 26.0 |
| 2004 | 22,368 | 7,691 | 25.6 | 20,405 | 7,281 | 26.3 |
| 2005 | 23,454 | 8,232 | 26.0 | 21,459 | 7,791 | 26.6 |
| 2006 | 24,536 | 8,796 | 26.4 | 22,504 | 8,314 | 27.0 |
| 2007 | 25,621 | 9,381 | 26.8 | 23,546 | 8,853 | 27.3 |
| 2008 | 26,694 | 9,985 | 27.2 | 24,563 | 9,415 | 27.7 |
| 2009 | 27,744 | 10,608 | 27.7 | 25,541 | 10,001 | 28.1 |
| 2010 | 28,785 | 11,246 | 28.1 | 26,498 | 10,604 | 28.6 |
| 2011 | 29,818 | 11,898 | 28.5 | 27,444 | 11,218 | 29.0 |
| **Behavioral** | | | | | | |
| 2001 | 113,997 | 3,469 | 3.0 | 99,146 | 3,047 | 3.0 |
| 2002 | 116,267 | 3,470 | 2.9 | 101,902 | 3,049 | 2.9 |
| 2003 | 118,368 | 3,465 | 2.8 | 104,256 | 3,046 | 2.8 |
| 2004 | 120,408 | 3,454 | 2.8 | 106,418 | 3,046 | 2.8 |
| 2005 | 122,375 | 3,438 | 2.7 | 108,416 | 3,041 | 2.7 |
| 2006 | 124,247 | 3,423 | 2.7 | 110,281 | 3,038 | 2.7 |
| 2007 | 125,960 | 3,411 | 2.6 | 111,957 | 3,036 | 2.6 |
| 2008 | 127,497 | 3,395 | 2.6 | 113,432 | 3,030 | 2.6 |
| 2009 | 128,868 | 3,376 | 2.6 | 114,729 | 3,018 | 2.6 |
| 2010 | 130,101 | 3,349 | 2.5 | 115,887 | 2,997 | 2.5 |
| 2011 | 131,154 | 3,312 | 2.5 | 116,874 | 2,966 | 2.5 |

SOURCE: NRC analysis.

pathologists. To compare with behavioral researchers, these categories are totaled without weighting.

In the last two BLS projections, the number of employed implies an average annual growth rate for biological scientists of 1.8 to 1.9 percent; for medical scientists a rate of 2.4 percent; and among psychologists, other social scientists, and speech-language pathologists a combined rate of 2.1 to 2.2 percent. These growth rates are reasonably close to those

estimated from 20-year trends. Note, however, that BLS constructs employment projections differently. BLS assumes a full-employment economy, takes labor supply into account, assesses growth in industries' outputs and intermediate inputs, and applies occupational staffing patterns by industry, coupled with expert assessments of likely trends.[6] The confluence of results from the BLS approach with at least our longer-term trend may provide some additional confidence.

In the past, BLS has underestimated growth in professional as well as service occupations.[7] For 1988-2000 the Bureau's projected annual growth rate for biological scientists of 2 percent was well below the actual growth rate of 3.3 percent, and the rate for psychologists of 2 percent was also well below the actual rate of 2.8 percent (for all occupations combined, the BLS projection was for 1.2 percent annual growth compared to the actual 1.6 percent growth rate). Furthermore, the BLS projected growth rates for 2000–2010 and 2002–2012 are even smaller than the rates projected for 1988–2000. If the new projections are similarly too conservative, the higher rates, at least for biomedical and clinical researchers, estimated from our five-year trend may be appropriate.

Applying BLS growth rates to the reported number of positions provides alternative projections of the positions to become available. These are shown in Table D-15. These projections do not represent actual BLS numbers but rather the numbers that would be obtained by applying their implied growth rates beginning in 2001. Estimates by sector are derived by partitioning total increases in proportion to increases in the 20-year trend projections.

The projections from the five-year trend clearly stand out. Over the decade the BLS growth rates, as well as the 20-year trend, imply an increase of about 20,000 biomedical researchers, but the five-year trend implies an increase of almost 30,000. Similarly, the BLS and the 20-year trend imply an increase of about 4,700 clinical researchers, as opposed to 7,700 from the five-year trend. How these projections compare with the projected workforce is the critical issue.

## WORKFORCE VERSUS POSITIONS

Comparisons are made with projected U.S.-trained researchers because research positions have been projected from survey data limited to U.S. graduates. (The BLS projections presumably allow for migrants, but their growth rates are applied to our own base-sector employment num-

[6]Finn, M. G. 2003. Stay rates of foreign doctorate recipients from U.S. universities, 2001. Paper prepared at the Oak Ridge Institute for Science and Education for the Division of Science Resources Studies, National Science Foundation.

[7]Alpert, A., and J. Auyer. 2003. The 1988–2000 employment projections: How accurate were they? *Occupational Outlook Quarterly* (Spring): 3–21.

TABLE D-13 Percent Foreign Trained in Alternative Scenarios, Projected 2011 Total Workforce, and Comparisons of Total to Medium Scenario, by Field

| Scenario | % Foreign Trained Among Entrants (2002–2011) | | | 2011 Total Workforce | | | Ratio to Medium Scenario Total Workforce | | |
|---|---|---|---|---|---|---|---|---|---|
| | Biomedical | Clinical | Behavioral | Biomedical | Clinical | Behavioral | Biomedical | Clinical | Behavioral |
| High | 23.3 | 31.2 | 4.5 | 198,703 | 48,181 | 139,863 | 1.13 | 1.15 | 1.04 |
| Rising | 15.8 | 26.6 | 2.0 | 178,203 | 42,011 | 135,139 | 1.01 | 1.01 | 1.01 |
| Medium | 15.8 | 26.6 | 2.0 | 176,400 | 41,716 | 134,466 | 1.00 | 1.00 | 1.00 |
| 90% | 13.2 | 21.5 | 1.8 | 172,702 | 39,843 | 134,180 | 0.98 | 0.96 | 1.00 |
| 50% | 8.7 | 14.2 | 1.0 | 163,699 | 36,886 | 133,105 | 0.93 | 0.88 | 0.99 |
| 0% | 0.0 | 0.0 | 0.0 | 152,346 | 33,184 | 131,791 | 0.86 | 0.80 | 0.98 |
| Low | 15.3 | 24.9 | 1.9 | 168,770 | 38,355 | 131,149 | 0.96 | 0.92 | 0.98 |

SOURCE: NRC analysis.

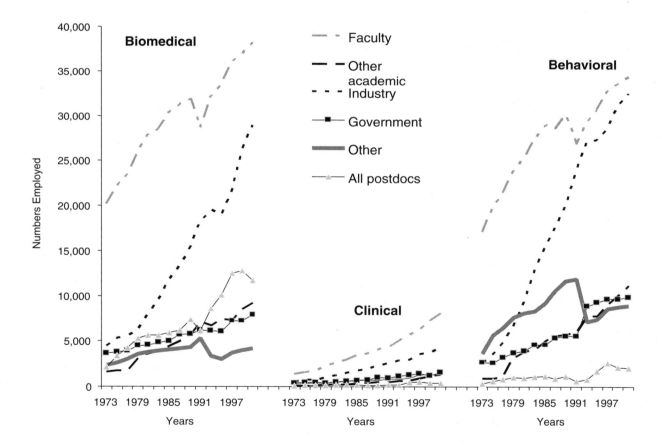

FIGURE D-15 Trends in employment by major field and sector, 1973–2001.
SOURCE: National Science Foundation Survey of Doctorate Recipients.

TABLE D-14 Linear Regressions for Trends in Employment in Various Sectors

| | 1997–2001 Data | | | | 1981–2001 Data | | | |
| | Constant | B | t-test | R² | Constant | B | t-test | R² |
|---|---|---|---|---|---|---|---|---|
| **Biomedical researchers** | | | | | | | | |
| Faculty | −1050820 | 544.25 | 8.44 | 0.986 | −943405 | 490.08 | 6.88 | 0.840 |
| Other academics | −961154 | 485.00 | 5.92 | 0.972 | −550611 | 279.69 | 15.65 | 0.965 |
| Industry | −3618579 | 1823.00 | 6.81 | 0.979 | −1942012 | 984.15 | 16.98 | 0.970 |
| Government | −329386 | 168.50 | 1.89 | 0.781 | −300883 | 154.16 | 12.02 | 0.941 |
| Other | −238397 | 121.25 | 12.18 | 0.993 | 20757 | −8.42 | −0.29 | 0.009 |
| Postdoctorates | 430600 | −209.25 | −1.02 | 0.511 | −784436 | 398.21 | 7.11 | 0.849 |
| All employed | −5773736 | 2935.75 | 7.12 | 0.981 | −4500066 | 2297.61 | 19.18 | 0.976 |
| **Clinical researchers** | | | | | | | | |
| Faculty | −891776 | 449.75 | 10.42 | 0.991 | −529538 | 268.42 | 15.27 | 0.963 |
| Other academics | −207292 | 104.25 | 4.49 | 0.953 | −103572 | 52.32 | 9.65 | 0.912 |
| Industry | −418385 | 211.25 | 2.82 | 0.888 | −292163 | 148.06 | 19.47 | 0.977 |
| Government | −67025 | 34.25 | 0.42 | 0.147 | −104107 | 52.80 | 11.18 | 0.933 |
| Other | −12660 | 7.00 | 1.01 | 0.505 | −85473 | 43.38 | 8.65 | 0.893 |
| Postdoctorates | 57922 | −28.75 | −1.52 | 0.698 | −33401 | 16.92 | 3.55 | 0.583 |
| All employed | −1539217 | 777.75 | 7.56 | 0.983 | −1148253 | 581.90 | 18.02 | 0.973 |
| **Behavioral researchers** | | | | | | | | |
| Faculty | −740856 | 387.50 | 11.09 | 0.992 | −750028 | 391.74 | 5.89 | 0.794 |
| Other academics | −1009329 | 510.00 | 46.49 | 1.000 | −716760 | 363.48 | 15.09 | 0.962 |
| Industry | −1881172 | 956.50 | 4.95 | 0.961 | −2296361 | 1164.63 | 19.79 | 0.978 |
| Government | −82699 | 46.25 | 1.81 | 0.766 | −683510 | 346.82 | 8.89 | 0.898 |
| Other | −192626 | 100.75 | 7.67 | 0.983 | 69222 | −30.17 | −0.38 | 0.016 |
| Postdoctorates | 247152 | −122.50 | −2.22 | 0.832 | −137383 | 69.70 | 3.06 | 0.509 |
| All employed | −3648552 | 1873.00 | 12.95 | 0.994 | −4512779 | 2305.16 | 31.26 | 0.991 |

SOURCE: Analysis based on National Science Foundation Survey of Earned Doctorates.

bers; consequently the resulting employment projections share the same limitation). Comparisons are made not with the potential workforce as a whole but with the numbers employed assuming that some proportion of the future workforce (as at present) will take jobs outside science, choose not to work, or be unemployed (possibly temporarily between jobs).

Table D-17 shows the comparisons between the projected numbers employed in the workforce and the projected numbers of positions from sector employment trends and BLS projections. Results vary by field, and Figure D-16 focuses on some key comparisons. On the one hand, U.S.-trained biomedical researchers will be close to the available number of positions in 2006 and 2011 if the five-year trend projections are correct. On the other hand, they will be about 4 percent too numerous in 2006 and 6 to 7 percent too numerous in 2011 if the 20-year projections and the BLS projections are correct. Possibly, a small deficit would not be an issue since it could presumably be filled by those projected

not to be active in science or by foreign-trained Ph.D.s. A possible excess, however, could be more of an issue, particularly since the foreign-trained Ph.D.s, who are not in the comparison, appear to be increasing more rapidly than U.S.-trained biomedical researchers.

Where clinical researchers are concerned, each comparison indicates that the workforce will exceed future available positions. By 2011 the excess will be 10 percent if the five-year trend continues and about 25 percent whether the 20-year trend continues or the BLS is accurate. This is a relatively small field that is growing rapidly. Some adjustment to slower workforce growth can be expected in the future but at what point and what level is not possible to say.

However, the situation for behavioral researchers is different. By 2006 little by way of excess or deficit will be evident. By 2011 this will still hold if the five-year trend is correct. If the 20-year trend or the BLS projections are accurate, there will be a deficit in the number of U.S.-trained Ph.D.s of around 5 percent. Because there are fewer foreign-

TABLE D-15 Positions by Sector and Increases from 2001–2011 In Alternative Projections, by Major Field

| Field and Sector | Positions in 2001 | 5-Year Trend | 20-Year Trend | Projected 10-Year Increase Based on BLS Rates for | |
|---|---|---|---|---|---|
| | | | | 2000–2010 | 2002–2012 |
| **Biomedical** | | | | | |
| Faculty[a] | 38,299 | 5,368 | 3,842 | 3,915 | 3,810 |
| Other academic | 9,236 | 4,945 | 2,612 | 2,662 | 2,591 |
| Industry | 28,935 | 18,539 | 8,170 | 8,325 | 8,103 |
| Government | 7,886 | 1,582 | 1,254 | 1,278 | 1,244 |
| Other | 4,213 | 1,224 | −385 | −392 | −382 |
| Postdoctorate | 11,655 | −1,856 | 4,716 | 4,806 | 4,678 |
| All sectors | 100,224 | 29,801 | 20,210 | 20,594 | 20,045 |
| **Clinical** | | | | | |
| Faculty[a] | 8,124 | 4,547 | 2,127 | 2,068 | 2,098 |
| Other academic | 1,285 | 1,069 | 364 | 354 | 359 |
| Industry | 4,413 | 2,026 | 1,171 | 1,138 | 1,155 |
| Government | 1,604 | 247 | 479 | 466 | 473 |
| Other | 1,339 | 78 | 429 | 417 | 423 |
| Postdoctorate | 415 | −309 | 207 | 201 | 204 |
| All sectors | 17,180 | 7,659 | 4,777 | 4,643 | 4,711 |
| **Behavioral** | | | | | |
| Faculty[a] | 34,491 | 3,915 | 3,263 | 3,251 | 3,324 |
| Other academic | 11,194 | 5,087 | 2,998 | 2,987 | 3,055 |
| Industry | 32,561 | 9,788 | 13,143 | 13,093 | 13,390 |
| Government | 9,877 | 433 | 4,073 | 4,058 | 4,149 |
| Other | 8,960 | 1,023 | −415 | −413 | −423 |
| Postdoctorate | 2,093 | −1,289 | 691 | 688 | 704 |
| All sectors | 99,176 | 18,958 | 23,754 | 23,663 | 24,199 |

NOTE: BLS rates are Bureau of Labor Statistics employment projections.

[a]Tenured or on tenure track—those on nontenure track are counted under "Other academic."

SOURCE: Analysis based on National Science Foundation Survey of Earned Doctorates and Bureau of Labor Statistics employment projections (Hecker, 2001, 2004).

trained migrant Ph.D.s, their numbers are unlikely to be sufficient to fill any gap. In principle, a deficit could be filled from the portion of the workforce with jobs outside science because this field is larger than the other two. However, whether this is practical would have to be investigated.

Therefore, the three fields have different prospects. Nor is each field homogeneous, being composed of a variety of specific disciplines and separate sectors. Although they deserve attention disciplines cannot be considered here. Instead sectoral trends are briefly examined.

## SECTORAL PROSPECTS AND POSTDOCTORATES

### Sectors

If employment grows according to the projections given here, the distribution by sector of those employed in science could show one important change: the balance could shift in the other direction of those employed as faculty (either tenured or on a tenure track) in the biomedical and social and behavioral fields in 2001 who outnumbered those in industry or self-employed by 2011. In the social and behavioral field this will happen whether growth is as slow as projected from the five-year trend or as fast as projected from the 20-year trend. But in the biomedical field it will happen only with the faster growth scenario from the five-year trend. However, academic employment in each field will still be higher than industrial employment if nonfaculty appointments and postdoctorates are taken into account.

Nontenure appointments are a growing part of academic employment. The growth has been steady since the 1970s. Those who are neither tenured nor on a tenure track are close to becoming half of all academic employees in the biomedical field. This proportion is lower in the other fields but is

TABLE D-16 Projected and Actual Growth Rates (%) for Various Occupational Groups

| 2001–2011 Projections | Biomedical Researchers | Clinical Researchers | Behavioral Researchers | | | |
|---|---|---|---|---|---|---|
| 1997–2001 Data | 2.60 | 3.69 | 1.75 | | | |
| 1981–2001 Data | 1.84 | 2.45 | 2.15 | | | |
| Bureau of Labor Statistics | Biological Scientists | Medical Scientists | All Social Scientists[a] | Psychologists | Other Social Scientists | Speech-Language Pathologists |
| 2002–2012 Projection | 1.82 | 2.42 | 2.18 | 2.19 | 0.57 | 2.44 |
| 2000–2010 Projection | 1.87 | 2.39 | 2.14 | 1.62 | 1.25 | 3.27 |
| 1988–2000 Projection | 1.95 | [b] | [b] | 1.99 | [b] | 2.08 |
| 1988–2000 Actual | 3.33 | [b] | [b] | 2.77 | [b] | 5.78 |

[a]Combines psychologists, other social scientists, and speech-language pathologists.

[b]No reported data.

SOURCES: Bureau of Labor Statistics rates are estimated from projections for 2002–2012 (Hecker, 2004), 2000–2010 (Hecker, 2001), and 1988–2000 (Alpert and Auyer, 2003) and data reported in Alpert and Auyer (2003).

TABLE D-17  Excess or Deficit of U.S.-Trained Researchers in Relation to Various Projections of Research Positions

| | Excess or Deficit Relative to Positions | | | | Excess or Deficit as % of Positions | | | |
|---|---|---|---|---|---|---|---|---|
| | Projected from Trend Over | | Based on BLS Growth Rates to | | Projected from Trend Over | | Based on BLS Growth Rates to | |
| Field and Year | 5 Years | 20 Years | 2010 | 2012 | 5 Years | 20 Years | 2010 | 2012 |
| **Biomedical** | | | | | | | | |
| 2002 | −483 | 3,395 | 1,033 | 1,080 | −0.5 | 3.4 | 1.0 | 1.1 |
| 2003 | −712 | 3,800 | 1,810 | 1,905 | −0.7 | 3.7 | 1.7 | 1.8 |
| 2004 | −952 | 4,196 | 2,541 | 2,685 | −0.9 | 4.0 | 2.4 | 2.5 |
| 2005 | −1,124 | 4,659 | 3,302 | 3,499 | −1.0 | 4.4 | 3.1 | 3.2 |
| 2006 | −1,215 | 5,203 | 4,107 | 4,357 | −1.1 | 4.8 | 3.7 | 4.0 |
| 2007 | −1,284 | 5,768 | 4,894 | 5,200 | −1.1 | 5.2 | 4.4 | 4.7 |
| 2008 | −1,352 | 6,335 | 5,644 | 6,008 | −1.1 | 5.6 | 4.9 | 5.3 |
| 2009 | −1,430 | 6,892 | 6,344 | 6,768 | −1.2 | 5.9 | 5.5 | 5.8 |
| 2010 | −1,529 | 7,428 | 6,983 | 7,468 | −1.2 | 6.3 | 5.9 | 6.3 |
| 2011 | −1,664 | 7,927 | 7,543 | 8,092 | −1.3 | 6.6 | 6.2 | 6.7 |
| **Clinical** | | | | | | | | |
| 2002 | 442 | 1,561 | 685 | 680 | 2.5 | 9.3 | 3.9 | 3.9 |
| 2003 | 727 | 2,042 | 1,322 | 1,311 | 3.9 | 11.8 | 7.3 | 7.3 |
| 2004 | 1,011 | 2,521 | 1,947 | 1,930 | 5.2 | 14.1 | 10.5 | 10.4 |
| 2005 | 1,287 | 2,993 | 2,554 | 2,530 | 6.4 | 16.2 | 13.5 | 13.4 |
| 2006 | 1,554 | 3,456 | 3,141 | 3,111 | 7.4 | 18.1 | 16.2 | 16.0 |
| 2007 | 1,818 | 3,916 | 3,714 | 3,678 | 8.4 | 20.0 | 18.7 | 18.5 |
| 2008 | 2,058 | 4,351 | 4,251 | 4,207 | 9.1 | 21.5 | 20.9 | 20.7 |
| 2009 | 2,258 | 4,747 | 4,737 | 4,686 | 9.7 | 22.8 | 22.8 | 22.5 |
| 2010 | 2,437 | 5,122 | 5,191 | 5,131 | 10.1 | 24.0 | 24.4 | 24.0 |
| 2011 | 2,605 | 5,487 | 5,621 | 5,553 | 10.5 | 25.0 | 25.8 | 25.4 |
| **Behavioral** | | | | | | | | |
| 2002 | 675 | −272 | 581 | 537 | 0.7 | −0.3 | 0.6 | 0.5 |
| 2003 | 1,150 | −224 | 744 | 653 | 1.1 | −0.2 | 0.7 | 0.6 |
| 2004 | 1,434 | −369 | 667 | 529 | 1.4 | −0.3 | 0.6 | 0.5 |
| 2005 | 1,553 | −677 | 378 | 189 | 1.5 | −0.6 | 0.3 | 0.2 |
| 2006 | 1,540 | −1,118 | −94 | −335 | 1.4 | −1.0 | −0.1 | −0.3 |
| 2007 | 1,337 | −1,748 | −805 | −1,100 | 1.2 | −1.5 | −0.7 | −1.0 |
| 2008 | 934 | −2,579 | −1,769 | −2,121 | 0.8 | −2.2 | −1.5 | −1.8 |
| 2009 | 352 | −3,589 | −2,964 | −3,375 | 0.3 | −3.0 | −2.5 | −2.9 |
| 2010 | −368 | −4,737 | −4,351 | −4,823 | −0.3 | −3.9 | −3.6 | −4.0 |
| 2011 | −1,260 | −6,056 | −5,965 | −6,501 | −1.1 | −4.9 | −4.9 | −5.3 |

SOURCE: NRC analysis.

rising just as insistently. The biomedical field is ahead in this trend mainly because of a high number of postdoctorates, which was rising until the late 1990s.

## Postdoctorates

A specific look at postdoctorates is warranted, first those who are U.S. trained, since the foreign-trained postdoctorates data are not included in the sectoral data. Though many Ph.D.

graduates may spend some time as postdoctorates, this period is generally short in comparison to other employment, so that at any given time postdoctorates are few relative to total employment. Among clinical and behavioral Ph.D.s, postdoctorates are only 1.5 to 3.5 percent of the total. In the biomedical field, though, they compose about 10 percent of total employment.

U.S.-trained postdoctorates are not necessarily young. Roughly 40 percent tend to be age 25 to 34, but about the

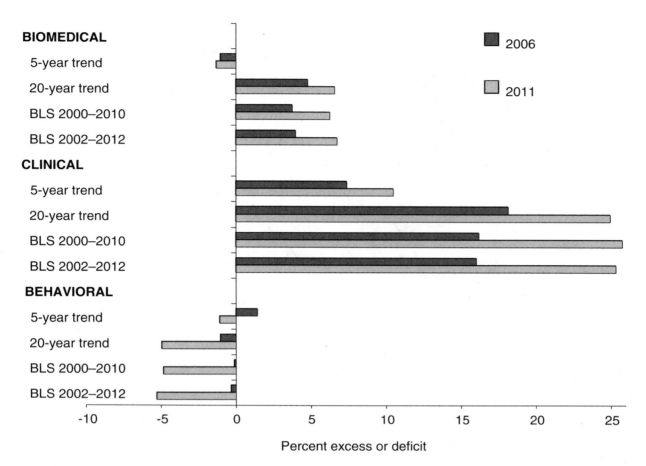

FIGURE D-16 Percent excess or deficit of U.S.-trained researchers in relation to various projections of research positions, 2006 and 2011.
SOURCE: NRC analysis and Bureau of Labor Statistics.

same proportion are 35 to 44. In the clinical and behavioral fields, about 20 to 25 percent are 45 and older. This is for years 1997, 1999, and 2001, across which there is little change. At younger ages, proportionally more of those employed are postdoctorates; this is particularly true in the biomedical field, where, under age 35, 50 percent of employed males and 60 percent of employed females are postdoctorates.

For the remainder of the postdoctoral pool, more limited information is available from department reports in the Graduate Student Survey, which was used to estimate the foreign-trained workforce. These reports indicate that postdoctorates with U.S. Ph.D.s, who have been considered first because of better information, are actually a minority in two fields, making up only 49 percent of biomedical postdoctorates and 40 percent of clinical postdoctorates in 2001. Among the much smaller contingent of behavioral postdoctorates they form a majority of 80 percent (see Figure D-17).

M.D.s and foreign-trained Ph.D.s take the remaining positions, M.D.s being more important among clinical post-

doctorates and foreign-trained Ph.D.s more important among biomedical and behavioral postdoctorates. The trends for M.D.s and foreign-trained Ph.D.s are opposite. The percentage of clinical postdoctorates taken by M.D.s has fallen by more than a third in two decades, from 59 percent in 1983 to 37 percent by 2001. Over the same period, the percentage of postdoctorates taken by foreign-trained Ph.D.s roughly doubled in each of the three fields, reaching 39 percent in biomedical research, 22 percent in clinical research, and 18 percent in behavioral research. The importance of noncitizen researchers may be even greater than these figures indicate. Among U.S.-trained Ph.D.s with postdoctorates, a number are on temporary resident visas: 25 percent in biomedical research, 23 percent in clinical research, and 8 percent in behavioral research. These percentages have risen about as fast as those for foreign-trained Ph.D.s.

Note, however, that department reports are not entirely consistent with sector data. Figure D-18 matches comparable groups: academic postdoctorates in sector data (who must, because of the survey sample, have U.S. Ph.D.s) and postdoctorates with U.S. Ph.D.s in department data (who

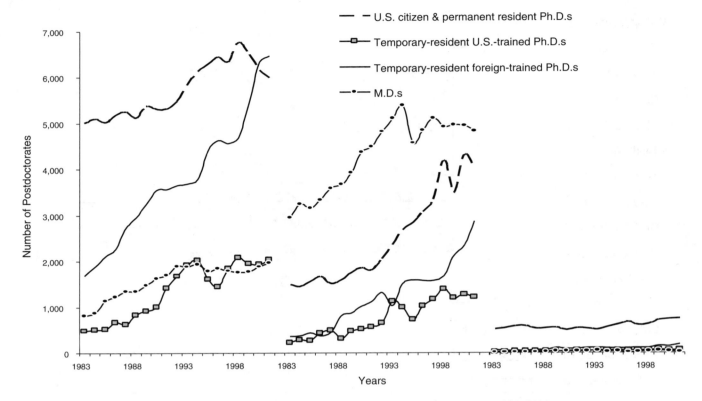

FIGURE D-17 Postdoctorates reported by graduate departments, by field, degree, and visa status, 1983–2001.
SOURCE: National Science Foundation Survey of Graduate Students and Postdoctorates in Engineering and Science, 2001.

must be academic). The sector data suggest a surge in academic postdoctorates in the 1990s that does not appear in the department data, except among clinical researchers. In the clinical field, however, the department data indicate far more postdoctorates (even with M.D.s excluded) than the sector data. The definition of clinical disciplines may be different between surveys, and some of the postdoctorates in clinical departments might have biomedical Ph.D.s. It is also possible that our partitioning of temporary residents into U.S. trained and foreign trained is inaccurate and that the foreign trained are even more common than they appear among clinical Ph.D.s. However, these possible explanations cannot be verified, and the inconsistencies need further investigation.

If sector data (which provide ages) is relied upon and it is assumed that the proportions of Ph.D.s on postdoctorates stay constant by age, these proportions can be applied to the projected workforce to estimate the number likely to be seeking postdoctorates in the near future. This can be done only for U.S.-trained Ph.D.s—a significant but unavoidable limitation. Table D-18 shows their numbers as well as the numbers of projected postdoctorate positions, taken from the preceding sectoral projections.

Numbers and positions are compared in Figure D-19. U.S.-trained graduates seeking postdoctorates may or may not outnumber the positions available for them. In the biomedical field, individuals and positions may in fact be in balance if the 20-year trend continues, but individuals will be far too numerous—by 5,600 by 2001 or 57 percent more than the available positions—if the more recent downturn reflected in the five-year trend continues. In clinical research, individuals will outnumber positions by 15 percent even given the more optimistic 20-year trend in positions, and if the more pessimistic five-year trend comes to pass, the number of individuals will be a startling eight times greater than the number of positions available. Similarly, in behavioral research, there will be either 13 percent more individuals than there are positions available or four times the number of positions, depending on which projection is used. A projected downturn in positions derived from the five-year trend is responsible for the large shortfalls; this essentially extrapolates from the recent decline in the number of positions taken by U.S.-trained Ph.D.s. This decline at least partly reflects the rising share of postdoctorates taken by foreign-trained Ph.D.s. Whether the foreign inflows—which also include

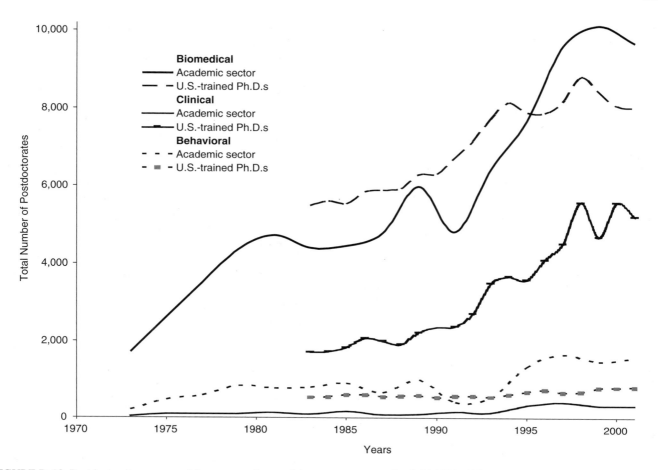

FIGURE D-18 Postdoctorates compared from sector data and department reports, by field 1973–2001.
SOURCES: National Science Foundation Survey of Earned Doctorates, 2001, and National Science Foundation Survey of Graduate Students and Postdoctorates in Engineering and Science, 2001.

rising U.S.-trained temporary residents—will continue is uncertain.

## CONCLUSION

This discussion began with the question of whether the right numbers of people are being trained for the future research workforce. To answer this question, first data on the workforce and its components were examined and then recent trends were modeled and projected into the future. Such workforce projections appear to have worked in the past. Projections from 1995 were generally accurate up to 2001, in the partial comparisons that are possible with current data.

Nevertheless, the projections have limitations, rooted especially in inadequate data. Projections have been made only for Ph.D. researchers and not for M.D. researchers since

there was only a rough estimate of the numbers of the latter. Our projections for foreign-trained Ph.D.s are based on dated and inconsistent data. Rates were assumed for movement between statuses that are constant within age groups, and adequate information was not available on trends in rates. A basic assumption could be made that future trends will resemble past trends. Trends in graduates (and to a degree in prior enrollment levels) are assumed to follow a future course modeled on past trends. Migration is assumed to follow previous trends, though alternatives were also modeled. Retirement ages are assumed to maintain their current distribution. Graduation, migration, and retirement are discretionary behaviors that could be postponed at will, within limits, or possibly accelerated, but no attempt was made to model the factors underlying such decisions.

The projections have been extended in another dimension

TABLE D-18 Projected U.S.-Trained Postdoctorates and Positions for U.S.-Trained Postdoctorates by Field, Alternative Scenarios, 2001–2011

| Field and Year | Postdocs in Workforce | | | Projected Positions from Trend Over | |
|---|---|---|---|---|---|
| | Medium | High | Low | 5 years | 20 years |
| **Biomedical** | | | | | |
| 2001 | 12,711 | 12,711 | 12,711 | 11,655 | 11,655 |
| 2002 | 12,726 | 12,820 | 12,627 | 11,682 | 12,787 |
| 2003 | 12,819 | 13,025 | 12,613 | 11,473 | 13,186 |
| 2004 | 12,950 | 13,278 | 12,617 | 11,263 | 13,584 |
| 2005 | 13,214 | 13,686 | 12,739 | 11,054 | 13,982 |
| 2006 | 13,515 | 14,149 | 12,882 | 10,845 | 14,380 |
| 2007 | 13,916 | 14,721 | 13,111 | 10,636 | 14,779 |
| 2008 | 14,291 | 15,282 | 13,309 | 10,426 | 15,177 |
| 2009 | 14,695 | 15,871 | 13,524 | 10,217 | 15,575 |
| 2010 | 15,052 | 16,416 | 13,690 | 10,008 | 15,973 |
| 2011 | 15,392 | 16,948 | 13,843 | 9,799 | 16,371 |
| **Clinical** | | | | | |
| 2001 | 507 | 507 | 507 | 415 | 415 |
| 2002 | 546 | 554 | 540 | 364 | 470 |
| 2003 | 585 | 601 | 570 | 336 | 487 |
| 2004 | 620 | 643 | 594 | 307 | 503 |
| 2005 | 659 | 694 | 623 | 278 | 520 |
| 2006 | 705 | 751 | 658 | 249 | 537 |
| 2007 | 750 | 808 | 690 | 221 | 554 |
| 2008 | 785 | 855 | 713 | 192 | 571 |
| 2009 | 813 | 895 | 727 | 163 | 588 |
| 2010 | 834 | 930 | 735 | 134 | 605 |
| 2011 | 859 | 967 | 744 | 106 | 622 |
| **Behavioral** | | | | | |
| 2001 | 2,391 | 2,391 | 2,391 | 2,093 | 2,093 |
| 2002 | 2,527 | 2,543 | 2,512 | 1,907 | 2,157 |
| 2003 | 2,651 | 2,685 | 2,617 | 1,784 | 2,226 |
| 2004 | 2,746 | 2,800 | 2,693 | 1,662 | 2,296 |
| 2005 | 2,842 | 2,917 | 2,765 | 1,539 | 2,366 |
| 2006 | 2,905 | 3,002 | 2,806 | 1,417 | 2,435 |
| 2007 | 2,968 | 3,090 | 2,845 | 1,294 | 2,505 |
| 2008 | 3,021 | 3,167 | 2,873 | 1,172 | 2,575 |
| 2009 | 3,072 | 3,245 | 2,900 | 1,049 | 2,645 |
| 2010 | 3,109 | 3,308 | 2,912 | 927 | 2,714 |
| 2011 | 3,144 | 3,369 | 2,919 | 804 | 2,784 |

SOURCE: NRC analysis.

to cover not only the workforce but also the positions that will become available. Positions are projected based on employment trends by sector and give results that appear comparable to occupational projections from the BLS. However, whether past employment trends will be sustained in the future is not known. Societal changes, such as the aging of the population, the increasing need for and complexity of health care, and the growing importance of science-based decision making could affect the demand for health research.

Without attempting to assess such factors, these projections of positions rely on past sectoral trends—which, it should be noted, presumably also reflect substantial and sometimes unexpected societal changes. Comparing these projections with workforce projections gives some limited and tentative answers to the initial question. The answers differ by field. Biomedical researchers are probably being graduated in sufficient numbers for the next decade (2001–2011), though perhaps they will be a few percentage points too numerous. Clinical Ph.D.s, however, seem to be headed for a situation of substantial oversupply. This field includes substantial numbers of M.D.s, who are not projected, that category is smaller but growing more rapidly than the other fields, so the trajectory is somewhat uncertain. Finally, behavioral researchers are on a trend that will lead largely to balance until the end of the decade, at which time a slight deficit is possible.

These statements refer only to U.S.-trained researchers. Foreign-trained researchers are an important and increasing part of the workforce in the biomedical and clinical fields. The research positions they fill are not distinguished from those taken by U.S.-trained researchers (but are not reflected in our sectoral employment data). Therefore the balance, or lack of balance, between the U.S.-trained workforce and positions filled by foreign-trained researchers presents a partial and somewhat artificial picture.

The complications introduced by foreign-trained researchers are evident from the perspective of postdoctorates. U.S.-trained researchers on postdoctorates declined in the late 1990s, and if this trend continues, a substantial oversupply of those seeking postdoctorates may emerge. However,

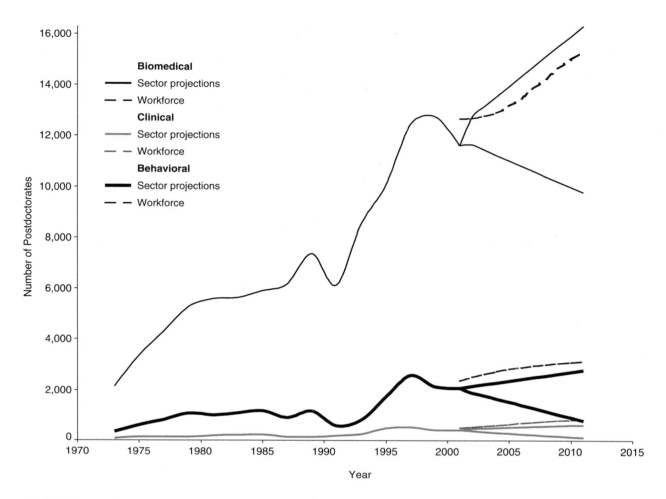

FIGURE D-19 Reported and projected U.S.-trained postdoctorates and postdoctorate positions, 1973–2011.
SOURCES: National Science Foundation Survey of Doctorate Recipients; and NRC analysis.

this decline may actually indicate a replacement of U.S.-trained with foreign-trained researchers, who are increasing rapidly in the postdoctorate pool in the biomedical and clinical fields. If this proves to be the case, the uncertain pros-pects for future migrants may substantially affect the prospects for bringing the numbers of U.S.-trained researchers seeking postdoctorates into balance with the numbers of positions that, from past trends, will be available to them.

# Appendix E

# Characteristics of Doctorates

TABLE E-1 Characteristics of Doctorates in the Biomedical Sciences, 1973–2003

| | 1970 | 1971 | 1972 | 1973 | 1974 | 1975 | 1976 | 1977 | 1978 | 1979 |
|---|---|---|---|---|---|---|---|---|---|---|
| Total Doctorates | 2,882 | 3,132 | 3,116 | 3,135 | 3,013 | 3,085 | 3,150 | 3,050 | 3,118 | 3,212 |
| Males | 2,420 | 2,572 | 2,530 | 2,474 | 2,340 | 2,347 | 2,424 | 2,351 | 2,311 | 2,351 |
| Females | 462 | 560 | 586 | 661 | 673 | 738 | 726 | 699 | 807 | 861 |
| Citizens | 2,385 | 2,591 | 2,573 | 2,582 | 2,381 | 2,556 | 2,610 | 2,528 | 2,628 | 2,738 |
| Permanent residents | 160 | 198 | 215 | 231 | 209 | 194 | 165 | 169 | 147 | 133 |
| Temporary residents | 312 | 266 | 256 | 253 | 283 | 256 | 277 | 261 | 259 | 253 |
| Unknown | 25 | 77 | 72 | 69 | 140 | 79 | 98 | 92 | 84 | 88 |
| Minorities | 2 | 1 | 3 | 80 | 84 | 86 | 80 | 78 | 108 | 79 |
| Postdoctoral training | | | | | | | | | | |
| Postdoctoral fellowship | 1,008 | 1,016 | 965 | 1,000 | 863 | 1,102 | 1,176 | 1,212 | 1,313 | 1,314 |
| Postdoctoral research | 317 | 389 | 402 | 435 | 505 | 536 | 503 | 528 | 535 | 500 |
| Postdoctoral traineeship | 64 | 84 | 83 | 46 | 39 | 54 | 56 | 69 | 75 | 100 |
| Other training | 78 | 89 | 148 | 160 | 173 | 199 | 202 | 157 | 163 | 213 |
| Total postdoctorates | 1,467 | 1,578 | 1,598 | 1,641 | 1,580 | 1,891 | 1,937 | 1,966 | 2,086 | 2,127 |
| Percent planning | 52.8% | 54.0% | 55.1% | 55.9% | 57.5% | 65.0% | 65.9% | 68.5% | 71.5% | 70.4% |
| Employment | 1,246 | 1,275 | 1,246 | 1,236 | 1,113 | 968 | 962 | 880 | 809 | 877 |
| Other | 63 | 70 | 59 | 61 | 54 | 49 | 42 | 25 | 24 | 17 |
| Ph.D. with plans | 2,776 | 2,923 | 2,903 | 2,938 | 2,747 | 2,908 | 2,941 | 2,871 | 2,919 | 3,021 |
| Time to degree | 5.92 | 6 | 6 | 6.17 | 6.17 | 6 | 6.17 | 6.25 | 6.33 | 6.41 |
| Registered time to degree | 5.41 | 5.42 | 5.67 | 5.75 | 5.67 | 5.59 | 5.75 | 5.75 | 5.91 | 5.91 |
| Age at time of degree | 28.92 | 29 | 29.42 | 29.58 | 29.42 | 29.25 | 29.25 | 29.34 | 29.38 | 29.41 |

| | 1987 | 1988 | 1989 | 1990 | 1991 | 1992 | 1993 | 1994 | 1995 | 1996 |
|---|---|---|---|---|---|---|---|---|---|---|
| Total Doctorates | 3,465 | 3,769 | 3,793 | 3,992 | 4,294 | 4,442 | 4,794 | 4,863 | 5,079 | 5,366 |
| Males | 2,214 | 2,377 | 2,348 | 2,477 | 2,655 | 2,740 | 2,864 | 2,887 | 2,955 | 3,102 |
| Females | 1,251 | 1,392 | 1,445 | 1,515 | 1,639 | 1,702 | 1,930 | 1,976 | 2,124 | 2,264 |
| Citizens | 2,670 | 2,858 | 2,850 | 2,899 | 3,050 | 3,072 | 3,264 | 3,203 | 3,278 | 3,291 |
| Permanent residents | 153 | 176 | 173 | 183 | 210 | 240 | 296 | 641 | 831 | 801 |
| Temporary residents | 455 | 515 | 570 | 814 | 987 | 1,078 | 1,165 | 980 | 918 | 1,173 |
| Unknown | 187 | 220 | 200 | 96 | 62 | 66 | 98 | 57 | 73 | 121 |
| Minorities | 128 | 123 | 135 | 135 | 159 | 162 | 190 | 223 | 243 | 246 |
| Postdoctoral training | | | | | | | | | | |
| Postdoctoral fellowship | 1,470 | 1,650 | 1,652 | 1,766 | 1,900 | 2,011 | 2,243 | 2,234 | 2,358 | 2,380 |
| Postdoctoral research | 657 | 704 | 679 | 811 | 879 | 894 | 940 | 968 | 994 | 1,031 |
| Postdoctoral traineeship | 75 | 81 | 65 | 76 | 87 | 81 | 99 | 111 | 107 | 115 |
| Other training | 217 | 216 | 260 | 233 | 294 | 307 | 332 | 313 | 346 | 406 |
| Total postdoctorates | 2,419 | 2,651 | 2,656 | 2,886 | 3,160 | 3,293 | 3,614 | 3,626 | 3,805 | 3,932 |
| Percent planning | 74.9% | 75.8% | 75.1% | 77.0% | 77.0% | 77.2% | 78.6% | 78.1% | 7.9% | 77.7% |
| Employment | 776 | 815 | 856 | 820 | 902 | 936 | 939 | 974 | 963 | 1,077 |
| Other | 36 | 32 | 27 | 43 | 40 | 35 | 45 | 40 | 48 | 52 |
| Ph.D. with plans | 3,231 | 3,498 | 3,539 | 3,749 | 4,102 | 4,264 | 4,598 | 4,640 | 4,816 | 5,061 |
| Time to degree | 7.33 | 7.42 | 7.42 | 7.58 | 7.5 | 7.59 | 7.67 | 7.75 | 7.83 | 7.67 |
| Registered time to degree | 6.5 | 6.58 | 6.5 | 6.59 | 6.58 | 6.75 | 6.75 | 6.75 | 6.83 | 6.83 |
| Age at time of degree | 30.5 | 30.83 | 30.92 | 31.17 | 31.08 | 31.17 | 31.17 | 31.17 | 31.25 | 31.25 |

| 1980 | 1981 | 1982 | 1983 | 1984 | 1985 | 1986 |
|------|------|------|------|------|------|------|
| 3,396 | 3,356 | 3,444 | 3,338 | 3,399 | 3,313 | 3,369 |
| 2,440 | 2,383 | 2,417 | 2,224 | 2,315 | 2,192 | 2,197 |
| 956 | 973 | 1,027 | 1,114 | 1,084 | 1,121 | 1,172 |
| 2,905 | 2,898 | 2,927 | 2,854 | 2,868 | 2,727 | 2,751 |
| 147 | 125 | 114 | 108 | 109 | 113 | 118 |
| 273 | 248 | 294 | 291 | 308 | 364 | 343 |
| 71 | 85 | 109 | 85 | 114 | 109 | 157 |
| 83 | 91 | 94 | 86 | 99 | 104 | 119 |
| 1,362 | 1,364 | 1,385 | 1,313 | 1,446 | 1,409 | 1,415 |
| 626 | 616 | 625 | 668 | 625 | 634 | 699 |
| 103 | 70 | 78 | 70 | 68 | 66 | 58 |
| 225 | 255 | 275 | 247 | 238 | 200 | 196 |
| 2,316 | 2,305 | 2,363 | 2,298 | 2,377 | 2,309 | 2,368 |
| 71.6% | 72.3% | 72.6% | 72.1% | 74.2% | 73.8% | 74.9% |
| 891 | 865 | 860 | 851 | 791 | 790 | 759 |
| 29 | 20 | 31 | 37 | 34 | 28 | 36 |
| 3,236 | 3,190 | 3,254 | 3,186 | 3,202 | 3,127 | 3,163 |
| 6.5 | 6.5 | 6.67 | 7 | 7.09 | 7.17 | 7.25 |
| 6 | 6 | 6 | 6.17 | 6.33 | 6.42 | 6.41 |
| 29.25 | 29.33 | 29.59 | 29.83 | 30.25 | 30.42 | 30.59 |

| 1997 | 1998 | 1999 | 2000 | 2001 | 2002 | 2003 |
|------|------|------|------|------|------|------|
| 5,459 | 5,465 | 5,340 | 5,547 | 5,397 | 5,375 | 5,412 |
| 3,110 | 3,113 | 3,074 | 3,060 | 2,984 | 3,015 | 2,960 |
| 2,349 | 2,352 | 2,266 | 2,478 | 2,403 | 2,358 | 2,439 |
| 3,451 | 3,492 | 3,438 | 3,620 | 3,623 | 3,563 | 3,534 |
| 562 | 533 | 477 | 364 | 341 | 315 | 266 |
| 1,233 | 1,213 | 1,224 | 1,336 | 1,202 | 1,222 | 1,341 |
| 243 | 241 | 218 | 227 | 231 | 275 | 366 |
| 261 | 277 | 308 | 315 | 364 | 367 | 358 |
| 2,293 | 2,312 | 2,223 | 2,340 | 2,170 | 2,269 | 2,343 |
| 979 | 1,027 | 977 | 931 | 882 | 884 | 932 |
| 87 | 69 | 75 | 148 | 102 | 109 | 172 |
| 193 | 250 | 476 | 362 | 387 | 273 | 311 |
| 3,552 | 3,658 | 3,751 | 3,781 | 3,541 | 3,535 | 3,758 |
| 71.1% | 73.0% | 75.8% | 73.6% | 71.0% | 71.3% | 75.0% |
| 1,288 | 1,257 | 1,152 | 1,276 | 1,373 | 1,368 | 1,193 |
| 156 | 93 | 43 | 83 | 76 | 58 | 60 |
| 4,996 | 5,008 | 4,946 | 5,140 | 4,990 | 4,961 | 5,011 |
| 7.92 | 7.83 | 7.59 | 7.75 | 7.83 | 7.59 | 7.59 |
| 6.92 | 6.92 | 6.75 | 6.84 | 6.92 | 6.75 | 6.67 |
| 31 | 30.92 | 30.83 | 30.91 | 30.83 | 30.67 | 30.58 |

TABLE E-2 Employment Characteristics of Biomedical Doctorates from U.S. Institutions, 1973–2001

| | 1973 | 1975 | 1977 | 1979 | 1981 | 1983 | 1985 | 1987 |
|---|---|---|---|---|---|---|---|---|
| Total employed in S&E | 34,367 | 39,661 | 43,411 | 48,591 | 53,357 | 56,481 | 61,810 | 65,800 |
| | 100.0% | 100.0% | 100.0% | 100.0% | 100.0% | 100.0% | 100.0% | 100.0% |
| Minority | 797 | 1,066 | 1,149 | 1,259 | 1,566 | 1,516 | 1,819 | 1,906 |
| | 2.3% | 2.7% | 2.6% | 2.6% | 2.9% | 2.7% | 2.9% | 2.9% |
| Citizens and permanent residents | 32,610 | 37,958 | 41,421 | 46,131 | 52,492 | 55,898 | 61,128 | 65,120 |
| | 94.9% | 95.7% | 95.4% | 94.9% | 98.4% | 99.0% | 98.9% | 99.0% |
| Temporary residents | 793 | 777 | 1,055 | 1,645 | 503 | 331 | 473 | 581 |
| | 2.3% | 2.0% | 2.4% | 3.4% | 0.9% | 0.6% | 0.8% | 0.9% |
| Total academics | 23,423 | 27,219 | 29,889 | 33,188 | 36,165 | 36,797 | 39,307 | 41,027 |
| | 68.2% | 68.6% | 68.9% | 68.3% | 67.8% | 65.1% | 63.6% | 62.4% |
| Faculty with rank appointments | 20,138 | 22,230 | 23,515 | 26,064 | 27,868 | 28,510 | 30,454 | 31,280 |
| | 58.6% | 56.1% | 54.2% | 53.6% | 52.2% | 50.5% | 49.3% | 47.5% |
| Tenured faculty | 4,567 | 13,376 | 14,345 | 15,636 | 17,836 | 18,884 | 20,114 | 19,157 |
| | 13.3% | 33.7% | 33.0% | 32.2% | 33.4% | 33.4% | 32.5% | 29.1% |
| Tenure-track faculty (not tenured) | 15,571 | 8,854 | 9,170 | 5,952 | 6,446 | 5,673 | 6,644 | 6,149 |
| | 45.3% | 22.3% | 21.1% | 12.2% | 12.1% | 10.0% | 10.7% | 9.3% |
| Academic postdoctorates | 1,713 | 2,615 | 3,507 | 4,358 | 4,722 | 4,405 | 4,450 | 4,784 |
| | 5.0% | 6.6% | 8.1% | 9.0% | 8.8% | 7.8% | 7.2% | 7.3% |
| Other academic appointments | 1,572 | 1,706 | 1,810 | 3,092 | 3,575 | 3,882 | 4,403 | 4,963 |
| | 4.6% | 4.3% | 4.2% | 6.4% | 6.7% | 6.9% | 7.1% | 7.5% |
| Industry (nonpostdoctorate) | 4,470 | 5,273 | 5,543 | 6,286 | 7,881 | 9,589 | 11,841 | 13,366 |
| | 1.3% | 13.3% | 12.8% | 12.9% | 14.8% | 17.0% | 19.2% | 20.3% |
| Industrial postdoctorates | 27 | 53 | 40 | 27 | 70 | 46 | 126 | 222 |
| | 0.1% | 0.1% | 0.1% | 0.1% | 0.1% | 0.1% | 0.2% | 0.3% |
| Government (nonpostdoctorate) | 3,675 | 3,785 | 3,914 | 4,449 | 4,545 | 4,843 | 5,026 | 5,725 |
| | 10.7% | 9.5% | 9.0% | 9.2% | 8.5% | 8.6% | 8.1% | 8.7% |
| Government postdoctorates | 156 | 245 | 336 | 327 | 286 | 444 | 373 | 529 |
| | 0.5% | 0.6% | 0.8% | 0.7% | 0.5% | 0.8% | 0.6% | 0.8% |
| Other sectors (nonpostdoctorate) | 2,303 | 2,624 | 3,029 | 3,551 | 3,778 | 3,909 | 4,082 | 4,199 |
| | 6.7% | 6.6% | 7.0% | 7.3% | 7.1% | 6.9% | 6.6% | 6.4% |
| Other-sector postdoctorates | 236 | 431 | 407 | 552 | 525 | 748 | 961 | 648 |
| | 0.7% | 1.1% | 0.9% | 1.1% | 1.0% | 1.3% | 1.6% | 1.0% |
| Doctorates with federal research support | 19,841 | 22,152 | 23,884 | 26,183 | 26,640 | 29,439 | 27,377 | 38,171 |
| | 57.7% | 55.9% | 55.0% | 53.9% | 49.9% | 52.1% | 44.3% | 58.0% |

*continues*

## TABLE E-2  Continued

|                                          | 1989     | 1991     | 1993     | 1995     | 1997     | 1999     | 2001     |
|------------------------------------------|----------|----------|----------|----------|----------|----------|----------|
| Total employed in S&E                    | 70,593   | 71,962   | 76,449   | 79,077   | 88,481   | 95,780   | 100,224  |
|                                          | 100.0%   | 100.0%   | 100.0%   | 100.0%   | 100.0%   | 100.0%   | 100.0%   |
| Minority                                 | 2,217    | 2,727    | 2,840    | 3,150    | 3,758    | 4,385    | 5,345    |
|                                          | 3.1%     | 3.8%     | 3.7%     | 4.0%     | 4.2%     | 4.6%     | 5.3%     |
| Citizens and permanent residents         | 69,709   | 70,834   | 75,023   | 77,826   | 87,105   | 93,100   | 97,126   |
|                                          | 98.7%    | 98.4%    | 98.1%    | 98.4%    | 98.4%    | 97.2%    | 96.9%    |
| Temporary residents                      | 884      | 945      | 1,410    | 1,251    | 1,376    | 2,680    | 3,098    |
|                                          | 1.3%     | 1.3%     | 1.8%     | 1.6%     | 1.6%     | 2.8%     | 3.1%     |
| Total academics                          | 43,572   | 40,581   | 45,258   | 48,622   | 53,026   | 55,682   | 57,227   |
|                                          | 61.7%    | 56.4%    | 59.2%    | 61.5%    | 59.9%    | 58.1%    | 57.1%    |
| Faculty with rank appointments           | 31,862   | 28,672   | 32,180   | 33,496   | 36,122   | 36,987   | 38,299   |
|                                          | 45.1%    | 39.8%    | 42.1%    | 42.4%    | 40.8%    | 38.6%    | 38.2%    |
| Tenured faculty                          | 19,755   | 17,106   | 19,070   | 19,516   | 20,326   | 21,535   | 21,695   |
|                                          | 28.0%    | 23.8%    | 24.9%    | 24.7%    | 23.0%    | 22.5%    | 21.6%    |
| Tenure-track faculty (not tenured)       | 5,872    | 7,556    | 7,722    | 8,259    | 8,974    | 8,909    | 8,784    |
|                                          | 8.3%     | 10.5%    | 10.1%    | 10.4%    | 10.1%    | 9.3%     | 8.8%     |
| Academic postdoctorates                  | 5,993    | 4,819    | 6,431    | 7,701    | 9,620    | 10,145   | 9,692    |
|                                          | 8.5%     | 6.7%     | 8.4%     | 9.7%     | 10.9%    | 10.6%    | 9.7%     |
| Other academic appointments              | 5,717    | 7,090    | 6,647    | 7,436    | 7,296    | 8,550    | 9,236    |
|                                          | 8.1%     | 9.9%     | 8.7%     | 9.4%     | 8.2%     | 8.9%     | 9.2%     |
| Industry (nonpostdoctorate)              | 15,376   | 18,309   | 19,538   | 18,949   | 21,643   | 26,216   | 28,935   |
|                                          | 21.8%    | 25.4%    | 25.6%    | 24.0%    | 24.5%    | 27.4%    | 28.9%    |
| Industrial postdoctorates                | 206      | 204      | 376      | 531      | 561      | 591      | 293      |
|                                          | 0.3%     | 0.3%     | 0.5%     | 0.7%     | 0.6%     | 0.6%     | 0.3%     |
| Government (nonpostdoctorate)            | 5,776    | 6,157    | 6,143    | 6,074    | 7,212    | 7,240    | 7,886    |
|                                          | 8.2%     | 8.6%     | 8.0%     | 7.7%     | 8.2%     | 7.6%     | 7.9%     |
| Government postdoctorates                 | 514      | 432      | 1057     | 1111     | 1437     | 1180     | 1050     |
|                                          | 0.7%     | 0.6%     | 1.4%     | 1.4%     | 1.6%     | 1.2%     | 1.1%     |
| Other sectors (nonpostdoctorate)         | 4,363    | 5,303    | 3,356    | 3,028    | 3,728    | 4,005    | 4,213    |
|                                          | 6.2%     | 7.4%     | 4.4%     | 3.8%     | 4.2%     | 4.2%     | 4.2%     |
| Other-sector postdoctorates              | 671      | 681      | 721      | 762      | 874      | 866      | 620      |
|                                          | 1.0%     | 0.9%     | 0.9%     | 1.0%     | 1.0%     | 0.9%     | 0.6%     |
| Doctorates with federal research support | 40,655   | 38,490   | 29,261   | 31,513   | 34,678   | 41,707   | 42,012   |
|                                          | 57.6%    | 53.5%    | 38.3%    | 39.9%    | 39.2%    | 43.5%    | 41.9%    |

TABLE E-3 Characteristics of Doctorates in the Behavioral and Social Sciences, 1973–2003

| | 1970 | 1971 | 1972 | 1973 | 1974 | 1975 | 1976 | 1977 | 1978 | 1979 |
|---|---|---|---|---|---|---|---|---|---|---|
| Total doctorates | 2,683 | 3,094 | 3,220 | 3,433 | 3,661 | 3,835 | 4,047 | 4,098 | 4,082 | 4,120 |
| Males | 2,079 | 2,352 | 2,391 | 2,452 | 2,549 | 2,611 | 2,733 | 2,634 | 2,554 | 2,445 |
| Females | 604 | 742 | 829 | 981 | 1,112 | 1,224 | 1,314 | 1,464 | 1,528 | 1,675 |
| Citizens | 2,458 | 2,812 | 2,928 | 3,128 | 3,231 | 3,461 | 3,722 | 3,724 | 3,676 | 3,728 |
| Permanent residents | 78 | 88 | 96 | 89 | 85 | 92 | 85 | 92 | 95 | 92 |
| Temporary residents | 121 | 150 | 140 | 157 | 165 | 214 | 183 | 167 | 152 | 161 |
| Unknown | 26 | 44 | 56 | 59 | 180 | 68 | 57 | 115 | 159 | 139 |
| Minorities | 0 | 3 | 11 | 84 | 115 | 172 | 202 | 234 | 235 | 266 |
| Postdoctoral training | | | | | | | | | | |
| Postdoctoral fellowship | 194 | 188 | 189 | 196 | 193 | 227 | 298 | 322 | 349 | 336 |
| Postdoctoral research | 59 | 67 | 67 | 84 | 84 | 106 | 100 | 114 | 120 | 127 |
| Postdoctoral traineeship | 22 | 43 | 36 | 35 | 49 | 58 | 51 | 75 | 98 | 78 |
| Other training | 21 | 40 | 37 | 52 | 64 | 61 | 85 | 74 | 72 | 63 |
| Total postdoctorates | 296 | 338 | 329 | 367 | 390 | 452 | 534 | 585 | 639 | 604 |
| Percent planning | 11% | 11% | 10% | 11% | 11% | 12% | 13% | 14% | 16% | 15% |
| Employment | 2,242 | 2,526 | 2,590 | 2,809 | 2,882 | 3,095 | 3,209 | 3,147 | 3,014 | 3,179 |
| Other | 49 | 70 | 87 | 68 | 80 | 68 | 83 | 66 | 75 | 53 |
| Ph.D. with plans | 2,587 | 2,934 | 3,006 | 3,244 | 3,352 | 3,615 | 3,826 | 3,798 | 3,728 | 3,836 |
| Time to degree | 6 | 6 | 6 | 6.17 | 6.25 | 6.25 | 6.33 | 6.59 | 6.83 | 7 |
| Registered time to degree | 5.59 | 5.5 | 5.58 | 5.67 | 5.67 | 5.75 | 5.92 | 5.96 | 6 | 6.25 |
| Age at time of degree | 29.66 | 29.58 | 29.75 | 30.08 | 30.08 | 30.25 | 30.25 | 30.58 | 30.59 | 31.16 |

| | 1987 | 1988 | 1989 | 1990 | 1991 | 1992 | 1993 | 1994 | 1995 | 1996 |
|---|---|---|---|---|---|---|---|---|---|---|
| Total doctorates | 3,988 | 3,844 | 3,975 | 4,064 | 4,087 | 4,080 | 4,289 | 4,185 | 4,162 | 4,224 |
| Males | 1,912 | 1,749 | 1,796 | 1,745 | 1,624 | 1,745 | 1,720 | 1,671 | 1,606 | 1,555 |
| Females | 2,076 | 2,095 | 2,179 | 2,319 | 2,463 | 2,335 | 2,569 | 2,514 | 2,556 | 2,669 |
| Citizens | 3,352 | 3,232 | 3,221 | 3,497 | 3,560 | 3,490 | 3,702 | 3,623 | 3,587 | 3,644 |
| Permanent residents | 111 | 107 | 95 | 107 | 124 | 132 | 146 | 155 | 177 | 170 |
| Temporary residents | 180 | 194 | 244 | 267 | 296 | 334 | 329 | 311 | 303 | 307 |
| Unknown | 345 | 312 | 415 | 193 | 112 | 133 | 123 | 104 | 101 | 111 |
| Minorities | 255 | 266 | 267 | 320 | 339 | 321 | 349 | 340 | 394 | 419 |
| Postdoctoral training | | | | | | | | | | |
| Postdoctoral fellowship | 413 | 414 | 432 | 480 | 568 | 585 | 684 | 676 | 725 | 700 |
| Postdoctoral research | 174 | 173 | 124 | 149 | 155 | 150 | 170 | 187 | 195 | 193 |
| Postdoctoral traineeship | 65 | 75 | 88 | 104 | 75 | 92 | 77 | 87 | 91 | 86 |
| Other training | 64 | 53 | 59 | 51 | 51 | 53 | 75 | 58 | 55 | 84 |
| Total postdoctorates | 716 | 715 | 703 | 784 | 849 | 880 | 1,006 | 1,008 | 1,066 | 1,063 |
| Percent planning | 18% | 19% | 18% | 19% | 21% | 22% | 24% | 24% | 26% | 25% |
| Employment | 2,785 | 2,688 | 2,720 | 2,842 | 2,834 | 2,784 | 2,888 | 2,780 | 2,646 | 2,675 |
| Other | 54 | 50 | 55 | 65 | 49 | 62 | 69 | 62 | 77 | 83 |
| Ph.D. with plans | 3,555 | 3,453 | 3,478 | 3,691 | 3,732 | 3,726 | 3,963 | 3,850 | 3,789 | 3,821 |
| Time to degree | 8.67 | 8.92 | 9.00 | 9.00 | 9.00 | 9.09 | 9.00 | 8.91 | 8.92 | 8.75 |
| Registered time to degree | 7.33 | 7.58 | 7.59 | 7.75 | 7.67 | 7.59 | 7.50 | 7.50 | 7.50 | 7.50 |
| Age at time of degree | 33.75 | 34.33 | 34.33 | 34.42 | 34.66 | 34.67 | 34.58 | 34.17 | 34.25 | 33.83 |

| 1980 | 1981 | 1982 | 1983 | 1984 | 1985 | 1986 |
|---|---|---|---|---|---|---|
| 4,015 | 4,339 | 4,023 | 4,263 | 4,141 | 3,964 | 3,979 |
| 2,315 | 2,461 | 2,240 | 2,265 | 2,087 | 1,993 | 1,962 |
| 1,700 | 1,878 | 1,783 | 1,998 | 2,054 | 1,971 | 2,017 |
| 3,630 | 3,935 | 3,600 | 3,799 | 3,662 | 3,487 | 3,426 |
| 98 | 85 | 82 | 90 | 75 | 91 | 108 |
| 152 | 173 | 151 | 182 | 190 | 179 | 185 |
| 135 | 146 | 190 | 192 | 214 | 207 | 260 |
| 244 | 256 | 269 | 271 | 272 | 261 | 278 |
| 380 | 389 | 339 | 403 | 396 | 427 | 438 |
| 118 | 146 | 134 | 132 | 135 | 133 | 139 |
| 91 | 104 | 95 | 104 | 109 | 97 | 101 |
| 61 | 76 | 56 | 69 | 59 | 49 | 63 |
| 650 | 715 | 624 | 708 | 699 | 706 | 741 |
| 16% | 17% | 16% | 17% | 17% | 18% | 19% |
| 3,068 | 3,311 | 3,063 | 3,191 | 3,096 | 2,910 | 2,837 |
| 55 | 65 | 60 | 60 | 42 | 55 | 54 |
| 3,773 | 4,091 | 3,747 | 3,959 | 3,837 | 3,671 | 3,632 |
| 7.25 | 7.5 | 7.92 | 8 | 8.17 | 8.5 | 8.59 |
| 6.42 | 6.59 | 6.91 | 7 | 7.16 | 7.25 | 7.25 |
| 31.33 | 31.92 | 32.08 | 32.5 | 32.75 | 33.08 | 33.58 |

| 1997 | 1998 | 1999 | 2000 | 2001 | 2002 | 2003 |
|---|---|---|---|---|---|---|
| 4,371 | 4,481 | 4,466 | 4,507 | 4,230 | 4,064 | 4,139 |
| 1,565 | 1,595 | 1,596 | 1,595 | 1,475 | 1,411 | 1,411 |
| 2,806 | 2,886 | 2,870 | 2,908 | 2,751 | 2,649 | 2,724 |
| 3,608 | 3,757 | 3,797 | 3,821 | 3,548 | 3,400 | 3,426 |
| 151 | 142 | 119 | 135 | 114 | 113 | 97 |
| 292 | 315 | 265 | 310 | 276 | 265 | 323 |
| 360 | 285 | 301 | 241 | 292 | 286 | 293 |
| 428 | 494 | 534 | 545 | 537 | 544 | 553 |
| 713 | 860 | 912 | 919 | 903 | 895 | 942 |
| 192 | 211 | 197 | 203 | 234 | 199 | 228 |
| 61 | 74 | 56 | 81 | 71 | 71 | 70 |
| 22 | 30 | 97 | 57 | 61 | 53 | 72 |
| 988 | 1,175 | 1,262 | 1,260 | 1,269 | 1,218 | 1,312 |
| 23% | 26% | 28% | 28% | 30% | 30% | 37% |
| 2,564 | 2,488 | 2,511 | 2,632 | 2,408 | 2,334 | 2,212 |
| 112 | 114 | 75 | 115 | 93 | 80 | 71 |
| 3,664 | 3,777 | 3,848 | 4,007 | 3,770 | 3,632 | 3,595 |
| 8.96 | 8.92 | 8.91 | 8.75 | 8.91 | 9.00 | 9.00 |
| 7.50 | 7.50 | 7.41 | 7.50 | 7.59 | 7.59 | 7.59 |
| 33.42 | 33.24 | 33 | 32.84 | 32.75 | 32.75 | 32.82 |

TABLE E-4 Employment Characteristics of Behavioral and Social Sciences Doctorates from U.S. Institutions, 1973–2001

| | 1973 | 1975 | 1977 | 1979 | 1981 | 1983 | 1985 | 1987 |
|---|---|---|---|---|---|---|---|---|
| Total employed in S&E | 74,570 | 34,360 | 39,237 | 45,532 | 51,743 | 58,458 | 64,616 | 68852 |
| | 100.0% | 100.0% | 100.0% | 100.0% | 100.0% | 100.0% | 100.0% | 100.0% |
| Minority | 520 | 842 | 1,066 | 1,517 | 2,059 | 2,546 | 2,897 | 3166 |
| | 0.7% | 2.5% | 2.7% | 3.3% | 4.0% | 4.4% | 4.5% | 4.6% |
| Citizens and permanent residents | 26,998 | 33,978 | 38,912 | 44,863 | 51,490 | 58,129 | 64,400 | 68761 |
| | 36.2% | 98.9% | 99.2% | 98.5% | 99.5% | 99.4% | 99.7% | 99.9% |
| Temporary residents | 107 | 172 | 122 | 369 | 168 | 247 | 156 | 59 |
| | 0.1% | 0.5% | 0.3% | 0.8% | 0.3% | 0.4% | 0.2% | 0.1% |
| Total academics | 18178 | 22333 | 24287 | 26972 | 29995 | 32267 | 34985 | 34911 |
| | 24.4% | 65.0% | 61.9% | 59.2% | 58.0% | 55.2% | 54.1% | 50.7% |
| Faculty with rank appointments | 17,095 | 19,917 | 21,383 | 23,888 | 25,364 | 27,442 | 29,079 | 28678 |
| | 22.9% | 58.0% | 54.5% | 52.5% | 49.0% | 46.9% | 4.5% | 41.7% |
| Tenured faculty | 3,560 | 11,606 | 13,139 | 14,812 | 16,982 | 19,302 | 19,833 | 18761 |
| | 4.8% | 33.8% | 33.5% | 32.5% | 32.8% | 33.0% | 30.7% | 27.2% |
| Tenure-track faculty (not tenured) | 13,535 | 8,311 | 8,244 | 5,336 | 5,204 | 4,963 | 5,623 | 4989 |
| | 18.2% | 24.2% | 21.0% | 11.7% | 10.1% | 8.5% | 8.7% | 7.2% |
| Academic postdoctorates | 205 | 481 | 594 | 836 | 775 | 798 | 901 | 664 |
| | 0.3% | 1.4% | 1.5% | 1.8% | 1.5% | 1.4% | 1.4% | 1.0% |
| Other academic appointments | 878 | 915 | 1,070 | 3,141 | 3,856 | 4,027 | 5,005 | 5569 |
| | 1.2% | 2.7% | 2.7% | 6.9% | 7.5% | 6.9% | 7.7% | 8.1% |
| Industry (nonpostdoctorate) | 2,682 | 3,666 | 4,883 | 6,695 | 9,357 | 12,891 | 15,469 | 17621 |
| | 3.6% | 10.7% | 12.4% | 14.7% | 18.1% | 22.1% | 23.9% | 25.6% |
| Industrial postdoctorates | 0 | 0 | 4 | 0 | 0 | 4 | 80 | 14 |
| | 0.0% | 0.0% | 0.0% | 0.0% | 0.0% | 0.0% | 0.1% | 0.0% |
| Government (nonpostdoctorate) | 2,680 | 2,603 | 3,216 | 3,718 | 3,938 | 4,627 | 4,632 | 5390 |
| | 3.6% | 7.6% | 8.2% | 8.2% | 7.6% | 7.9% | 7.2% | 7.8% |
| Government postdoctorates | 22 | 15 | 53 | 49 | 88 | 85 | 22 | 51 |
| | 0.0% | 0.0% | 0.1% | 0.1% | 0.2% | 0.1% | 0.0% | 0.1% |
| Other sectors (nonpostdoctorate) | 3,647 | 5,609 | 6,431 | 7,600 | 8,134 | 8,299 | 9,205 | 10561 |
| | 4.9% | 16.3% | 16.4% | 16.7% | 15.7% | 14.2% | 14.2% | 15.3% |
| Other-sector postdoctorates | 113 | 91 | 151 | 180 | 125 | 201 | 177 | 158 |
| | 0.2% | 0.3% | 0.4% | 0.4% | 0.2% | 0.3% | 0.3% | 0.2% |
| Doctorates with federal research support | 10,881 | 12,965 | 13,790 | 15,213 | 15,689 | 16,648 | 13,651 | 21864 |
| | 14.6% | 37.7% | 35.1% | 33.4% | 30.3% | 28.5% | 21.1% | 31.8% |

*continues*

## TABLE E-4  Continued

| | 1989 | 1991 | 1993 | 1995 | 1997 | 1999 | 2001 |
|---|---|---|---|---|---|---|---|
| Total employed in S&E | 74,570 | 75,420 | 81,126 | 84,408 | 91,662 | 95,909 | 99,154 |
| | 100.0% | 100.0% | 100.0% | 100.0% | 100.0% | 100.0% | 100.0% |
| Minority | 3,713 | 4,542 | 4,943 | 5,609 | 6,482 | 7,045 | 8,534 |
| | 5.0% | 6.0% | 6.1% | 6.6% | 7.1% | 7.3% | 8.6% |
| Citizens and permanent residents | 74,348 | 75,178 | 80,894 | 84,200 | 91,333 | 95,531 | 98,725 |
| | 99.7% | 99.7% | 99.7% | 99.8% | 99.6% | 99.6% | 99.6% |
| Temporary residents | 194 | 164 | 190 | 195 | 329 | 378 | 429 |
| | 0.3% | 0.2% | 0.2% | 0.2% | 0.4% | 0.4% | 0.4% |
| Total academics | 36961 | 33280 | 37617 | 39905 | 43736 | 45402 | 47206 |
| | 49.6% | 44.1% | 46.4% | 47.3% | 47.7% | 47.3% | 47.6% |
| Faculty with rank appointments | 30,239 | 26,852 | 29,402 | 30,787 | 32,941 | 33,837 | 34,491 |
| | 40.6% | 35.6% | 36.2% | 36.5% | 35.9% | 35.3% | 34.8% |
| Tenured faculty | 20,041 | 18,201 | 19,858 | 20,720 | 22,266 | 22,032 | 22,196 |
| | 26.9% | 24.1% | 24.5% | 24.5% | 24.3% | 23.0% | 22.4% |
| Tenure-track faculty (not tenured) | 5,379 | 5,400 | 5,956 | 5,991 | 6,032 | 6,364 | 6,510 |
| | 7.2% | 7.2% | 7.3% | 7.1% | 6.6% | 6.6% | 6.6% |
| Academic postdoctorates | 993 | 416 | 534 | 1,329 | 1,641 | 1,458 | 1,543 |
| | 1.3% | 0.6% | 0.7% | 1.6% | 1.8% | 1.5% | 1.6% |
| Other academic appointments | 5,729 | 6,012 | 7,681 | 7,789 | 9,154 | 10,136 | 11,194 |
| | 7.7% | 8.0% | 9.5% | 9.2% | 10.0% | 10.6% | 11.3% |
| Industry (nonpostdoctorate) | 19,998 | 23,995 | 27,236 | 27,348 | 28,735 | 31,318 | 32,561 |
| | 26.8% | 31.8% | 33.6% | 32.4% | 31.3% | 32.7% | 32.8% |
| Industrial postdoctorates | 5 | 20 | 50 | 151 | 462 | 211 | 201 |
| | 0.0% | 0.0% | 0.1% | 0.2% | 0.5% | 0.2% | 0.2% |
| Government (nonpostdoctorate) | 5,557 | 5,565 | 8,867 | 9,310 | 9,692 | 9,696 | 9,877 |
| | 7.5% | 7.4% | 10.9% | 11.0% | 10.6% | 10.1% | 10.0% |
| Government postdoctorates | 11 | 84 | 147 | 176 | 267 | 210 | 165 |
| | 0.0% | 0.1% | 0.2% | 0.2% | 0.3% | 0.2% | 0.2% |
| Other sectors (nonpostdoctorate) | 11,697 | 11,865 | 7,129 | 7,423 | 8,557 | 8,804 | 8,960 |
| | 15.7% | 15.7% | 8.8% | 8.8% | 9.3% | 9.2% | 9.0% |
| Other-sector postdoctorates | 166 | 66 | 80 | 95 | 213 | 268 | 184 |
| | 0.2% | 0.1% | 0.1% | 0.1% | 0.2% | 0.3% | 0.2% |
| Doctorates with federal research support | 23,831 | 20,902 | 12,686 | 15,385 | 16,308 | 20,487 | 22,549 |
| | 32.0% | 27.7% | 15.6% | 18.2% | 17.8% | 21.4% | 22.7% |

TABLE E-5 Characteristics of Doctorates in the Clinical Sciences, 1973–2003

| | 1970 | 1971 | 1972 | 1973 | 1974 | 1975 | 1976 | 1977 | 1978 | 1979 |
|---|---|---|---|---|---|---|---|---|---|---|
| Total doctorates | 273 | 329 | 306 | 323 | 339 | 340 | 357 | 385 | 387 | 432 |
| Males | 218 | 271 | 245 | 249 | 252 | 233 | 248 | 266 | 256 | 271 |
| Females | 55 | 58 | 61 | 74 | 87 | 107 | 109 | 119 | 131 | 161 |
| Citizens | 210 | 263 | 219 | 250 | 239 | 258 | 273 | 296 | 305 | 339 |
| Permanent residents | 19 | 20 | 40 | 34 | 37 | 35 | 32 | 41 | 26 | 39 |
| Temporary residents | 37 | 30 | 29 | 31 | 33 | 35 | 40 | 42 | 38 | 37 |
| Unknown | 7 | 16 | 18 | 8 | 30 | 12 | 12 | 6 | 18 | 17 |
| Minorities | 0 | 3 | 0 | 8 | 11 | 12 | 14 | 22 | 15 | 22 |
| Postdoctoral training | | | | | | | | | | |
| Postdoctoral fellowship | 22 | 21 | 37 | 27 | 16 | 29 | 39 | 44 | 31 | 50 |
| Postdoctoral research | 7 | 7 | 17 | 19 | 26 | 13 | 16 | 24 | 21 | 24 |
| Postdoctoral traineeship | 2 | 3 | 3 | . | 1 | 1 | 2 | 3 | 3 | 3 |
| Other training | 7 | 5 | 9 | 12 | 7 | 6 | 7 | 7 | 7 | 14 |
| Total postdoctoral | 38 | 36 | 66 | 58 | 50 | 49 | 64 | 78 | 62 | 91 |
| Percent planning | 14% | 11% | 22% | 18% | 15% | 14% | 18% | 20% | 16% | 21% |
| Employment | 201 | 247 | 200 | 225 | 224 | 255 | 264 | 269 | 285 | 297 |
| Other | 6 | 9 | 8 | 10 | 10 | 7 | 8 | 7 | 4 | 12 |
| Ph.D. with plans | 245 | 292 | 274 | 293 | 284 | 311 | 336 | 354 | 351 | 400 |
| Time to degree | 6.59 | 6.21 | 6.42 | 6.34 | 6.75 | 7 | 6.63 | 6.5 | 7.09 | 6.92 |
| Registered time to degree | 5.25 | 5.75 | 5.42 | 5.59 | 5.83 | 5.92 | 5.75 | 5.8 | 6 | 6.08 |
| Age at time of degree | 31.21 | 29.96 | 30.33 | 30.59 | 30.67 | 31.83 | 31.58 | 30.75 | 31.67 | 31.75 |

| | 1987 | 1988 | 1989 | 1990 | 1991 | 1992 | 1993 | 1994 | 1995 | 1996 |
|---|---|---|---|---|---|---|---|---|---|---|
| Total doctorates | 699 | 788 | 881 | 840 | 950 | 1022 | 1100 | 1208 | 1225 | 1237 |
| Males | 290 | 302 | 313 | 322 | 333 | 363 | 396 | 420 | 456 | 435 |
| Females | 409 | 486 | 568 | 518 | 617 | 659 | 704 | 788 | 769 | 802 |
| Citizens | 527 | 573 | 656 | 630 | 706 | 739 | 803 | 897 | 857 | 865 |
| Permanent residents | 33 | 38 | 29 | 34 | 58 | 48 | 63 | 91 | 102 | 87 |
| Temporary residents | 84 | 108 | 118 | 145 | 161 | 213 | 202 | 214 | 236 | 253 |
| Unknown | 55 | 69 | 78 | 31 | 29 | 30 | 44 | 15 | 41 | 41 |
| Minorities | 38 | 50 | 38 | 41 | 56 | 49 | 79 | 70 | 90 | 83 |
| Postdoctoral training | | | | | | | | | | |
| Postdoctoral fellowship | 64 | 71 | 60 | 85 | 79 | 111 | 107 | 156 | 138 | 136 |
| Postdoctoral research | 27 | 39 | 38 | 51 | 40 | 44 | 50 | 43 | 70 | 70 |
| Postdoctoral traineeship | 4 | 9 | 6 | 12 | 5 | 12 | 9 | 11 | 11 | 7 |
| Other training | 14 | 14 | 12 | 17 | 17 | 25 | 19 | 16 | 17 | 26 |
| Total postdoctoral | 109 | 133 | 116 | 165 | 141 | 192 | 185 | 226 | 236 | 239 |
| Percent planning | 16% | 17% | 13% | 20% | 15% | 19% | 17% | 19% | 19% | 19% |
| Employment | 506 | 561 | 659 | 589 | 725 | 746 | 820 | 840 | 850 | 855 |
| Other | 16 | 14 | 11 | 14 | 16 | 12 | 14 | 15 | 23 | 30 |
| Ph.D. with plans | 631 | 708 | 786 | 768 | 882 | 950 | 1019 | 1081 | 1109 | 1124 |
| Time to degree | 9.00 | 9.00 | 9.08 | 9.59 | 9.17 | 9.92 | 9.63 | 9.50 | 9.91 | 9.75 |
| Registered time to degree | 7.00 | 7.00 | 7.17 | 7.25 | 7.25 | 7.33 | 7.75 | 7.42 | 7.50 | 7.63 |
| Age at time of degree | 35.92 | 36.42 | 36.75 | 37.17 | 37.83 | 37.75 | 38.42 | 37.79 | 38.08 | 38.46 |

| 1980 | 1981 | 1982 | 1983 | 1984 | 1985 | 1986 |
|------|------|------|------|------|------|------|
| 464 | 524 | 575 | 526 | 621 | 619 | 677 |
| 273 | 303 | 319 | 249 | 262 | 244 | 259 |
| 191 | 221 | 256 | 277 | 359 | 375 | 418 |
| 370 | 429 | 457 | 401 | 492 | 458 | 489 |
| 32 | 33 | 33 | 30 | 36 | 32 | 30 |
| 53 | 48 | 64 | 70 | 66 | 85 | 93 |
| 9 | 14 | 21 | 25 | 27 | 44 | 65 |
| 14 | 19 | 30 | 23 | 34 | 31 | 32 |
| 58 | 45 | 54 | 37 | 64 | 55 | 48 |
| 27 | 30 | 29 | 21 | 22 | 29 | 38 |
| 4 | 5 | 6 | 3 | 6 | 2 | 7 |
| 16 | 19 | 7 | 8 | 12 | 3 | 16 |
| 105 | 99 | 96 | 69 | 104 | 89 | 109 |
| 23% | 19% | 17% | 13% | 17% | 14% | 16% |
| 332 | 388 | 435 | 398 | 465 | 461 | 478 |
| 6 | 10 | 14 | 15 | 10 | 6 | 9 |
| 443 | 497 | 545 | 482 | 579 | 556 | 596 |
| 7.17 | 7.67 | 7.5 | 7.92 | 8.17 | 8.83 | 8.91 |
| 6 | 6.29 | 6.17 | 6.59 | 6.75 | 6.87 | 7.00 |
| 32 | 32.37 | 32.87 | 34.08 | 34.33 | 35.58 | 35.92 |

| 1997 | 1998 | 1999 | 2000 | 2001 | 2002 | 2003 |
|------|------|------|------|------|------|------|
| 1354 | 1425 | 1338 | 1527 | 1558 | 1579 | 1574 |
| 469 | 474 | 480 | 518 | 566 | 510 | 528 |
| 885 | 951 | 858 | 1007 | 981 | 1069 | 1039 |
| 911 | 1003 | 925 | 1070 | 1036 | 1058 | 1115 |
| 77 | 85 | 81 | 74 | 76 | 63 | 60 |
| 256 | 266 | 250 | 275 | 293 | 300 | 299 |
| 126 | 77 | 92 | 108 | 153 | 158 | 100 |
| 85 | 97 | 105 | 116 | 112 | 106 | 137 |
| 131 | 145 | 137 | 139 | 190 | 201 | 219 |
| 75 | 66 | 70 | 65 | 85 | 74 | 90 |
| 10 | 10 | 18 | 14 | 11 | 12 | 24 |
| 9 | 9 | 38 | 26 | 21 | 16 | 36 |
| 225 | 230 | 263 | 244 | 307 | 303 | 369 |
| 17% | 16% | 20% | 16% | 20% | 19% | 26% |
| 910 | 943 | 906 | 1095 | 1017 | 1024 | 1019 |
| 30 | 48 | 24 | 37 | 26 | 49 | 38 |
| 1165 | 1221 | 1193 | 1376 | 1350 | 1376 | 1426 |
| 10.09 | 10.50 | 10.00 | 10.00 | 10.00 | 10.75 | 10.00 |
| 7.92 | 8.00 | 7.75 | 7.92 | 7.59 | 8.00 | 7.92 |
| 38.58 | 38.25 | 37.24 | 38.33 | 36.92 | 38.17 | 37.08 |

**TABLE E-6** Employment Characteristics of Clinical Sciences Doctorates from U.S. Institutions, 1973–2001

|  | 1973 | 1975 | 1977 | 1979 | 1981 | 1983 | 1985 | 1987 |
|---|---|---|---|---|---|---|---|---|
| Total employed in S&E | 2,682 | 3,475 | 3,748 | 4,489 | 5,312 | 6,003 | 7,188 | 7,669 |
|  | 100.0% | 100.0% | 100.0% | 100.0% | 100.0% | 100.0% | 100.0% | 100.0% |
| Minority | 95 | 132 | 146 | 183 | 198 | 250 | 273 | 342 |
|  | 3.5% | 3.8% | 3.9% | 4.1% | 3.7% | 4.2% | 3.8% | 4.5% |
| Citizens and permanent residents | 2,522 | 3,320 | 3,585 | 4,266 | 5,261 | 5,986 | 7,106 | 7,614 |
|  | 94.0% | 95.5% | 95.7% | 95.0% | 99.0% | 99.7% | 98.9% | 99.3% |
| Temporary residents | 69 | 83 | 86 | 133 | 44 | 8 | 79 | 55 |
|  | 2.6% | 2.4% | 2.3% | 3.0% | 0.8% | 0.1% | 1.1% | 0.7% |
| Total academics | 1,478 | 1,856 | 2,064 | 2,564 | 2,963 | 3,225 | 3,938 | 4,164 |
|  | 55.1% | 53.4% | 55.1% | 57.1% | 55.8% | 53.7% | 54.8% | 54.3% |
| Faculty with rank appointments | 1,359 | 1,615 | 1,774 | 2,259 | 2,642 | 2,922 | 3,413 | 3,675 |
|  | 50.7% | 46.5% | 47.3% | 50.3% | 49.7% | 48.7% | 47.5% | 47.9% |
| Tenured faculty | 276 | 931 | 1,031 | 1,271 | 1,424 | 1,516 | 1,968 | 1,960 |
|  | 10.3% | 26.8% | 27.5% | 28.3% | 26.8% | 25.3% | 27.4% | 25.6% |
| Tenure-track faculty (not tenured) | 1,083 | 684 | 743 | 565 | 780 | 921 | 1,002 | 931 |
|  | 40.4% | 19.7% | 19.8% | 12.6% | 14.7% | 15.3% | 13.9% | 12.1% |
| Academic postdoctorates | 40 | 107 | 108 | 105 | 139 | 100 | 177 | 90 |
|  | 1.5% | 3.1% | 2.9% | 2.3% | 2.6% | 1.7% | 2.5% | 1.2% |
| Other academic appointments | 79 | 78 | 104 | 231 | 182 | 203 | 348 | 399 |
|  | 2.9% | 2.2% | 2.8% | 5.1% | 3.4% | 3.4% | 4.8% | 5.2% |
| Industry (nonpostdoctorate) | 536 | 739 | 733 | 992 | 1,259 | 1,485 | 1,793 | 1,940 |
|  | 20.0% | 21.3% | 19.6% | 22.1% | 23.7% | 24.7% | 24.9% | 25.3% |
| Industrial postdoctorates | 0 | 0 | 0 | 0 | 0 | 8 | 5 | 14 |
|  | 0.0% | 0.0% | 0.0% | 0.0% | 0.0% | 0.1% | 0.1% | 0.2% |
| Government (nonpostdoctorate) | 383 | 491 | 462 | 446 | 527 | 585 | 689 | 745 |
|  | 14.3% | 14.1% | 12.3% | 9.9% | 9.9% | 9.7% | 9.6% | 9.7% |
| Government postdoctorates | 5 | 9 | 8 | 11 | 35 | 34 | 14 | 8 |
|  | 0.2% | 0.3% | 0.2% | 0.2% | 0.7% | 0.6% | 0.2% | 0.1% |
| Other sectors (nonpostdoctorate) | 257 | 358 | 437 | 422 | 489 | 585 | 724 | 747 |
|  | 9.6% | 10.3% | 11.7% | 9.4% | 9.2% | 9.7% | 10.1% | 9.7% |
| Other-sector postdoctorates | 23 | 22 | 18 | 14 | 12 | 60 | 25 | 13 |
|  | 0.9% | 0.6% | 0.5% | 0.3% | 0.2% | 1.0% | 0.3% | 0.2% |
| Doctorates with federal research support | 1,416 | 1,804 | 1,836 | 2,041 | 2,179 | 2,416 | 2,307 | 3,272 |
|  | 52.8% | 51.9% | 49.0% | 45.5% | 41.0% | 40.2% | 32.1% | 42.7% |

*continues*

## TABLE E-6 Continued

| | 1989 | 1991 | 1993 | 1995 | 1997 | 1999 | 2001 |
|---|---|---|---|---|---|---|---|
| Total employed in S&E | 8,736 | 9,506 | 10,748 | 11,996 | 14,069 | 15,268 | 17,180 |
| | 100.0% | 100.0% | 100.0% | 100.0% | 100.0% | 100.0% | 100.0% |
| Minority | 533 | 574 | 760 | 899 | 1,092 | 1,347 | 1,497 |
| | 6.1% | 6.0% | 7.1% | 7.5% | 7.8% | 8.8% | 8.7% |
| Citizens and permanent residents | 8,669 | 9,422 | 10,573 | 11,938 | 13,875 | 14,933 | 16,822 |
| | 99.2% | 99.1% | 98.4% | 99.5% | 98.6% | 97.8% | 97.9% |
| Temporary residents | 53 | 84 | 175 | 58 | 194 | 335 | 358 |
| | 0.6% | 0.9% | 1.6% | 0.5% | 1.4% | 2.2% | 2.1% |
| Total academics | 4,600 | 5,065 | 5,827 | 6,684 | 7,609 | 8,855 | 9,730 |
| | 52.7% | 53.3% | 54.2% | 55.7% | 54.1% | 58.0% | 56.6% |
| Faculty with rank appointments | 4,046 | 4,402 | 5,084 | 5,705 | 6,325 | 7,374 | 8,124 |
| | 46.3% | 46.3% | 47.3% | 47.6% | 45.0% | 48.3% | 47.3% |
| Tenured faculty | 1,925 | 2,156 | 2,341 | 2,770 | 3,081 | 3,507 | 3,647 |
| | 22.0% | 22.7% | 21.8% | 23.1% | 21.9% | 23.0% | 21.2% |
| Tenure-track faculty (not tenured) | 1,424 | 1,339 | 1,784 | 1,988 | 1,878 | 2,138 | 2,384 |
| | 16.3% | 14.1% | 16.6% | 16.6% | 13.3% | 1.4% | 13.9% |
| Academic postdoctorates | 99 | 169 | 144 | 342 | 416 | 324 | 321 |
| | 1.1% | 1.8% | 1.3% | 2.9% | 3.0% | 2.1% | 1.9% |
| Other academic appointments | 455 | 494 | 599 | 637 | 868 | 1,157 | 1,285 |
| | 5.2% | 5.2% | 5.6% | 5.3% | 6.2% | 7.6% | 7.5% |
| Industry (nonpostdoctorate) | 2,341 | 2,530 | 2,869 | 2,923 | 3,568 | 3,731 | 4,413 |
| | 26.8% | 26.6% | 26.7% | 24.4% | 25.4% | 24.4% | 25.7% |
| Industrial postdoctorates | 3 | 4 | 4 | 17 | 49 | 10 | 21 |
| | 0.0% | 0.0% | 0.0% | 0.1% | 0.3% | 0.1% | 0.1% |
| Government (nonpostdoctorate) | 1,034 | 946 | 1,144 | 1,309 | 1,467 | 1,250 | 1,604 |
| | 11.8% | 10.0% | 10.6% | 10.9% | 10.4% | 8.2% | 9.3% |
| Government postdoctorates | 18 | 0 | 67 | 101 | 47 | 50 | 30 |
| | 0.2% | 0.0% | 0.6% | 0.8% | 0.3% | 0.3% | 0.2% |
| Other sectors (nonpostdoctorate) | 717 | 890 | 816 | 936 | 1,311 | 1,349 | 1,339 |
| | 8.2% | 9.4% | 7.6% | 7.8% | 9.3% | 8.8% | 7.8% |
| Other-sector postdoctorates | 8 | 10 | 21 | 26 | 18 | 23 | 43 |
| | 0.1% | 0.1% | 0.2% | 0.2% | 0.1% | 0.2% | 0.3% |
| Doctorates with federal research support | 3,896 | 4,125 | 3,016 | 3,323 | 3,849 | 5,172 | 5,822 |
| | 44.6% | 43.4% | 28.1% | 27.7% | 27.4% | 33.9% | 33.9% |